Thieme

The Temporal Bone: Anatomical Dissection and Surgical Approaches

Mario Sanna, MD
Professor of Otolaryngology
Department of Head and Neck Surgery
University of Chieti
Chieti, Italy
Director
Gruppo Otologico
Piacenza and Rome, Italy

Alessandra Russo, MD
Otologist and Skull Base Surgeon
Gruppo Otologico
Piacenza and Rome, Italy

Abdelkader Taibah, MD
Neurosurgeon, Otologist, and Skull Base Surgeon
Gruppo Otologico
Piacenza and Rome, Italy

Gianluca Piras, MD
Otologist and Skull Base Surgeon
Gruppo Otologico
Piacenza and Rome, Italy

Wenlong Tang, MD
Otologist and Skull Base Surgeon
Shenzhen Longgang ENT Hospital
Shenzhen ENT Institute
Guangdong, China

With the collaboration of
Antonio Caruso, Annalisa Giannuzzi, Enrico Piccirillo, Lorenzo Lauda,
Sampath Chandra Prasad Rao

827 illustrations

Thieme
Stuttgart • New York • Delhi • Rio de Janeiro

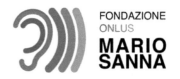

Library of Congress Cataloging-in-Publication Data is available from the publisher

© 2018 by Georg Thieme Verlag KG

Thieme Publishers Stuttgart
Rüdigerstrasse 14, 70469 Stuttgart, Germany
+49 [0]711 8931 421, customerservice@thieme.de

Thieme Publishers New York
333 Seventh Avenue, New York, NY 10001 USA
+1 800 782 3488, customerservice@thieme.com

Thieme Publishers Delhi
A-12, Second Floor, Sector-2, Noida-201301
Uttar Pradesh, India
+91 120 45 566 00, customerservice@thieme.in

Thieme Publishers Rio, Thieme Publicações Ltda.
Edifício Rodolpho de Paoli, 25º andar
Av. Nilo Peçanha, 50 – Sala 2508
Rio de Janeiro 20020-906 Brasil
+55 21 3172 2297 / +55 21 3172 1896

Cover design: Thieme Publishing Group
Typesetting by DiTech Process Solutions

Printed in Germany by CPI Books GmbH

5 4 3 2 1

ISBN 978-3-13-241934-6

Also available as an e-book:
eISBN 978-3-13-241935-3

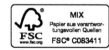

Contents

Preface

The anatomy of the temporal bone represents one of the most complicated areas in the human body. The vital structures, the three-dimensional relationships involved, and the fact that these structures are hidden within bony canals and a drill is needed to expose them make the understanding of the anatomy a difficult task. To add to the complexity, a pathology involving the area generally leads to some degree of alteration of the anatomy. For this reason, it is essential for any physician interested in otology–neurotology or skull base surgery to be perfectly familiar with the anatomy. The best way is to study the anatomy in a temporal bone dissection laboratory creating a situation as close as possible to live surgery.

At the beginning of my training, such an opportunity was easier said than done due to the scarcity of well-equipped laboratories and the difficulty of acquiring temporal bones. Seeking a good-quality training, I travelled to different places all over the world, in particular Los Angeles and Zurich. Despite the paucity of such centers at the time, I was fortunate enough to get high-quality training at some of the leading centers in the world.

Nevertheless, after each course I was left only with the memories of what I have seen, supplemented only by some notes. As a beginner, I always felt the need for something tangible to remind me of what I have learnt in these few days and to serve as a guide for further training. This dream has accompanied me during all my clinical life, and kept growing every time a training course was held at our center.

Today, this book represents a dream come true. With the help of my hardworking coworkers, we dedicated a major share of our time and efforts to create this book to serve as a guide for young trainees. It contains comprehensive, high-quality, full-color pictures of the detailed steps of all the major approaches that can be performed in a temporal bone, supplemented at the end by a set of pictures of cadaveric dissections to help understand the intracranial anatomy where indicated by the approach. For each approach, left- and right-sided dissections are shown.

I would like to express special thanks to my great teachers. Carlo Zini introduced me to the secrets of microsurgery of the middle ear. Jim Sheehy had a great influence in developing my understanding of middle ear surgery that he passed on to me through his art of teaching. William House taught me how to go beyond the bone and introduced me to the world of skull base surgery. Ugo Fisch helped me refine my surgical technique, understanding the importance of the infratemporal fossa approaches.

Also, thanks to the lesson of these masters, the "Gruppo Otologico" is one of the most important internationally acclaimed centers for advanced otology, neurotology, and skull base surgery.

This work will certainly serve as a sufficient and satisfactory guide for helping fresh trainees in overcoming the obstacles we faced earlier.

Mario Sanna, MD

Contributors

Antonio Caruso, MD
Otologist and Skull Base Surgeon
Gruppo Otologico
Piacenza and Rome, Italy

Annalisa Giannuzzi, MD, PhD
Otologist and Skull Base Surgeon
Gruppo Otologico
Piacenza and Rome, Italy

Lorenzo Lauda, MD
ENT and Skull Base Surgeon
Gruppo Otologico
Piacenza and Rome, Italy

Enrico Piccirillo, MD
ENT and Skull Base Surgeon
Gruppo Otologico
Piacenza and Rome, Italy

Gianluca Piras, MD
Otologist and Skull Base Surgeon
Gruppo Otologico
Piacenza and Rome, Italy

Sampath Chandra Prasad Rao, MS, DNB,
FEB-ORLHNS
ENT and Skull Base Surgeon
Gruppo Otologico
Piacenza and Rome, Italy

Alessandra Russo, MD
Otologist and Skull Base Surgeon
Gruppo Otologico
Piacenza and Rome, Italy

Mario Sanna, MD
Professor of Otolaryngology
Department of Head and Neck Surgery
University of Chieti
Chieti, Italy
Director
Gruppo Otologico
Piacenza and Rome, Italy

Abdelkader Taibah, MD
Neurosurgeon, Otologist, and Skull Base Surgeon
Gruppo Otologico
Piacenza and Rome, Italy

Wenlong Tang, MD
Otologist and Skull Base Surgeon
Shenzhen Longgang ENT Hospital
Shenzhen ENT Institute
Guangdong, China

1 Temporal Bone Dissection Laboratory

Abstract

In this chapter, all the equipment needed for the dissection laboratory is described. Also, the details on how to prepare the specimen and use the surgical drill will be provided.

Keywords: microscope, drill, suction irrigation, specimen

1.1 Surgical Instruments

A minimum set of surgical instruments is needed in order to carry out a temporal bone dissection that imitates live surgery as much as possible:

- A good-quality microscope (▶ Fig. 1.1).
- A nonsterilizable micromotor with various sizes of diamond and cutting burrs (▶ Fig. 1.2).
- Suction tubes and suction irrigation tubes of different sizes.
- Surgical knives.
- Tissue scissors and microsurgery scissors.
- Tissue elevators and dissectors. The following set is recommended: Lempert's periosteal elevator, two Freer's elevators, three straight dissectors, four round dissectors (right-angled), five round dissectors (straight), six fine dissector hooks (right-angled), and a fine dissector needle.
- Self-retaining retractor.
- Rongeur.

1.2 General Guidelines for Drilling

In general, a lower level of magnification is preferable to provide comprehensive orientation in relation to the relevant anatomy. On the other hand, a higher magnification level is important for appreciating minute details. Magnification by four is rarely needed in temporal bone dissections, though it does become important in extensive skull base procedures in order to provide a general view of the whole approach.

- Use the largest possible burr; small burrs are very dangerous.
- Adjust the length of the burr according to the depth of the area to be drilled. In general, the shorter the burr, the better the control you have.
- Most bone work is done using cutting burrs. Diamond burrs are reserved for working near delicate structures such as the facial nerve, dura, or sigmoid sinus, or for stopping bleeding originating from the bone.
- Straight handpieces are preferable to angulated ones, since the surgeon has much better control with the former.
- Hold the drill like a pen, and always try to make the direction of the drill strike in a tangential direction rather than perpendicular to the structures you are drilling, so that the drilling is carried out with the side rather than the tip of the burr.
- Drilling should start from the most dangerous areas and progress to the least dangerous ones, always parallel to the important structures, and always in one direction.
- Apply minimal pressure or no pressure during drilling, especially near important structures.
- In delicate work near important structures, the direction of rotation can be adjusted so that the burr rotates away from the structure rather than toward it.
- In fine work, the little finger is placed on the patient's head to support the hand while drilling.

1.3 Suction Irrigation

Ensuring adequate suction irrigation is indispensable in otologic and neuro-otologic surgery. Suction irrigation removes bone dust that impedes vision and becomes clogged between the flukes of the burr end, making it less sharp. It also cools the surface being drilled, avoiding thermal injury. Ample irrigation is important when the facial nerve is being identified, or during blue-lining of a semicircular canal.

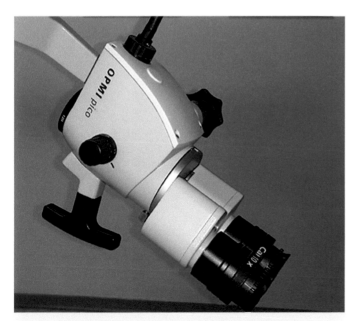

Fig. 1.1 A good quality microscope used for our dissections.

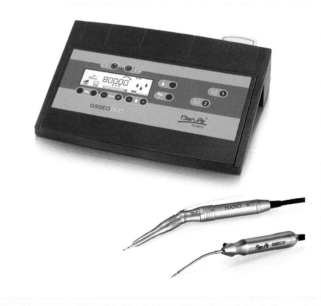

Fig. 1.2 A nonsterilizable micromotor with various sizes of diamond and cutting burrs.

The suction irrigator should not be held steady during burring. Instead, it should wander around the burr. A useful trick is to place the sucker between a structure of importance (especially when already exposed) and the burr. In this way, if control of the burr is lost, it strikes the sucker instead of going through the structure.

There is a special type of suction tip called the Brackmann sucker. The tip of this is blunt, and it has side holes to avoid direct suction being applied to neurovascular structures during neuro-otologic work in the cerebellopontine angle.

1.4 Preparation of the Specimen

We prefer freshly obtained bones preserved in formalin. Older bone is subject to color changes, and the vessels are usually obliterated by hard, difficult-to-remove coagula. Before dissection, the bones are immersed in water for 2 hours to remove the unpleasant odor of formalin. The specimens should never be left exposed overnight, since this causes the dura and soft tissues to become dry, resulting in color changes and increased fragility.

The injection technique described here was developed at our center by Dr. M. Landolfi. The internal jugular vein and internal carotid artery are identified in the neck. The vessels are washed with tap water repeatedly, using a 20-mL syringe, to remove all the small coagula. Once the water begins to flow freely, colored silicone is injected. In cadaver heads, we prefer to inject into the transverse sinus rather than the internal jugular vein in the neck, while the internal carotid and external carotid arteries are injected in the neck. The dye is left to harden before dissection is started.

Preparation of colored silicone. The materials used are as follows:
• Transparent silicone.
• Coloring agent (water or oil colors).
• A solvent—for example, any commercially available benzene solution.
• Syringes, catheters, butterflies, etc.

The density of the solution injected can be varied by modifying the relative amounts of the components used:
• Dense solution: 20-mL silicone, 10-mL solvent, and 5-mL coloring agent.
• Medium-density solution: 10-mL silicone, 10-mL solvent, and 5-mL coloring agent.
• Fluid solution: 15-mL silicone, 20-mL solvent, and 5 mL of coloring agent.

A dense solution has the advantage of providing rapid hardening, with better filling of large vessels that have relatively thin walls—for example, the lateral sinus and jugular bulb. In addition, minor injuries to the sinus or bulb during dissection will not involve any risk of the dye spreading all over the bone, producing a poor appearance. The disadvantage of a dense solution, however, is that the dye sometimes fails to pass through the smaller venous channels (e.g., the superior petrosal sinus). A medium-density dye is used when injecting the internal carotid artery, while a more fluid dye is used when injecting the small intracranial vessels when carrying out a cadaveric dissection.

The dye is injected using a 20-mL syringe with a mounted catheter. The catheter is then withdrawn while the injection is still continuing.

1.5 Temporal Bone Holder

To facilitate dissection in the temporal bone laboratory, the bones are mounted on a House–Urban temporal bone holder (▶ Fig. 1.3). For half-head preparations used for skull base approaches, we use a special temporal bone holder that we designed ourselves. This has a larger diameter and five fixing rods, making it suitable for these large specimens (▶ Fig. 1.4).

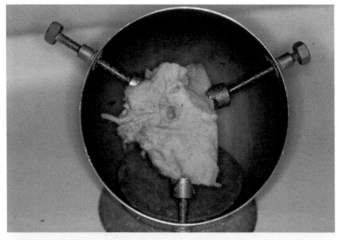

Fig. 1.3 A temporal bone mounted on a House–Urban temporal bone holder.

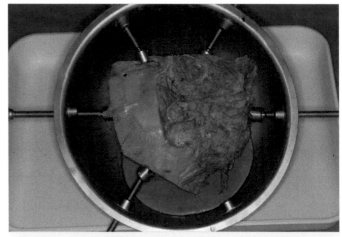

Fig. 1.4 For half-head preparations, we use this holder that we designed ourselves.

2 Anatomy of the Temporal Bone

Abstract

In this chapter, a description of the temporal bone anatomy is provided. The relationship between the key structures of the middle ear, mastoid compartment, and lateral skull base is described. At the end of the chapter, high-resolution endoscopic anatomical images are shown.

Keywords: squamous bone, tympanic bone, mastoid, petrous bone, middle ear, facial nerve, carotid artery, sigmoid sinus, jugular bulb

The temporal bone actually consists of four fused parts—the squamous, tympanic, mastoid, and petrous bones. See ▶ Fig. 2.1, ▶ Fig. 2.2, ▶ Fig. 2.3, ▶ Fig. 2.4, ▶ Fig. 2.5, ▶ Fig. 2.6, ▶ Fig. 2.7, ▶ Fig. 2.8, ▶ Fig. 2.9, ▶ Fig. 2.10, ▶ Fig. 2.11.

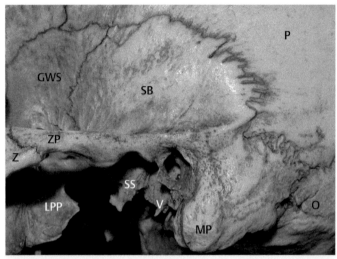

Fig. 2.1 Lateral view of the articulated temporal bone. LPP, lateral pterygoid process; MP, mastoid process; O, occipital bone; P, parietal bone; GWS, greater wing of the sphenoid; SB, squamous bone; SS, spine of the sphenoid; V, vaginal process of the tympanic bone; Z, zygomatic bone; ZP, zygomatic process.

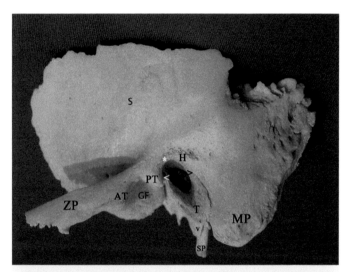

Fig. 2.2 The lateral surface of a left temporal bone. *, roof of the external auditory canal (squamous bone); <, tympanosquamous suture line; >, tympanomastoid suture line; AT, anterior zygomatic tubercle; GF, glenoid fossa; H, spine of Henle; MP, mastoid process; PT, posterior zygomatic tubercle; S, vertical portion of the squamous bone; SP, styloid process; T, tympanic bone; V, vaginal process; ZP, zygomatic process.

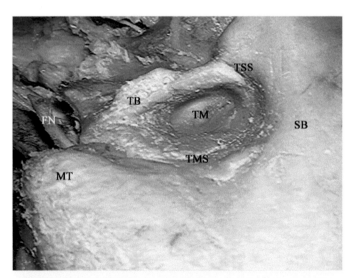

Fig. 2.3 A closer view of the external auditory canal and tympanic ring area. FN, facial nerve; MT, mastoid tip; SB, squamous bone; TB, tympanic bone; TM, tympanic membrane; TMS, tympanomastoid suture; TSS, tympanosquamous suture.

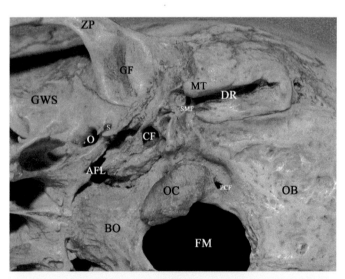

Fig. 2.4 An inferior view of an articulated temporal bone. AFL, anterior foramen lacerum; BO, basilar part of the occipital bone; CF, carotid foramen; DR, digastric ridge; FM, foramen magnum; GF, glenoid fossa; GWS, greater wing of the sphenoid; MT, mastoid tip; O, foramen ovale; OB, occipital bone; OC, occipital condyle; PCF, posterior condylar foramen; S, foramen spinosum; SMF, stylomastoid foramen; ZP, zygomatic process.

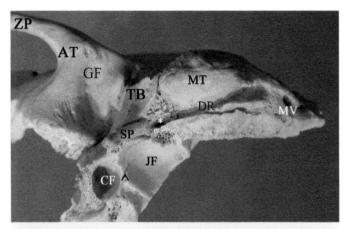

Fig. 2.5 An inferior view of a left temporal bone. *, stylomastoid foramen; ^, Jacobson's nerve canal; AT, anterior zygomatic tubercle; CF, carotid foramen; DR, digastric ridge; GF, glenoid fossa; JF, jugular foramen; MT, mastoid tip; MV, mastoid emissary vein foramen; SP, styloid process; TB, tympanic bone; ZP, zygomatic process.

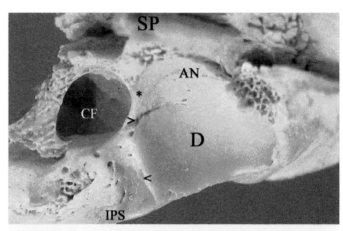

Fig. 2.6 A close-up view of the jugular foramen–carotid foramen area on the inferior aspect of a left temporal bone. *, jugulocarotid spine; <, cochlear aqueduct canal; >, Jacobson's nerve canal; AN, Arnold's nerve canal; CF, carotid foramen; D, dome of the jugular bulb; IPS, groove for the inferior petrosal sinus; SP, styloid process.

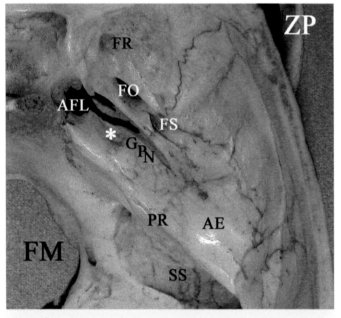

Fig. 2.7 A superior view of an articulated temporal bone. *, Meckel's cave impression; AE, arcuate eminence; AFL, anterior foramen lacerum; FM, foramen magnum; FO, foramen ovale; FR, foramen rotundum; FS, foramen spinosum; GPN, groove for the greater petrosal nerve; PR, petrous ridge; SS, sigmoid sinus sulcus; ZP, zygomatic process.

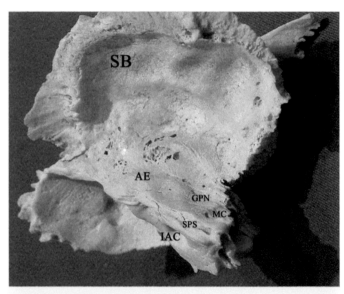

Fig. 2.8 An anterosuperior view of a left temporal bone. AE, arcuate eminence; GPN, groove for the greater petrosal nerve; IAC, internal auditory canal; MC, Meckel's cave impression; SB, squamous bone; SPS, groove for the superior petrosal sinus.

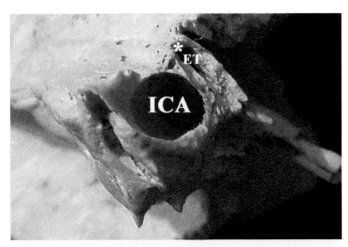

Fig. 2.9 A view of the petrous apex component of the anterior foramen lacerum of a left temporal bone. *, canal of the tensor tympani muscle; ET, isthmus of the eustachian tube; ICA, internal carotid artery canal.

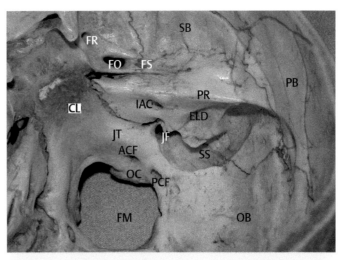

Fig. 2.10 A view of the posterior surface of an articulated temporal bone. ACF, anterior condylar foramen; CL, clivus; ELD, endolymphatic duct foramen; FM, foramen magnum; FO, foramen ovale; FR, foramen rotundum; FS, foramen spinosum; IAC, internal auditory canal; JF, jugular foramen; JT, jugular tubercle; OB, occipital bone; OC, occipital condyle; PB, parietal bone; PCF, posterior condylar foramen; PR, petrous ridge; SB, squamous bone; SS, sigmoid sinus groove.

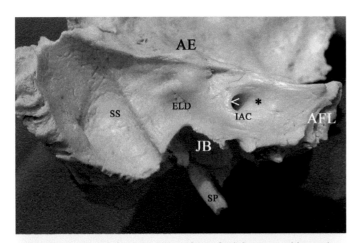

Fig. 2.11 A view of the posterior surface of a left temporal bone. *, anterior lip; <, posterior lip; AE, arcuate eminence; AFL, anterior foramen lacerum component of the petrous apex; ELD, endolymphatic duct foramen; IAC, internal auditory canal; JB, jugular bulb; SP, styloid process; SS, sigmoid sinus groove.

2.1 Squamous Bone

The squamous part of the bone represents the major part of the lateral surface of the bone. Above the level of the zygomatic process, the vertical portion of the squamous bone extends upward to cover part of the temporal lobe of the brain. The zygomatic process is actually part of the squamous portion of the bone. It originates anterior to the external auditory canal at the level of the junction of the vertical and horizontal parts of the squamous bone. The root of the zygomatic process shows an initial swelling known as the posterior zygomatic tubercle. Traced anteriorly, the root thins out to form the glenoid fossa for the articulation of the head of the mandible, and then thickens again to form the anterior zygomatic tubercle. The zygomatic process then thins out and flattens as it separates from the squamous bone and ends by articulation with the zygomatic bone. Posterior to the external auditory canal, the zygomatic process can be traced as a somewhat faint line, the supramastoid crest, indicating the level of the middle cranial fossa. The squamous bone then extends inferiorly in its retromeatal portion, forming the flattened

lateral part of the mastoid process. The squamous part of the temporal bone also forms the superior parts of both the anterior and posterior walls of the bony external auditory canal. On the posterosuperior border of the canal, the spine of Henle can be seen.

2.2 Tympanic Bone

The gutter-shaped tympanic bone forms the inferior wall and major parts of the anterior and posterior walls of the bony external auditory canal. Two sutures between the elementary structures that form the temporal bone appear in the canal. The tympanosquamous suture is located anterosuperiorly, and the tympanomastoid suture posteroinferiorly. Connective tissue enters these suture lines, and sharp dissection may be required during meatal skin elevation. The temporomandibular joint is located just anterior to the canal and is separated from the canal only by a thin bony shell. The lateral border of the tympanic bone is roughened for the attachment of the cartilaginous part of the external auditory canal, which forms the outer two-thirds of the canal. The inferior edge of the tympanic bone expands to form the vaginal process where the styloid process lies.

2.3 Mastoid Process

The mastoid process can be seen at the posterior and inferior border of the temporal bone, protruding anteroinferiorly to variable levels, depending on the pneumatization of the mastoid. The process serves as the anterior part of the attachment of the sternocleidomastoid muscle. On its medial surface lies the digastric groove, from which the posterior belly of the digastric muscle originates. On the posteromedial end of the groove, an impression of the occipital artery can be seen. The stylomastoid foramen, from which the main trunk of the facial nerve exits the temporal bone, can be seen at the anterior border of the digastric ridge posterior to the styloid process.

The temporal component of the jugular foramen can be seen anteromedial to the stylomastoid foramen and medial to both the tympanic bone and the styloid process. From the lateral border of the foramen, the jugular spine of the temporal bone can be seen extending into the foramen toward its occipital counterpart and separating the foramen into what are known as the vascular and nervous compartments. Through the fossa and at a more superior level, the dome of the jugular bulb can be seen. Posteriorly lies the small canal for the passage of Arnold's nerve (the auricular branch of the vagus nerve), while anteriorly the end of the groove of the inferior petrosal sinus can be seen lateral and anterior to the opening of the cochlear aqueduct. The foramen of the internal carotid artery is separated from the anterior border of the jugular foramen by a thin wedge of bone called the jugulocarotid spine, through which a canal for the passage of Jacobson's nerve (the tympanic nerve) to the tympanic cavity lies.

2.4 Petrous Bone

The most prominent feature of the medial aspect of the temporal bone is the petrous part. Shaped like a pyramid, this part protrudes in an anteromedial direction, with the base located laterally and formed by the semicircular canals, vestibule, cochlea, and carotid artery. The apex of this bone forms part of the anterior foramen lacerum. Through the apex, the internal carotid artery exits the petrous bone to the anterior foramen lacerum, where it curves superiorly on its way to the cavernous sinus. The end of the bony part of the eustachian tube, the isthmus, is also located in the apex anterior to the carotid opening and just medial to the spine of the sphenoid. The superior surface of the petrous bone forms part of the middle cranial fossa. It begins from the arcuate eminence and ends at the foramen lacerum. The groove of the greater petrosal nerve can be seen coursing close to the bone near the anterior border of this surface; in 10% of cases, the nerve can be traced posteriorly into a dehiscent geniculate ganglion. The bisection of the angle is formed by this groove and the arcuate eminence marks the position of the internal auditory canal. Near the foramen lacerum, the impression of Meckel's cavity can be seen. The posterior border of this surface is marked by the groove for the superior petrosal sinus, which separates the superior and posterior surfaces.

The posterior surface of the petrous bone forms part of the posterior cranial fossa. The opening for endolymphatic duct and sac can be seen at the lateral end of this surface. This opening represents an important landmark for the posterior semicircular canal in procedures using the retrosigmoid approach. The most important feature of the posterior surface is the internal auditory meatus.

2.5 The Middle Ear

2.5.1 The Tympanic Membrane

The conically shaped tympanic membrane is tilted anteroinferiorly. As a result of this, the anteroinferior bony wall is longer than the posterosuperior one, and the anterior tympanomeatal angle is more acute than the posterior. The anterior angle is often obstructed by a bony protrusion of the anterior wall. Adequate visualization of this angle is the key to successful tympanic membrane reconstruction. The tympanic membrane is composed of three layers. Laterally, it is covered with an epidermal layer, and medially with a mucosal layer. Between these two layers, there is a fibrous layer, the lamina propria. The tympanic membrane is divided into two parts. The pars tensa, located inferior to the lateral process of the malleus and the anterior and posterior malleal folds, represents the majority of the tympanic membrane. The lamina propria thickens in the periphery of the pars tensa to form the tympanic annulus. The tympanic annulus is attached to a groove on the bony canal, called the tympanic sulcus. The pars flaccida is located superior to the lateral process of the malleus and is delineated superiorly by a bony notch in the superior canal wall, called the Rivinus notch. Medial to the pars flaccida and lateral to the neck of the malleus is Prussak's space, in which epitympanic cholesteatomas start to invaginate medially from the pars flaccida. See ▶ Fig. 2.12, ▶ Fig. 2.13, ▶ Fig. 2.14, ▶ Fig. 2.15, ▶ Fig. 2.16, ▶ Fig. 2.17.

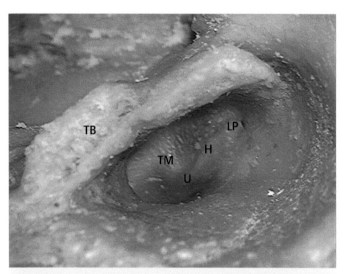

Fig. 2.12 A microscopic view of the left tympanic membrane. H, handle of the malleus; LP, lateral process of the malleus; TB, tympanic bone; TM, tympanic membrane; U, umbo.

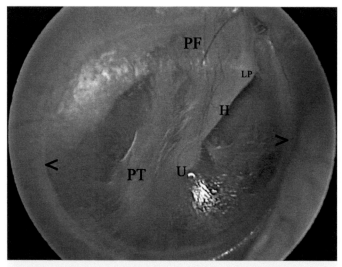

Fig. 2.13 A right normal tympanic membrane as seen by the endoscope. <>, annulus; H, handle of the malleus; LP, lateral process of the malleus; PF, pars flaccida; PT, pars tensa; U, umbo.

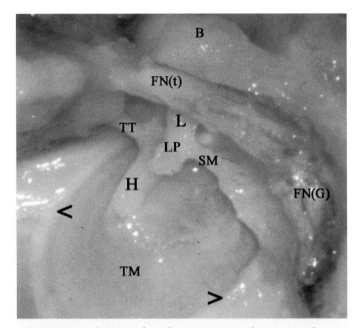

Fig. 2.14 A medial view of a right tympanic membrane. Note the membrane's cone shape. <>, annulus; B, body of the incus; FN(G), genu of the facial nerve; FN(t), tympanic segment of the facial nerve; H, handle of the malleus; L, long process of the incus; LP: lenticular process of the incus; SM, stapedius muscle; TM, tympanic membrane; TT, tensor tympani muscle.

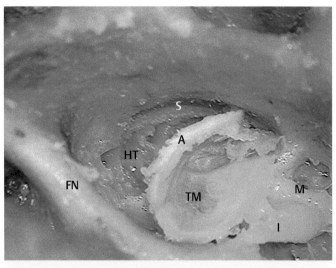

Fig. 2.15 In this left temporal bone, the annulus (A) has been detached from its sulcus (S) to show the relationship between the two. FN, mastoid segment of the facial nerve; HT, hypotympanum; I, incus; M, malleus; TM, tympanic membrane.

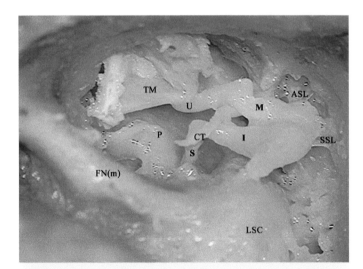

Fig. 2.16 A view of the articulated ossicular chain of the left ear. ASL, anterior suspensory ligament; CT, chorda tympani; FN(m), mastoid segment of the facial nerve; I, incus; LSC, lateral semicircular canal; M, malleus; P, promontory; S, stapes; SSL, superior suspensory ligament; TM, tympanic membrane; U, umbo.

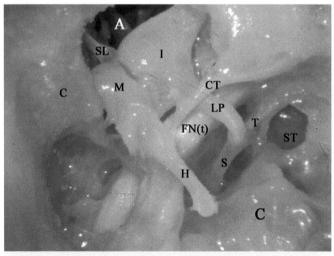

Fig. 2.17 Another view of the articulated ossicular chain. A, attic; C, cochlea; C, cog; CT, chorda tympani; FN(t), tympanic segment of the facial nerve; H, handle of the malleus; I, incus; LP, long process of the incus; M, malleus; S, stapes; SL, superior suspensory ligament; ST, sinus tympani; T, tendon of the stapedius muscle.

2.5.2 The Ossicular Chain

The Malleus

The manubrium of the malleus is firmly attached to the tympanic membrane. Its tip corresponds to the umbo of the tympanic membrane, which is the bottom of its conical shape. The lateral process is located at the superolateral end of the manubrium. Because of its proximity to the superolateral canal wall, meticulous care should be taken not to touch this process with burrs during canalplasty. The head of the malleus is located in the attic, and its neck connects the head and the manubrium. The tendon of the tensor tympani muscle attaches to the medial surface of the neck. Contraction of the muscle pulls the ossicle medially, and the resulting tension on the tympanic membrane limits sound transmission to the inner ear to some extent. The head of the malleus is supported by the superior and anterior suspensory ligaments. See ▶ Fig. 2.18, ▶ Fig. 2.19, ▶ Fig. 2.20.

The Incus

The anterior surface of the body of the incus forms an articulation with the head of the malleus. The short process of the incus projects posteriorly. The short process is lodged in the fossa incudis. The long process projects into the tympanic cavity, and forms an articulation with the stapes at its lenticular process. The incus is supported by the malleus anteriorly and the posterior incudal ligament posteriorly (▶ Fig. 2.21, ▶ Fig. 2.22).

The Stapes

The smallest bone in the human body, the stapes, is located in the oval window. The head of the stapes forms an articulation with the incus. The stapedius muscle inserts onto the head and the posterior crus. The footplate is accommodated in the oval window, which opens into the vestibule. The connective tissue lying between the footplate and the edge of the oval window is called the annular ligament. Contraction of the stapedius muscle tilts the stapes and its footplate, and the resulting tension on the annular ligament limits sound transmission into the inner ear to some extent (▶ Fig. 2.23).

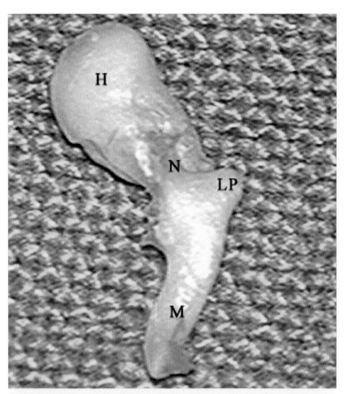

Fig. 2.18 A view of the lateral left malleus bone. H, head, LP, lateral process; M, manubrium or handle; N, neck.

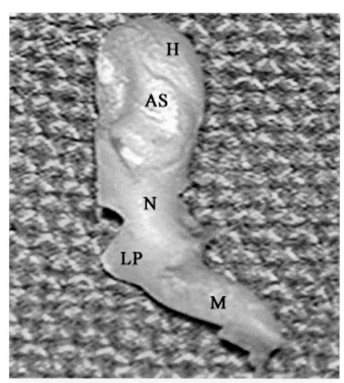

Fig. 2.19 A view of the medial surface of a left malleus bone. AS, articular surface; H, head; LP, lateral process; M, manubrium or handle; N, neck.

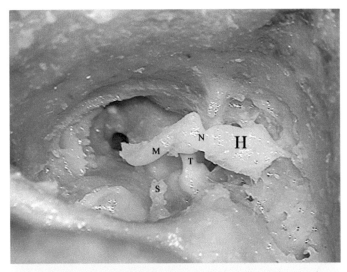

Fig. 2.20 A view of an articulated left malleus, showing the attachment of the tendon of the tensor tympani (T) to the medial aspect of the neck of the malleus (N). H, head of the malleus; M, manubrium or handle of the malleus; S, stapes head.

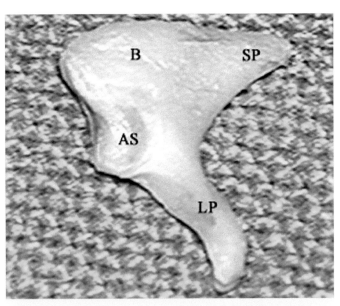

Fig. 2.21 A lateral view of a left incus bone. AS, articular surface; B, body; LP, long process; SP, short process.

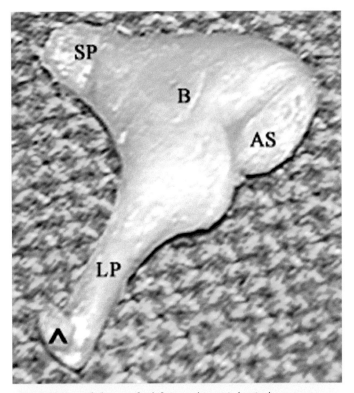

Fig. 2.22 A medial view of a left incus bone. ^, lenticular process; AS, articular surface; B, body; LP, long process; SP, short process.

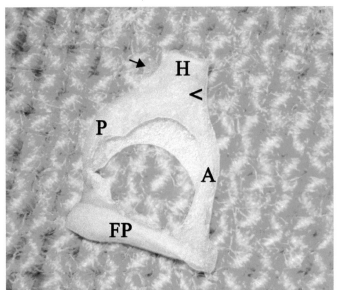

Fig. 2.23 A view of the stapes bone. →, tendon of the stapedius muscle; <, neck; A, anterior crus; FP, footplate; H, head; P, posterior crus.

2.5.3 The Tympanic Cavity

The mesotympanum is a portion located just medial to the tympanic membrane. Superior to the epitympanum (attic), it is bordered by the tympanic segment of the facial nerve. A recess inferior to the tympanic membrane is the hypotympanum. The protympanum, located anteriorly to the tympanic membrane, has the tympanic orifice of the eustachian tube, just inferior to the semicanal of the tensor tympani muscle. A branch of the facial nerve, the chorda tympani, courses lateral to the long process of the incus and medially to the manubrium of the malleus after emerging from the posterior wall. The nerve contains sensory fibers for taste and secretory fibers innervating the submandibular and sublingual glands (▶ Fig. 2.24, ▶ Fig. 2.25, ▶ Fig. 2.26).

Medial Wall

The Facial Nerve

See later in this chapter.

The Cochleariform Process

The cochleariform process lodges the tendon of the tensor tympani. It is located just medial to the neck of the malleus, anterosuperior to the oval window, and just inferior to the tympanic segment of the facial nerve. At this bony process, the tendon of the tensor tympani muscle makes a right angle and courses laterally to attach to the neck of the malleus.

The Promontory

The promontory is a prominent eminence located anteroinferior to the oval window and anterior to the round window. It corresponds to the basal turn of the cochlea. The axis of the cochlea is directed anteriorly and laterally.

The Oval Window

The stapes footplate is lodged in this window to transmit mechanical energy to the scala vestibuli of the cochlea. The window edge and the stapes footplate are connected by connective tissue known as the annular ligament. The tympanic segment of the facial nerve runs just superior to the window, and near its posterior edge, the nerve turns inferiorly toward the stylomastoid foramen.

The Round Window

The round window is located in the round window niche, inferior to the oval window. The round window is the other opening of

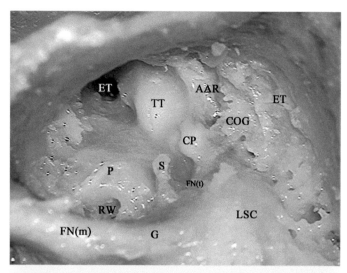

Fig. 2.24 A view of the tympanic cavity of a left ear after removal of the superior and posterior canal walls, the malleus and incus bones. AAR, anterior attic recess; COG, cog; CP, cochleariform process, ET (white), epitympanum; ET (black), eustachian tube; FN(m), mastoid segment of the facial nerve; FN(t), tympanic segment of the facial nerve; G, second genu of the facial nerve; LSC, lateral semicircular canal; P, promontory; RW, round window; S, head of the stapes; TT, tensor tympani muscle.

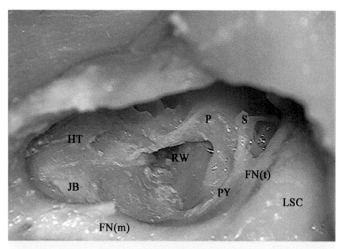

Fig. 2.25 In this left temporal bone, the anterior and posterior crura of the stapes (S) can be clearly seen. The air cells in the hypotympanic area (HT) have been partially drilled to show the relationship of the jugular bulb (JB) to the hypotympanum. FN(m), mastoid segment of the facial nerve; FN(t), tympanic segment of the facial nerve; LSC, lateral semicircular canal; P, promontory; PY, pyramidal process; RW, round window.

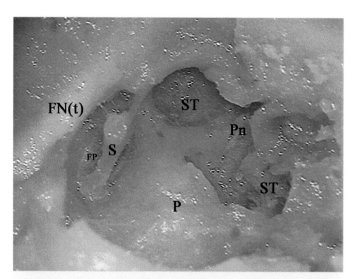

Fig. 2.26 A microscopic view of the sinus tympani (ST) area in a left ear. FN(t), tympanic segment of the facial nerve; FP, footplate; P, promontory; Pn, ponticulus; S, stapes.

the labyrinth to the middle ear. With this window, the cochlear fluid packed into the bony structure is vulnerable to mechanical vibration. The round window membrane lies in the roof of the round window niche, and lies mostly in the horizontal plane. It is therefore difficult to see the membrane directly without removing the superior overhang of the niche.

Posterior Wall

The posterior tympanum contains deep recesses. The facial nerve running in the middle divides them into the tympanic sinus medially and the facial recess laterally.

The Facial Recess

The facial recess is bordered by the bony annulus laterally and the facial canal medially. This is the portion to be drilled for posterior tympanotomy in canal wall–up tympanoplasty. The facial recess is also subdivided into two segments by a bony bridge called the chordal crest that connects with the pyramidal eminence and the emergence of the chorda tympani called the chordal eminence.

The Tympanic Sinus

The sinus is located medial to the facial nerve. The posterior extension of the tympanic sinus is variable, and it may extend far medially to the facial nerve. Since direct visualization of its base is impossible in the majority of cases, eradication of disease from this sinus requires considerable experience. The tympanic sinus is subdivided into two segments, located superiorly and inferiorly, by a bony bridge known as the ponticulus, which connects the pyramidal eminence and the promontory. The tympanic sinus is bordered inferiorly by another bony bridge lying between the posterior wall and the round window niche, called the subiculum.

The Attic

A bony spur known as the cog extends vertically from the tegmen to a point just anterior to the head of the malleus. With this structure, the attic is divided into a posterior division and an anterior division, known as the supratubal recess. Cholesteatoma often advances into the recess, and the recess often becomes a site of residual disease if it is not fully opened during surgery. Since the cog is located superior to the facial nerve, with its tip pointing to it, the structure serves as one of the landmarks for the nerve. The floor of the anterior attic recess contains the postgeniculate portion of the facial nerve. An opening of the antrum called the aditus ad antrum is located posterior to the attic.

2.5.4 The Antrum

The antrum connects the mastoid air cells with the attic. It is located just posterior to the epitympanum, inferior to the middle fossa plate, and lateral to the labyrinth. Since the antrum is very consistent and there are no important structures lateral to it, the antrum serves as one of the most important landmarks in the initial stage of mastoidectomy. The prominence of the lateral semicircular canal is one of the most important landmarks for the facial nerve (▸ Fig. 2.27, ▸ Fig. 2.28).

2.5.5 The Labyrinth

Semicircular Canals

The prominence of the lateral semicircular canal in the medial wall of the antrum slopes at about 30 degrees, running from anterosuperior to posteroinferior. The bony capsule of the labyrinth is compact and hard, and more resistant to bone erosion. However, due to its proximity to the antrum, the lateral semicircular canal is the most vulnerable labyrinth to pathologies that erode the medial wall of the antrum, such as cholesteatoma. At the anterior end of the lateral semicircular canal lies the ampulla, which accommodates sensory cells and opens to the utricles. The ampulla is located in the medial wall of the posterior attic.

The other two semicircular canals are sited nearly perpendicularly to the lateral semicircular canal. The posterior semicircular canal lies just posterior to the lateral semicircular canal, and the

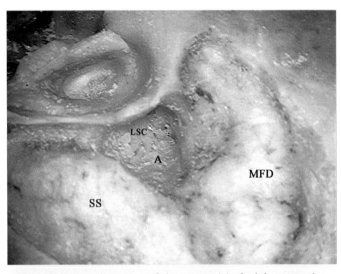

Fig. 2.27 A microscopic view of the antrum (A) of a left temporal bone. LSC, lateral semicircular canal; MFD, middle fossa dura; SS, sigmoid sinus.

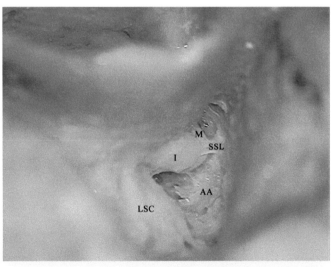

Fig. 2.28 A closer view, showing the aditus ad antrum (AA) in a left temporal bone. I, incus; LSC, lateral semicircular canal; M, malleus; SSL, superior suspensory ligament.

posterior edge of the lateral semicircular canal points almost to the center of the posterior semicircular canal. The posterior semicircular canal courses nearly in parallel with the posterior fossa dura. Its ampulla is located at its inferior end, just medial to the mastoid segment of the facial nerve. The superior end of the posterior semicircular canal joins the superior semicircular canal, forming the common crus.

The superior semicircular canal is located just beneath the middle cranial fossa plate. Its ampulla is at the anterior end, just superomedial to the ampulla of the lateral semicircular canal. It courses nearly perpendicular to the long axis of the pyramis, which places the canal deeper and farther from the antrum

posteriorly. The canal is therefore not seen in the majority of cases, and the entire canal may be exposed in limited cases in which intensive removal of perilabyrinthine cells is required, such as petrous bone cholesteatoma. In rare cases, the canal is dehiscent and is directly in contact with the middle fossa dura.

The ampullae of the superior and lateral semicircular canals are located in the medial wall of the posterior attic. If it is necessary to drill deeply into the medial wall of the attic, great care should therefore be taken not to open these two ampullae. The labyrinth is less resistant to an insult to the ampulla than to the semicircular canals. See ▶ Fig. 2.29, ▶ Fig. 2.30, ▶ Fig. 2.31, ▶ Fig. 2.32, ▶ Fig. 2.33, ▶ Fig. 2.34, ▶ Fig. 2.35, ▶ Fig. 2.36.

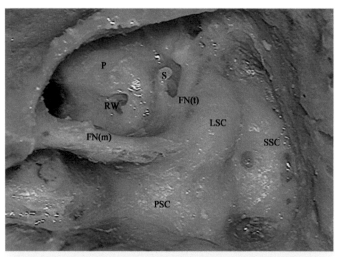

Fig. 2.29 In this left temporal bone, the superior semicircular canal (SSC), lateral semicircular canal (LSC), posterior semicircular canal (PSC), and cochlea have been identified to show their anatomy. FN(m), mastoid segment of the facial nerve; FN(t), tympanic segment of the facial nerve; P, promontory; RW, round window; S, stapes.

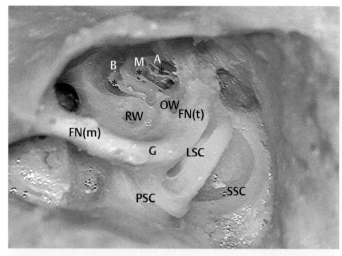

Fig. 2.30 The labyrinth has been opened. *, basilar membrane; <, modiolus; A, apical turn of the cochlea; B, basal turn of the cochlea; FN(m), mastoid segment of the facial nerve; FN(t), tympanic segment of the facial nerve; G, genu; LSC, lateral semicircular canal; M, middle turn of the cochlea; OW, oval window; PSC, posterior semicircular canal; RW, round window; SSC, superior semicircular canal.

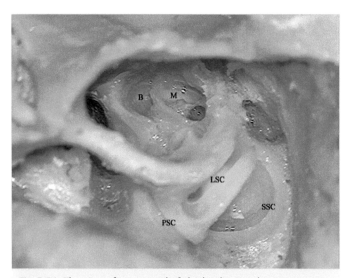

Fig. 2.31 The view after removal of the basilar membrane. <, modiolus; B, basal turn of the cochlea; LSC, lateral semicircular canal; M, middle turn of the cochlea; PSC, posterior semicircular canal; SSC, superior semicircular canal.

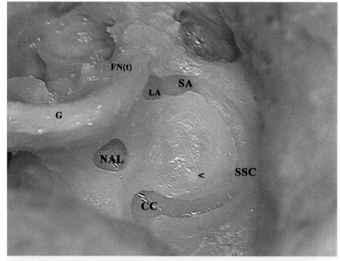

Fig. 2.32 In this view, the lateral and posterior semicircular canals have been drilled out. The intimate relationship between the ampullae of the lateral (LA) and superior (SA) canals and the tympanic segment of the facial nerve (FN[t]) can be appreciated. <, subarcuate artery; CC, common crus; G, genu; NAL, nonampullated end of the lateral canal; SSC, superior semicircular canal.

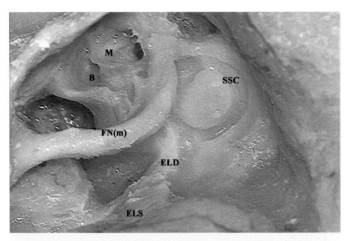

Fig. 2.33 The endolymphatic duct (ELD) of a left temporal bone can be seen passing from behind the posterior semicircular canal to the posterior fossa dura. B, basal turn of the cochlea; ELS, endolymphatic sac; FN(m), mastoid segment of the facial nerve; M, middle turn of the cochlea; SSC, semicircular canal.

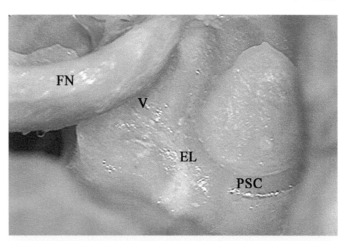

Fig. 2.34 The lower part of the posterior semicircular canal (PSC) has been drilled away here, and the endolymphatic duct (EL) can be followed proximally to the vestibule (V). FN, facial nerve.

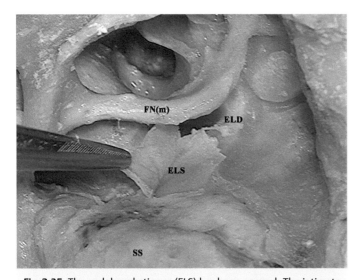

Fig. 2.35 The endolymphatic sac (ELS) has been opened. The intimate relationship between the sac and the posterior fossa dura can be appreciated. ELD, endolymphatic duct; FN(m), mastoid segment of the facial nerve; SS, sigmoid sinus.

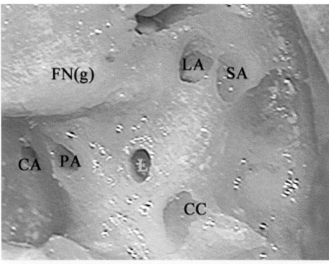

Fig. 2.36 The semicircular canals of a left temporal bone have been drilled out, and the five openings into the vestibule can be seen. CA, cochlear aqueduct; CC, common crus; FN(g), facial nerve genu; L, nonampullated end of the lateral semicircular canal; LA, ampulla of the lateral semicircular canal; PA, ampulla of the posterior canal; SA, ampulla of the superior semicircular canal.

Vestibule

The vestibule is a hollow space within the petrous bone that contains the utricle and the saccule. This space lies anterior to the semicircular canals, medial to the oval window, lateral to the fundus of the internal auditory canal, and posterior to the cochlea. Its posterior surface receives the five openings of the semicircular canals. Anteriorly, the ductus reuniens connects the vestibule to the scala vestibuli of the cochlea.

Cochlea

The cochlea, a spirally curved tube that forms two and a half turns, lies in front of the vestibule. It has a wide base and a narrow apex. The basal turn of the cochlea projects into the middle ear, forming the promontory bulge. The coils of the cochlea curve around a central cone of bone known as the modiolus, which arises from the fundus of the internal auditory canal and carries

within it the fibers of the cochlear nerve. From the modiolus, a shelf-like bony projection known as the bony spiral lamina extends halfway into the cavity of the cochlear turns. The membranous spiral lamina or basilar membrane connects the edge of the bony spiral lamina to the lateral surface of the cochlear turns, thus dividing the space into two compartments—the scala vestibule superiorly and the scala tympani inferiorly.

2.6 Internal Auditory Canal

The internal auditory canal is a canal almost 1 cm in length that runs in a lateral direction from the cerebellopontine angle through the petrous bone. The meatus of the internal auditory canal can be seen in the posterior surface of the petrous bone. Its posterior border is formed by an acute angle, while the anterior border is flatter. The dura of the posterior cranial fossa continues into the internal auditory canal, lining the whole length, and ends by merging with the contained nerves as these enter their corresponding foramina. The long axis of the canal lies in line with the long axis of the external auditory canal.

At the lateral end of the internal auditory canal lies the fundus. The horizontal crest divides this area into a smaller upper zone and a larger lower zone. The upper zone is further divided by the vertical bar ("Bill's bar") into an anterior foramen for the passage of the facial nerve and a posterior one for the passage of the superior vestibular nerve. The cochlear nerve passes to the cochlea through a central canal surrounded by multiple small foramina located anteriorly in the lower zone of the fundus. The inferior vestibular nerve passes from the posterior part of this zone. Posteroinferior to this nerve lies the canal for the singular nerve, which supplies the ampulla of the posterior semicircular canal. In addition to these nerve, the canal also contains the internal auditory artery and vein, and a loop of the anterior inferior cerebellar artery may also be present.

2.6.1 The Carotid Artery

The carotid artery enters the temporal bone through the carotid foramen. It ascends vertically and emerges in the medial wall of the hypotympanum at the area just beneath the cochlea. It then turns anteromedially nearly at a right angle toward the petrous apex, forming a horizontal segment just posteroinferior to the eustachian tube and anterior to the cochlea. In 2% of cases, a bony shell separating the carotid artery and the eustachian tube is absent. The distance between the cochlea and the carotid artery ranges from 1 to 5 mm.

2.6.2 The Sigmoid Sinus and Jugular Bulb

The sigmoid sinus is a space lying between the inner and outer layer of the dura. Starting at the end of the transverse sinus, the sigmoid sinus curves downward and forward, leaving a deep impression on the inner surface of the mastoid bone. At its upper end, the superior sigmoid sinus receives the superior petrosal sinus. Near its middle, the mastoid emissary vein connects the sigmoid sinus to the posterior auricular vein. The sigmoid sinus ends at the posterior margin of the jugular foramen, where it expands to form the jugular bulb. This structure is located in the posterior and largest compartment of the foramen jugulare, connecting the sigmoid sinus and the internal jugular vein. The jugular bulb is located medial to the mastoid segment of the facial nerve and inferior to the semicircular canals. The distance from the facial nerve and the labyrinth varies, and the bulb is variably positioned in the hypotympanum. In some cases, the bulb is dehiscent in the hypotympanum. It should be remembered that the ninth to eleventh cranial nerves (the glossopharyngeal, vagus, and accessory nerves) pass the skull base with this venous system.

2.7 The Intratemporal Facial Nerve

This part of the facial nerve (FN) is encased within a bony canal and is divided into three segments that are separated from each other by two genua.

See ► Fig. 2.37, ► Fig. 2.38, ► Fig. 2.39, ► Fig. 2.40, ► Fig. 2.41, ► Fig. 2.42, ► Fig. 2.43, ► Fig. 2.44, ► Fig. 2.45, ► Fig. 2.46, ► Fig. 2.47, ► Fig. 2.48, ► Fig. 2.49, ► Fig. 2.50, ► Fig. 2.51, ► Fig. 2.52, ► Fig. 2.53, ► Fig. 2.54, ► Fig. 2.55, ► Fig. 2.56, ► Fig. 2.57, ► Fig. 2.58, ► Fig. 2.59, ► Fig. 2.60, ► Fig. 2.61, ► Fig. 2.62, ► Fig. 2.63, ► Fig. 2.64, ► Fig. 2.65, ► Fig. 2.66, ► Fig. 2.67, ► Fig. 2.68, ► Fig. 2.69, ► Fig. 2.70, ► Fig. 2.71.

2.7.1 Labyrinthine Segment

The labyrinthine segment is the thinnest and shortest segment of the FN. Its base runs from medial to lateral, from the fundus to the geniculate ganglion (GG). The borders of the narrow canal containing this segment are formed by the cochlea anteriorly, the

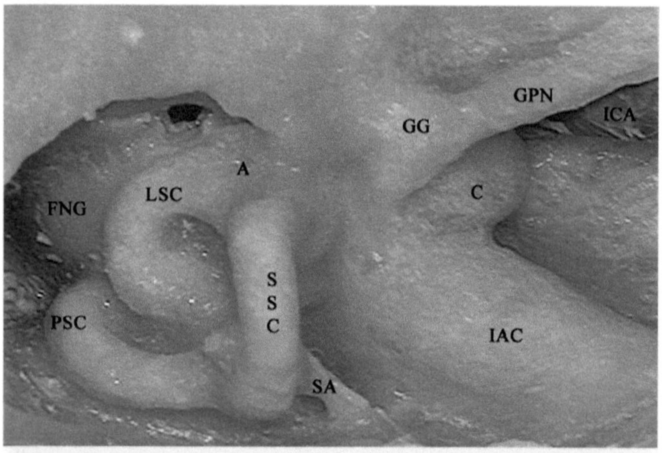

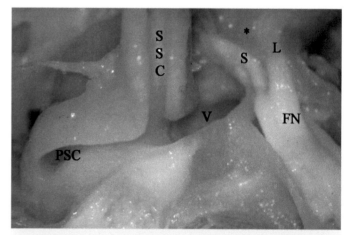

Fig. 2.37 A view of the inner ear components as seen from the middle cranial fossa of a left temporal bone. A, ampulla of the lateral semicircular canal; C, cochlea; FNG, facial nerve genu; GG, geniculate ganglion; GPN, greater petrosal nerve; IAC, internal auditory canal; ICA, internal carotid artery; LSC, lateral semicircular canal; PSC, posterior semicircular canal; SA, subarcuate artery; SSC, superior semicircular canal.

Fig. 2.38 A view from the middle cranial fossa of a left temporal bone, showing the superior semicircular canal (SSC) and posterior semicircular canal (PSC) as these join together, forming the common crus, to enter the vestibule (V). *, Bill's bar; FN, internal auditory canal segment of the facial nerve; L, labyrinthine segment of the facial nerve; S, superior vestibular nerve.

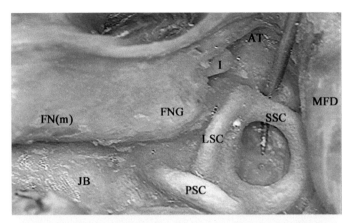

Fig. 2.39 A view of the labyrinth as seen from the mastoid cavity of a left temporal bone. The tip of the instrument is pointing to the subarcuate artery. AT, attic; FN(m), mastoid segment of the facial nerve; FNG, facial nerve genu; I, incus; JB, jugular bulb; LSC, lateral semicircular canal; MFD, middle fossa dura; PSC, posterior semicircular canal; SSC, superior semicircular canal.

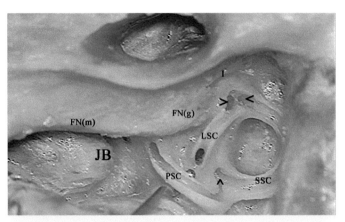

Fig. 2.40 The semicircular canals have been opened. Note the joint lateral (>) and superior (<) ampullae, and the union of the non-ampullated ends of the superior and posterior semicircular canals into the common crus (^). The tip of the instrument is pointing to the nonampullated end of the lateral semicircular canal. FN(m), mastoid segment of the facial nerve; FN(g), facial nerve genu; I, incus; JB, jugular bulb; LSC, lateral semicircular canal; PSC, posterior semicircular canal; SSC, superior semicircular canal.

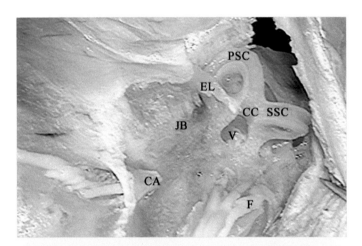

Fig. 2.41 Via a retrosigmoid approach, the posterior (PSC) and superior (SSC) semicircular canals of a left temporal bone have been opened and followed to the common crus (CC) as it enters the vestibule (V). Note the endolymphatic duct (EL) passing posterior to the posterior canal and the common crus, serving as a landmark to their location in the retrosigmoid approach. Note also the high jugular bulb (JB) in this case. CA, cochlear aqueduct; F, facial nerve.

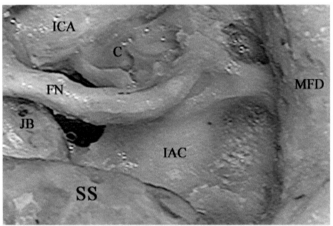

Fig. 2.42 Skeletonization of the internal auditory canal (IAC) of a left temporal bone has been started. The color of the canals' dura can be seen through the bone. C, cochlea; FN, facial nerve; ICA, internal carotid artery; JB, jugular bulb; MFD, middle fossa dura; SS, sigmoid sinus.

superior semicircular canal posteriorly, the vestibule inferiorly, and a thin plate of bone separating the nerve from the middle cranial fossa dura superiorly. The GG is a swelling that marks the first genu of the FN and contains the cell bodies of all the sensory fibers of the FN. The thin plate of bone separating the geniculate ganglion form the middle cranial fossa dura may be absent in 10 to 15% of cases, putting the FN at risk during middle cranial fossa surgery. The first branch of the FN, the greater superficial petrosal nerve, leaves the anterior surface of the geniculate ganglion.

2.7.2 Tympanic Segment

Curving posteriorly at an angle ranging between 60 and 90 degrees, the FN continues as the tympanic segment. This segment lies on the medial wall of the tympanum and protrudes into the cavity covered by a thin shell of bone. The beginning of this segment is marked by the cog superiorly and by the cochleariform process inferiorly. As the nerve passes posteriorly, it can be seen slanting inferiorly to assume an inferior position under the protrusion of the lateral semicircular canal on the medial wall of the middle ear. Underneath the nerve at this level lie the bulge of the promontory and the oval window. The incidence of dehiscence of the fallopian canal covering this segment is high, and in some series it has been reported to be up to 50%. When the nerve reaches the level of the oval window, it starts to curve inferiorly, forming the second genu, which lies within the curvature of the lateral semicircular canal. Just before the nerve reaches the genu, the ampullae of the superior and lateral semicircular canal lie medial to the FN, separated from it by a thin plate of bone.

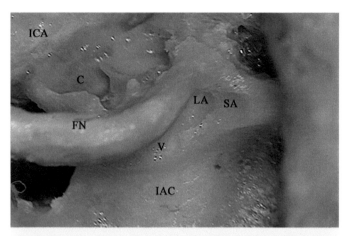

Fig. 2.43 A closer view, showing the relationship between the ampulla of the superior canal (SA) and the upper surface of the internal auditory canal (IAC). The superior canal ampulla serves as a landmark to the level of the upper surface of the internal auditory canal. C, cochlea; FN, facial nerve; ICA, internal carotid artery; LA, lateral canal ampulla; V, vestibule.

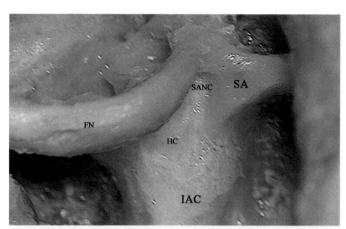

Fig. 2.44 The bone overlying the internal auditory canal (IAC) has been completely removed, and the superior ampullary nerve canal (SANC) has been followed into the ampulla of the lateral semicircular canal. FN, facial nerve; HC, horizontal crest; SA, ampulla of the superior canal.

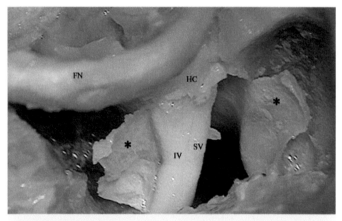

Fig. 2.45 The dura of the internal auditory canal (*) has been opened. The superior vestibular (SV) and inferior vestibular (IV) nerves can be seen lying posteriorly in the canal, separated by the horizontal crest (HC). FN, facial nerve.

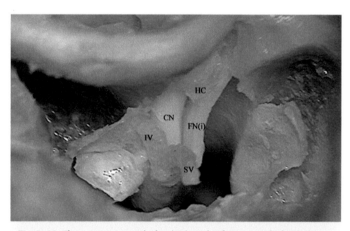

Fig. 2.46 The superior vestibular (SV) and inferior vestibular (IV) nerves have been dislocated from their entrances into the fundi and reflected posteriorly. The cochlear nerve (CN) and the internal auditory canal segment of the facial nerve (FNi) can be seen lying anteriorly, separated by the horizontal crest (HC).

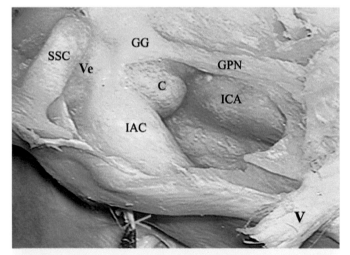

Fig. 2.47 From a middle cranial fossa view of a left temporal bone, the internal auditory canal (IAC) has been skeletonized. The relationship of the canal to the cochlea (C) and vestibule (Ve) can be seen. The canal can also be seen lying in the orientation of the bisection of the angle between the superior semicircular canal (SSC) and the greater petrosal nerve (GPN). <, acousticofacial bundle, GG, geniculate ganglion; ICA, internal carotid artery; V, trigemninal nerve.

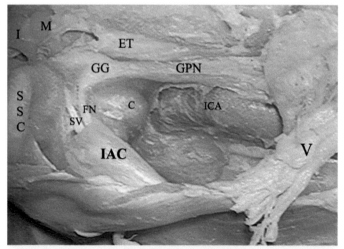

Fig. 2.48 The bone overlying the internal auditory canal has been removed and the dura of the canal has been removed near the fundus. The facial nerve (FN)can be seen entering its labyrinthine segment to form the geniculate ganglion (GG) more laterally. <, acousticofacial bundle; C, cochlea; ET, eustachian tube; GPN, greater petrosal nerve; I, incus; IAC, internal auditory canal; ICA, internal carotid artery; M, malleus; SSC, superior semicircular canal; SV, superior vestibular nerve; V, trigeminal nerve.

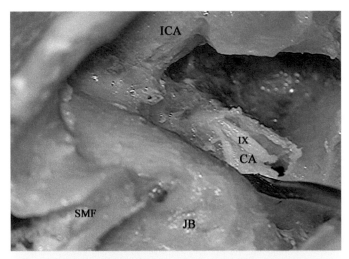

Fig. 2.49 After rerouting the facial nerve and drilling away the fallopian canal of a left temporal bone, the cochlear aqueduct (CA) has been opened. The proximity of the glossopharyngeal nerve (IX) can be well appreciated. Since the nerve lies just inferior to the cochlear aqueduct, the latter is used as a landmark to the nerve in the translabyrinthine approach, indicating the lower limit of drilling in order to avoid injury to the glossopharyngeal nerve. ICA, internal carotid artery; JB, jugular bulb; SMF, stylomastoid foramen.

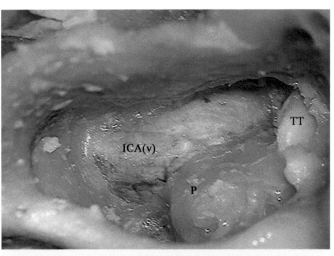

Fig. 2.50 In a left temporal bone, the hypotympanic air cells have been drilled out and the vertical segment of the internal carotid artery (ICA[v]) skeletonized. P, promontory; TT, tensor tympani.

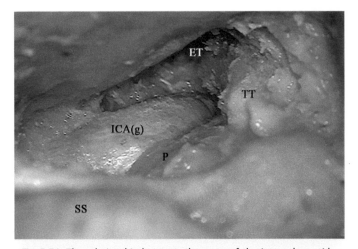

Fig. 2.51 The relationship between the genu of the internal carotid artery (ICA[g]), the promontory (P), and the eustachian tube (ET) can be appreciated. TT, tensor tympani muscle; SS, sigmoid sinus.

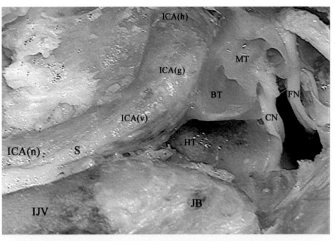

Fig. 2.52 The full length of the intratemporal internal carotid artery has been skeletonized. BT, basal turn of the cochlea; CN, cochlear nerve; FN, facial nerve; HT, hypotympanum; ICA(g), genu of the internal carotid artery; ICA(h), horizontal segment of the intratemporal internal carotid artery; ICA(n), internal carotid artery in the neck; ICA(v), vertical segment of the intratemporal internal carotid artery; IJV, internal jugular vein; JB, jugular bulb; MT, middle turn of the cochlea; S, sympathetic chain.

2.7.3 Mastoid Segment

Medial to the short process of the incus, the nerve assumes a descending course starting the mastoid segment of the nerve. The pyramid, a bony protrusion that houses the stapedius muscle, lies few millimeters inferior to the short process of the incus, in contact with the anterior surface of the nerve. At this level (the pyramidal turn), the FN protrudes posterolateral to the lateral semicircular canal, putting the nerve at risk of injury during mastoid surgery. The descending or mastoid segment of the FN can be traced from the second genu to the anterior edge of the digastric ridge, where the stylomastoid foramen lies, marking the end of the intratemporal part of the FN. The relationship of this segment to the tympanic annulus is important in external auditory canal surgery. The posteromedial relationship of the FN to the annulus is more constant near the posterosuperior quadrant

of the annulus. When the posteroinferior quadrant is reached, however, there is a high probability that the nerve may cross anterolateral to the plane of the annulus, making it susceptible to injury there.

The ampulla of the posterior semicircular canal lies medial to the midportion of this segment, forming a useful landmark in translabyrinthine surgery. The lower part of this segment is centered on the lateral surface of the jugular bulb, the superior extension of which determines the space available for a subfacial tympanotomy between the FN, jugular bulb, and inferior semicircular canal. The first muscular branch is the nerve to the stapedius. This nerve emerges from the anterior surface of the FN at the level of the pyramidal process. After branching out from the

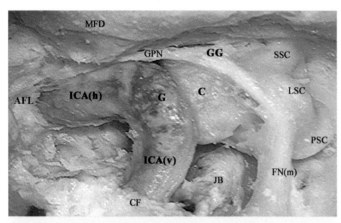

Fig. 2.53 All the bone surrounding the intratemporal internal carotid artery of a left temporal bone has been drilled out. AFL, anterior foramen lacerum; C, cochlea; CF, carotid foramen; FN(m), mastoid segment of the facial nerve; G, genu; GG, geniculate ganglion; GPN, greater petrosal nerve; ICA(h), horizontal segment of the internal carotid artery; ICA(v), vertical segment of the internal carotid artery; JB, jugular bulb; LSC, lateral semicircular canal; MFD, middle fossa dura; PSC, posterior semicircular canal; SSC, superior semicircular canal.

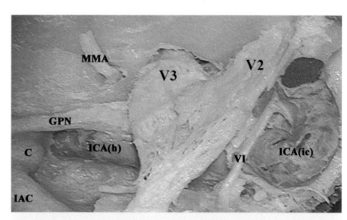

Fig. 2.54 The course of the horizontal segment of the internal carotid artery (ICA[h]), as seen from the middle cranial fossa of a left temporal bone. VI, abducent nerve; C, cochlea; GPN, greater petrosal nerve; IAC, internal auditory canal; ICA(ic), intracranial internal carotid artery; V3, mandibular nerve; MMA, middle meningeal artery; V2, maxillary nerve.

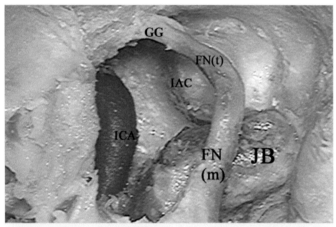

Fig. 2.55 Another case of a left transotic approach, with the bone in a vertical orientation. Note that the jugular bulb (JB) is very high in this case, and is almost lying in contact with the internal auditory canal (IAC). FN(m), mastoid segment of the facial nerve; FN(t), tympanic segment of the facial nerve; GG, geniculate ganglion; ICA, internal carotid artery.

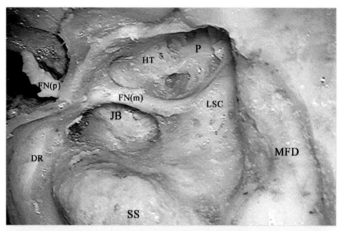

Fig. 2.56 In this left temporal bone, the sigmoid sinus (SS) has been skeletonized and followed to the jugular bulb (JB), which lies medial to the mastoid segment of the facial nerve (FN[m]). DR, digastric ridge; FN(p), intraparotid portion of the facial nerve; HT, hypotympanum; LSC, lateral semicircular canal; MFD, middle fossa dura; P, promontory.

FN, it passes in a small canal within the pyramid to reach the stapedius muscle, which originates from within the pyramid. The chorda tympani is the branch that carries the secretomotor fibers to the sublingual and submandibular glands and the taste fibers from the anterior two-thirds of the tongue and the soft palate. The point of origin of this branch from the FN may lie anywhere between the lateral semicircular canal and the stylomastoid foramen. An origin from the extratemporal part of the FN has also been reported. In such instances, the chorda tympani travels back to enter the stylomastoid foramen. After originating from the FN, the chorda travels for a short distance within the posterior wall of the tympanic cavity and enters the tympanic cavity, passing in an anterior direction medial to the neck of the malleus, to exit through the tympanosquamous fissure (the gasserian fissure) at the anterior border of the tympanic membrane.

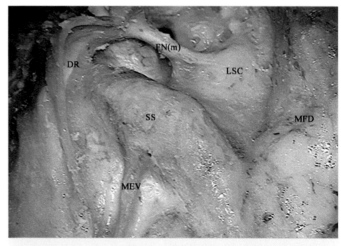

Fig. 2.57 The mastoid emissary vein (MEV) can be seen branching from the sigmoid sinus (SS). DR, digastric ridge; FN(m), mastoid segment of the facial nerve; LSC, lateral semicircular canal; MFD, middle fossa dura.

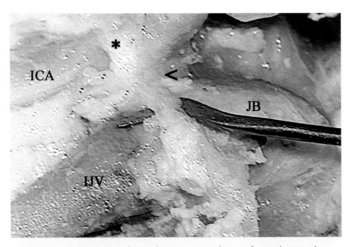

Fig. 2.58 The bone overlying the transitional zone from the jugular bulb (JB) to the internal jugular vein (IJV) has been drilled away. The hook can be seen underneath the fibrous band covering the exit of the bulb from the bone. The jugulocarotid spine of bone (<) can be seen lying between the internal carotid artery (ICA) and the jugular bulb. *, the fibrous band covering the entrance of the internal carotid artery into the temporal bone.

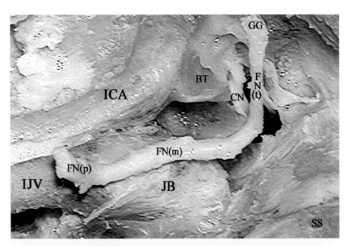

Fig. 2.59 The relationship of the mastoid segment of the facial nerve (FN[m]) to the jugular bulb (JB) after the removal of all the surrounding bone. BT, basal turn of the cochlea; CN, cochlear nerve; FN(p), intraparotid segment of the facial nerve; FN(t), tympanic segment of the facial nerve; GG, geniculate ganglion; ICA, internal carotid artery; IJV, internal jugular vein; SS, sigmoid sinus.

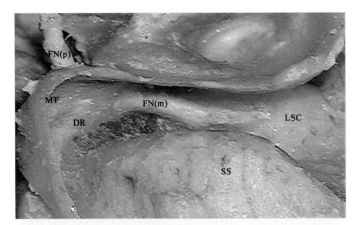

Fig. 2.60 In a left temporal bone, the digastric ridge (DR) has been identified. At its anterior end, the mastoid segment of the facial nerve (FN[m]) can be seen. FN(p), intraparotid portion of the facial nerve; LSC, lateral semicircular canal; MT, mastoid tip; SS, sigmoid sinus.

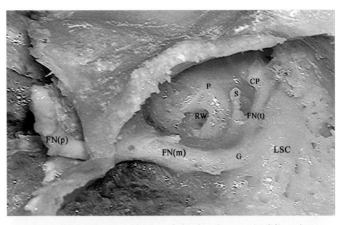

Fig. 2.61 The tympanic segment of the facial nerve (FN[t]) and its landmarks can be seen. The cochleariform process can be seen lying at the anteroinferior end; the stapes can be seen inferiorly, and the lateral semicircular canal superiorly. CP, cochleariform process; FN(m), mastoid segment of the facial nerve; FN(p), intraparotid portion of the facial nerve; G, genu; LSC, lateral semicircular canal; P, promontory; S, stapes; RW, round window.

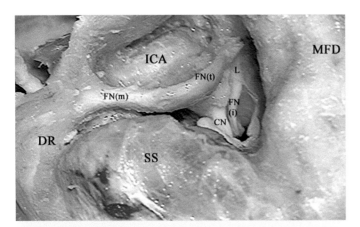

Fig. 2.62 The full length of the intratemporal facial nerve can be seen. CN, cochlear nerve; DR, digastric ridge; FN(i), internal auditory canal segment of the facial nerve; FN(m), mastoid segment of the facial nerve; FN(t), tympanic segment of the facial nerve; ICA, internal carotid artery; L, labyrinthine segment of the facial nerve; MFD, middle fossa dura; SS, sigmoid sinus.

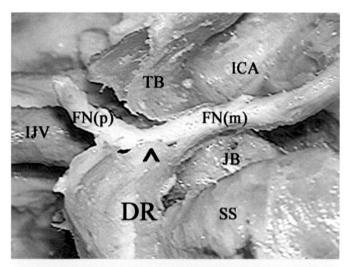

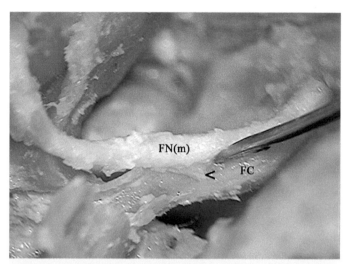

Fig. 2.63 This figure shows the exit of the facial nerve from the stylomastoid foramen (^) of a left temporal bone. DR, digastric ridge; FN(m), mastoid segment of the facial nerve; FN(p), intraparotid facial nerve; ICA, internal carotid artery; IJV, internal jugular vein; JB, jugular bulb; SS, sigmoid sinus; TB, tympanic bone.

Fig. 2.64 The fibrovascular attachments (<) of the mastoid segment of the facial nerve (FN[m]) to the fallopian canal (FC) can be appreciated.

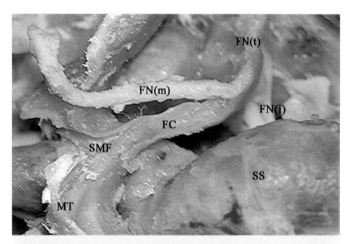

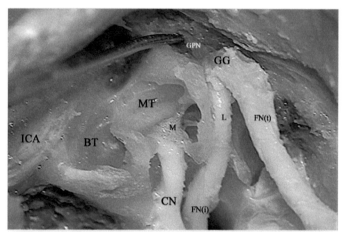

Fig. 2.65 The fibrovascular attachment has been sharply cut, and the mastoid segment of the facial nerve (FN[m]) has been freed from the fallopian canal (FC). FN(i), internal auditory canal segment of the facial nerve; FN(t), tympanic segment of the facial nerve; MT, mastoid tip; SMF, stylomastoid foramen; SS, sigmoid sinus.

Fig. 2.66 The cochlear nerve (CN) can be seen here passing from the internal auditory canal to the modiolus (M), and the relationship between this part of the cochlear nerve and the internal auditory canal (FN[i]) and labyrinthine (L) segments of the facial nerve can be appreciated. BT, basal turn of the cochlea; FN(t), tympanic segment of the facial nerve; GG, geniculate ganglion; GPN, greater petrosal nerve; ICA, internal carotid artery; MT, middle turn of the cochlea.

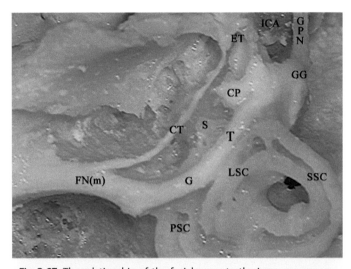

Fig. 2.67 The relationship of the facial nerve to the inner ear as seen from a lateral view of a left temporal bone. CP, cochleariform process; CT, chorda tympani; ET, eustachian tube; FN(m), mastoid segment of the facial nerve; G, genu; GG, geniculate ganglion; GPN, greater petrosal nerve; ICA, internal carotid artery; LSC, lateral semicircular canal; PSC, posterior semicircular canal; S, stapes; SSC, superior semicircular canal; T, tympanic segment of the facial nerve.

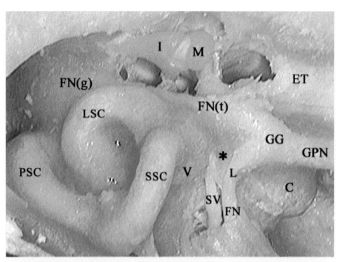

Fig. 2.68 The relationship of the facial nerve to the inner ear seen from a left middle cranial fossa. *, Bill's bar; C, cochlea; ET, eustachian tube; FN, tympanic segment of the facial nerve; FN(g), facial nerve genu; FN(t), tympanic segment of the facial nerve; GG, geniculate ganglion; GPN, greater petrosal nerve; I, incus; L, labyrinthine segment of the facial nerve; LSC, lateral semicircular canal; M, malleus; PSC, posterior semicircular canal; SSC, superior semicircular canal; SV, superior vestibular nerve; V, vestibule.

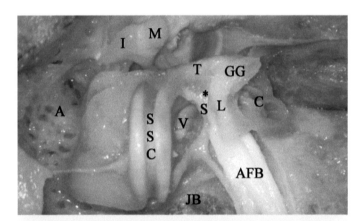

Fig. 2.69 The relationship of the facial nerve to the inner ear, seen from a left middle cranial fossa. In this case, the labyrinth has been opened. *, Bill's bar; AFB, acousticofacial bundle; A, antrum; C, cochlea; GG, geniculate ganglion; I, incus; JB, jugular bulb; L, labyrinthine segment of the facial nerve; M, malleus; S, superior vestibular nerve; SSC, superior semicircular canal; T, tympanic segment of the facial nerve; V, vestibule.

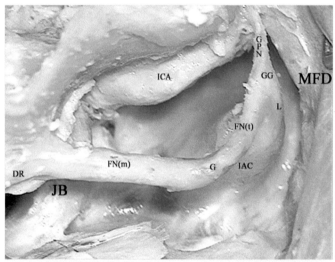

Fig. 2.70 A transotic approach has been used in a left temporal bone, and the whole course of the facial nerve has been skeletonized. Note the wide distance between the low jugular bulb (JB) and the internal auditory canal (IAC). Note also that the mastoid segment of the facial nerve (FN[m]) is centered on the lateral surface of the jugular bulb. DR, diastric ridge; FN(t), tympanic segment of the facial nerve; G, second genu of the facial nerve; GG, geniculate ganglion; GPN, greater petrosal nerve; ICA, internal carotid artery; L, labyrinthine segment of the facial nerve; MFD, middle fossa dura.

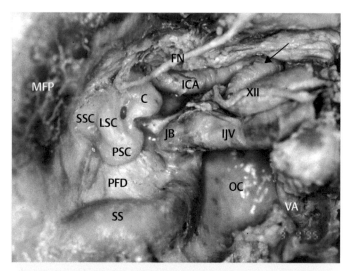

Fig. 2.71 Right ear. Infratemporal fossa type A approach with transcondylar transtubercolar extension. The relationship between the cochlea (C), the internal carotid artery (ICA), the facial nerve (FN), the jugular bulb (JB) and internal jugular vein (IJV), the hypoglossal nerve (XII), and the semicircular canals can be appreciated. The ICA shows a kinking on its cervical portion (*arrow*), which precludes arterial stenting. Note the extent of bone removal toward the occipital condyle (OC). LSC, lateral semicircular canal; MFP, middle fossa dura plate; PFD, posterior fossa dura; PSC, posterior semicircular canal; SS, sigmoid sinus; SSC, superior semicircular canal; VA, vertebral artery.

2.8 Endoscopic Surgical Anatomy

See ▶ Fig. 2.72, ▶ Fig. 2.73, ▶ Fig. 2.74, ▶ Fig. 2.75, ▶ Fig. 2.76, ▶ Fig. 2.77, ▶ Fig. 2.78, ▶ Fig. 2.79, ▶ Fig. 2.80, ▶ Fig. 2.81, ▶ Fig. 2.82, ▶ Fig. 2.83, ▶ Fig. 2.84, ▶ Fig. 2.85.

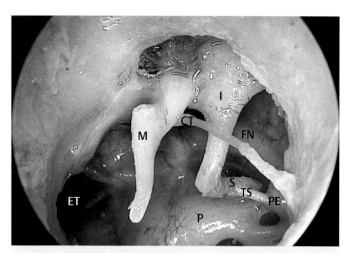

Fig. 2.72 Endoscopic view of a left middle ear (45-degree endoscope). The tympanic membrane has been removed. CT, chorda tympani; ET, eustachian tube; FN, facial nerve; I, icus; M, malleus; P, promontory; PE, pyramidal eminence; S, stapes; TS, tendon of the stapedius muscle.

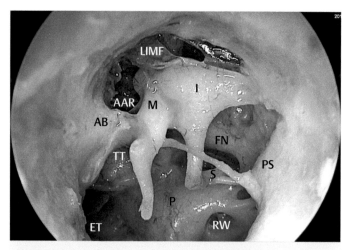

Fig. 2.73 Removal of the scutum exposes the whole incudomalleolar joint and the attic. AAR, anterior attic recess; AB, anterior buttress; ET, eustachian tube; FN, facial nerve; I, icus; M, malleus; P, promontory; PS, posterior spine; RW, round window; S, stapes; LIMF, lateral incudomalleolar fold;, TT tensor tympani muscle.

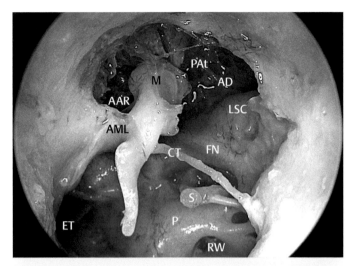

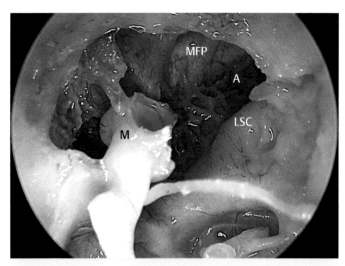

Fig. 2.74 Removal of the incus exposes the posterior attic (PAt) and the aditus ad antrum (AD). AAR, anterior attic recess; AML, anterior malleolar ligament; CT, chorda tympani; ET, eustachian tube; FN, facial nerve; LSC, lateral semicircular canal; M, malleus; P, promontory; RW, round window; S, stapes.

Fig. 2.75 The endoscope is tilted to show the antrum (A). LSC, lateral semicircular canal; M, malleus; MFP, middle fossa dura plate.

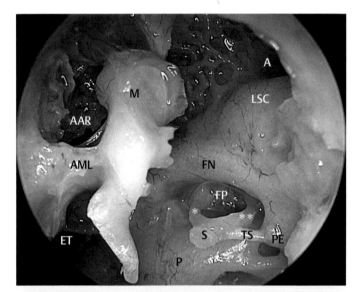

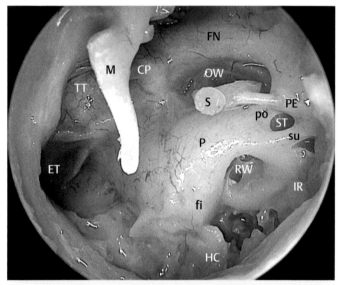

Fig. 2.76 The chorda tympani has been cut. *, anterior crus of the stapes; **, posterior crus of the stapes; A, antrum; AAR, anterior attic recess (also known as "supratubal recess"); AML, anterior malleolar ligament; ET, eustachian tube; FN, facial nerve; FP, footplate; LSC, lateral semicircular canal; M, malleus; P, promontory; PE, pyramidal eminence; S, stapes (head); TS, tendon of the stapedius muscle.

Fig. 2.77 Closer view of the protympanum, hypotympanum, and retrotympanum. CP, cochleariform process; ET, eustachian tube; FN, facial nerve; fi, finiculus; HC, hypotympanic cells, IR, inferior retrotympanum (or sinus subtympanicus); M, malleus; OW, oval window; P, promontory; PE, pyramidal eminence; po, ponticulus; RW, round window; S, stapes; ST, sinus tympani; su, subiculum; TT, tensor tympani muscle;

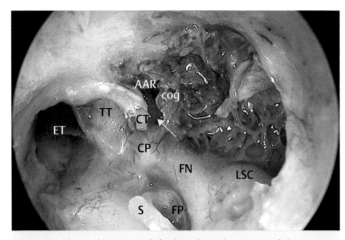

Fig. 2.78 The endoscope is shifted to show the course of the tympanic portion of the facial nerve (FN). The arrow indicates the direction of the geniculate ganglion. The malleus has been removed. The cog is a bony septum which divides the anterior from the posterior attic. AAR, anterior attic recess; CP, cochleariform process; CT, chorda tympani (cut); ET, eustachian tube; FP, footplate; LSC, lateral semicircular canal; S, stapes; TT tensor tympani muscle.

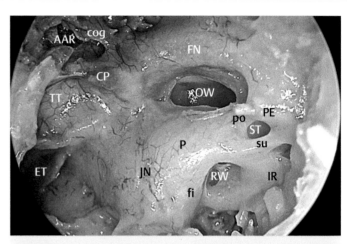

Fig. 2.79 Removal of the stapes shows the oval window (OW). AAR, anterior attic recess; CP, cochleariform process; ET, eustachian tube; FN, facial nerve; fi, finiculus; IR, inferior retrotympanum (or sinus subtympanicus); JN, Jacobson's nerve; P, promontory; PE, pyramidal eminence; po, ponticulus; RW, round window; ST sinus tympani; su, subiculum; TT, tensor tympani muscle.

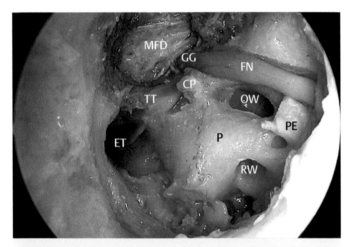

Fig. 2.80 The tympanic portion of the facial nerve (FN) has been uncovered from the overlying bone. CP, cochleariform process; ET, eustachian tube; GG, geniculate ganglion; MFD, middle fossa dura; OW, oval window; P, promontory; PE, pyramidal eminence; RW, round window; TT, tensor tympani muscle.

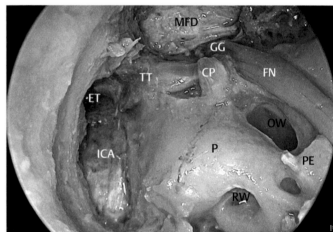

Fig. 2.81 Closer view. The bone over the vertical portion of the petrous internal carotid artery (ICA) has been removed. CP, cochleariform process; ET, eustachian tube; FN, facial nerve; GG, geniculate ganglion; MFD, middle fossa dura; OW, oval window; P, promontory; PE, pyramidal eminence; RW, round window; TT, tensor tympani muscle.

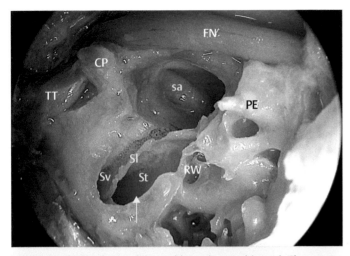

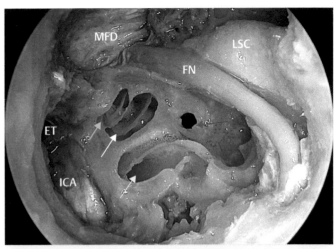

Fig. 2.82 The basal turn of the cochlea is dissected (*arrow*). The recess of the saccule (sa) is visible after the oval window is expanded. CP, cochleariform process; FN, facial nerve; PE, pyramidal eminence; RW, round window membrane; Sl, osseous spiral lamina; St, scala tympani; Sv scala vestibuli; TT, tensor tympani muscle.

Fig. 2.83 The middle (*white arrow*) and apical (*green arrow*) turns of the cochlea are dissected. The spherical recess has been removed, so the internal auditory canal is starting to appear (*red arrow*). ET, eustachian tube; FN, facial nerve; ICA, internal carotid artery; LSC, lateral semicircular canal; MFD, middle fossa dura; yellow arrow, basal turn of the cochlea.

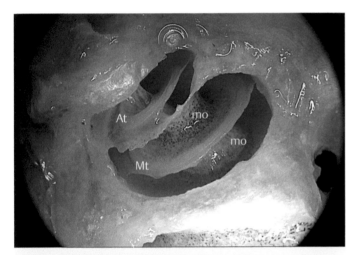

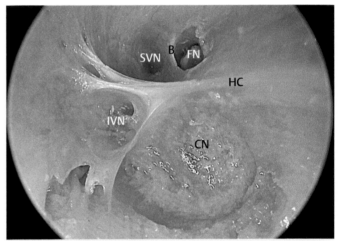

Fig. 2.84 Closer view. At, apical turn of the cochlea; mo, modiolus; Mt, middle turn of the cochlea.

Fig. 2.85 An endoscopic view of the fundus of a left internal auditory canal. The opening of the fallopian canal for the passage of the facial nerve (FN) can be seen lying anterior to Bill's bar (B). CN, cochlear nerve; HC, horizontal crest; IVN, inferior vestibular nerve; SVN, superior vestibular nerve.

3 Transmastoid Approaches

Abstract

This chapter illustrated all the procedures of tympanoplasty that can be performed in case of chronic otitis media with cholesteatoma. Special consideration goes to subtotal petrosectomy. In some patients, obliteration of the middle ear using abdominal fat with blind sac closure of the external auditory canal and closure of the eustachian tube is required. Such cases include chronically inflamed ear, usually open cavity, with no hearing, sustained cerebrospinal fluid (CSF) leak into the middle ear with or without meningitis, and a large meningoencephalocele in the middle ear in which resection or reposition is impractical.

An overview on lateral temporal bone resection, which is the surgery of choice in case of malignant tumors of the external auditory canal, will also be described.

At the end of the chapter the surgical steps of endolymphatic sac decompression and cochlear implantation will be provided.

Keywords: closed tympanoplasty, open tympanoplasty, modified Bondy's technique, radical mastoidectomy, subtotal petrosectomy, lateral temporal bone resection, endolymphatic sac decompression, cochlear implantation

3.1 Closed Tympanoplasty

3.1.1 Indications

- Cholesteatoma in children and in patients with highly pneumatized mastoids.
- Chronic otitis media without cholesteatoma, when exploration of the mastoid cavity is required.
- Minor epitympanic erosion.
- Mesotympanic cholesteatoma.
- Cochlear implants.
- Facial nerve decompression.
- Some cases of class B tympanomastoid paragangliomas.

3.1.2 Surgical Steps

See the steps listed below and also refer ▶ Fig. 3.1, ▶ Fig. 3.2, ▶ Fig. 3.3, ▶ Fig. 3.4, ▶ Fig. 3.5, ▶ Fig. 3.6, ▶ Fig. 3.7, ▶ Fig. 3.8, ▶ Fig. 3.9, ▶ Fig. 3.10, ▶ Fig. 3.11, ▶ Fig. 3.12, ▶ Fig. 3.13, ▶ Fig. 3.14, ▶ Fig. 3.15, ▶ Fig. 3.16, ▶ Fig. 3.17, ▶ Fig. 3.18, ▶ Fig. 3.19, ▶ Fig. 3.20, ▶ Fig. 3.21, ▶ Fig. 3.22, ▶ Fig. 3.23, ▶ Fig. 3.24, ▶ Fig. 3.25, ▶ Fig. 3.26, ▶ Fig. 3.27.

1. Drilling of the mastoid cortex is begun using a large cutting burr to identify the middle fossa dura. Drilling is started at the level of the temporalis ridge, which more or less corresponds to the level of the dura. The movement of the drill should be anteroposterior, parallel to the expected orientation of the middle fossa dura, and never perpendicular to it. Drilling is carried on carefully using continuous suction irrigation to provide adequate visualization. In live surgery, the signal that the level of the dura is close is provided by the appearance of the pink color of the dura through the bone, in addition to a change in the noise produced by drilling to a high-pitched sound when the dura is reached.

2. Drilling is now started at the expected level of the sigmoid sinus. As there is no solid external landmark for the position of the sigmoid sinus, the drill is moved in an oblique manner, joining the posterior edge of the upper margin of the drilling to the tip of the mastoid bone. The same principles apply here—the drill should always be moved parallel to the structure being looked for (the sigmoid sinus, in this case), and ample irrigation and suction should be used to identify the appearance of the blue color which signals that there is only a thin shell of bone separating us from the sigmoid sinus.

3. The two lines of drilling created until now are joined together by drilling the posterior tangent of the external auditory canal, thus creating a triangle of attack.

4. The bone in the center of the triangle can now be safely drilled out using the same large cutting burr. During this step, the cavity should be deepened evenly and gradually, avoiding the creation of a deep, narrow hole. The edges of the cavity should be rounded in order to provide the maximum visualization. A diamond burr is then used to thin out the remaining bone over the sigmoid sinus, the dura, and the posterior canal wall.

5. In the area of the sinodural angle, the drill should be moved in a medial to lateral direction in order to avoid injury to important structures if the drill slips medially.

6. Following the middle fossa dural plate, the antrum can be identified and opened. Once it has been opened, the lateral semicircular canal can be seen. Tilting the specimen away from the surgeon, the short process of the incus can be identified lateral to the canal, and care should be taken to avoid touching it with the rotating burr. These two structures are the first landmarks of the facial nerve (FN) to be encountered.

7. The next landmark to be identified is the digastric ridge. In the area of the mastoid tip, drilling is started in a posterior to anterior direction until the whole digastric ridge is developed. The FN will be found lying anteriorly.

8. Identification of the mastoid segment of the FN is started using a large cutting burr, which is moved in a direction parallel to the nerve and never crossing it. Once the whole length of the nerve can be seen through the bone, a smaller diamond burr is used to drill open the facial recess. While this step is being carried out, care should be taken not to move the drill too far anterolaterally, jeopardizing the annulus and tympanic membrane. On the other hand, drilling more medially would endanger the FN. For this reason, the right size of the burr should be used. Superiorly, a thin strut of bone should be left covering the short process of the incus to protect it from inadvertent injury with the burr. This strut of bone can be removed later on using a curette.

9. Epitympanotomy is started from a posterior position. A burr of a size sufficient to fit into the space between the middle fossa dural plate and the superior canal wall is used. A drill larger than the space provided will lead to injury to the dural

plate, the superior canal wall, or both. On the other hand, using a smaller drill will lead to a prolonged operation. The direction of drilling is from medial to lateral, leaving a thin plate of bone overlying the ossicular chain in order to avoid touching it with the rotating burr. The anterior extent of the atticotomy should be sufficient to expose the anterior attic recess.

10. The inferior extension of the tympanotomy depends on what type of pathology is being treated and on its extent. In surgery for cochlear implantation, an attempt to preserve the chorda tympani must be made, and the inferior extension of drilling should be stopped once the chorda starts to show through the bone. The adequacy of the approach is checked, and further inferior extension can then be performed if required. However, if the pathology being treated is a cholesteatoma, middle ear tumor, a type B paraganglioma, or a facial nerve tumor, the seriousness of the condition requires the sacrifice of the chorda tympani in order to obtain adequate control of the whole extent of the pathology and allow for its complete removal. In these cases, the posterior tympanotomy should be extended to the hypotympanum.

11. Particularly in type B paragangliomas, further exposure to the hypotympanum is needed. This exposure can be achieved by a retrofacial tympanotomy. The bone medial to the FN in the area limited superiorly by the lower limit of the posterior semicircular canal and inferiorly by the jugular bulb is now drilled using a large diamond burr. In addition to the posterior canal and the jugular bulb, the posterior fossa dura forms the medial relation to this area and the FN forms the lateral limit. Extreme attention should be paid at this step to avoid injuring any of these important structures.

3.1.3 Hints and Pitfalls

- Adequate saucerization of the mastoid cavity, with complete drilling of the sinodural angle and bony overhang on the cavity edges, should be carried out before posterior epitympanotomy and posterior tympanotomy are performed. The saucerized cavity provides a maximum surgical view and surgical angle.
- Canalplasty is required whenever the canal wall impedes complete view of the tympanic membrane. The canal wall should therefore not be thinned from the beginning.
- The utmost care should be taken not to touch the ossicular chain with the burr when the chain is intact.
- Care should be taken not to perforate the superior wall of the external auditory canal. If this occurs, reconstruction with cartilage and bone paste is necessary.
- Care should be taken not to injure the middle fossa dura in order to avoid possible cerebrospinal fluid leakage or meningoencephalic herniation. To avoid injuring any of these structures, drilling in the area of the attic should be conducted from medial to lateral, never pressing the burr heads against the superior and inferior bony wall in this area.
- Positive identification of the facial nerve is the most effective way of avoiding injuring it.
- Dissection of pathology from fragile structures in the tympanic cavity is carried out using the combined approach, with one instrument introduced from the external auditory canal and the other from the posterior cavity. In this way, the instruments do not obscure the required view of the delicate structures.
- Dissection of the pathology from the area of the windows is started after all of the bone work has been completed. All maneuvers on the stapes superstructure should be carried out with extreme care. Dissection is conducted along with its long axis, never perpendicular to it. If the pathology is adherent underneath the arch of the superstructure, the superstructure can be removed with long and straight malleable scissors, with care being taken not to fracture the footplate. Do not use the crurotomy scissors, which can damage the footplate.
- If the hypotympanic cells are infiltrated by the pathology, the area between the jugular bulb and the carotid artery is carefully drilled with a diamond burr. Care should be taken not to damage the jugular bulb, since the structure is extremely fragile.

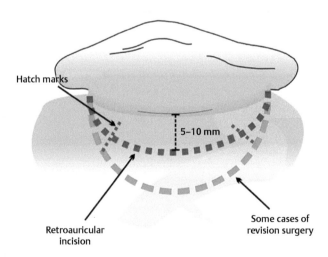

Fig. 3.1 Retroauricular skin incision.

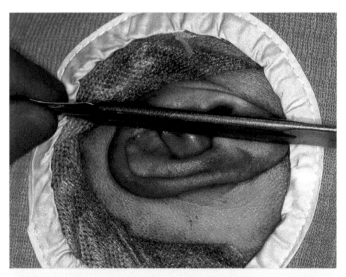

Fig. 3.2 To allow maximum flexion of the auricle, the retroauricular incision is planned in such way that the incision covers 180 degrees of the external auditory canal.

Left Ear

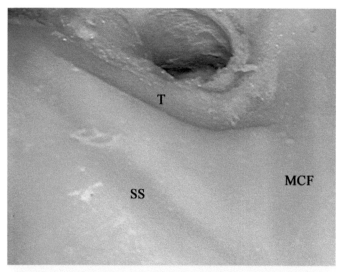

Fig. 3.3 The triangle of attack has been created in a left temporal bone. MCF, level of the middle cranial fossa; SS, expected level of the sigmoid sinus; T, posterior tangent to the external auditory canal.

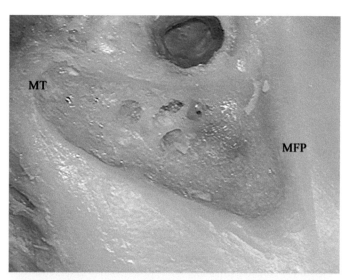

Fig. 3.4 Mastoidectomy has been started. MFP, middle fossa plate; MT, mastoid tip.

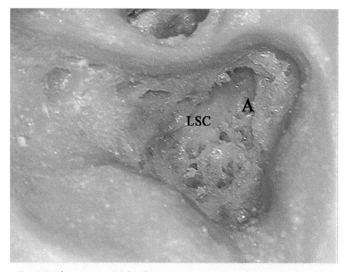

Fig. 3.5 The antrum (A) has been opened, and the lateral semicircular canal (LSC) has been identified.

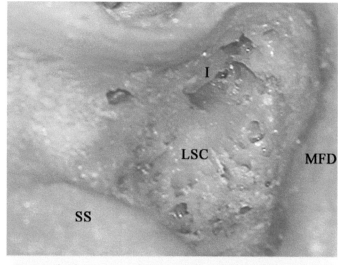

Fig. 3.6 The short process of the incus (I) has been identified. LSC, lateral semicircular canal; MFD, middle fossa dura; SS, sigmoid sinus.

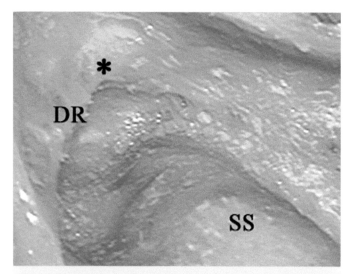

Fig. 3.7 The digastric ridge (DR) has been identified; the facial nerve lies at its anterior edge (*), at the stylomastoid foramen level. SS, sigmoid sinus.

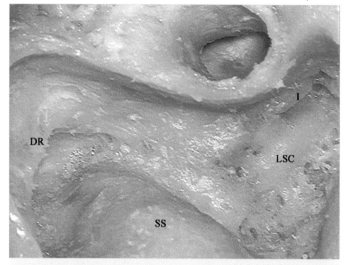

Fig. 3.8 The digastric ridge (DR), the short process of the incus (I), and the lateral semicircular canal (LSC) are the landmarks for the mastoid segment of the facial nerve. SS, sigmoid sinus.

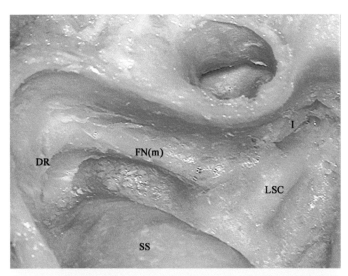

Fig. 3.9 The mastoid segment of the facial nerve (FN[m]) has been skeletonized. DR, digastric ridge; I, incus; LSC, lateral semicircular canal; SS, sigmoid sinus.

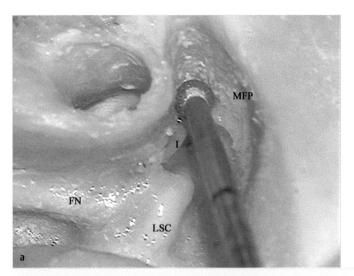 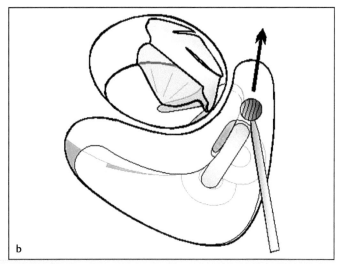

Fig. 3.10 Atticotomy is being carried out. (a) Note the size of the diamond burr used for this step. (b) The direction of movement should be from medial to lateral. FN, facial nerve; I, incus; LSC, lateral semicircular canal; MFP, middle fossa plate.

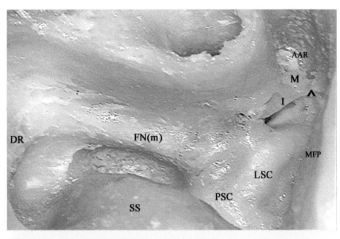 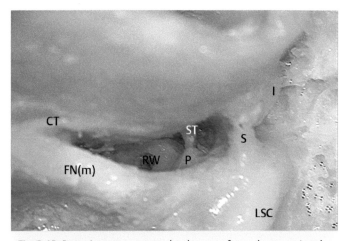

Fig. 3.11 Atticotomy has been completed. ^, superior suspensor ligament; AAR, anterior attic recess; DR, digastric ridge; FN(m), mastoid segment of the facial nerve; I, incus; LSC, lateral semicircular canal; M, malleus; MFP, middle fossa plate; PSC, posterior semicircular canal; SS, sigmoid sinus.

Fig. 3.12 Posterior tympanotomy has been performed, conserving the chorda tympani (CT). A strut of bone (S) has been left behind to protect the incus (I) from the rotating burr. Note that in this case, the round window exposure is complete, making this amount of posterior tympanotomy sufficient for a cochlear implant procedure.
FN(m), mastoid segment of the facial nerve; LSC, lateral semicircular canal; P, pyramidal process; RW, round window; ST, stapes.

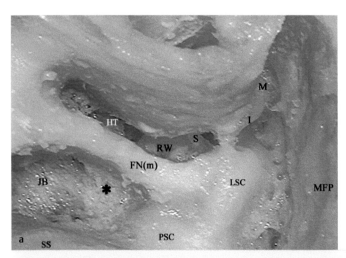

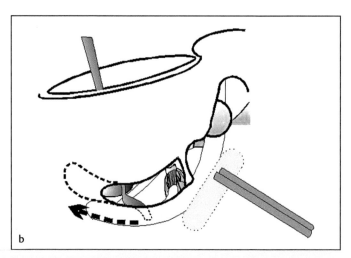

Fig. 3.13 (a) The posterior tympanotomy has been extended inferiorly toward the hypotympanum (HT). The bone medial to the facial nerve (*) is to be removed next. FN(m), mastoid segment of the facial nerve; I, incus; JB, jugular bulb; LSC, lateral semicircular canal; M, malleus; MFP, middle fossa plate; PSC, posterior semicircular canal; RW, round window; S, stapes; SS, sigmoid sinus. (b) The extended posterior tympanotomy allows management of the hypotympanum and middle ear through two different angles.

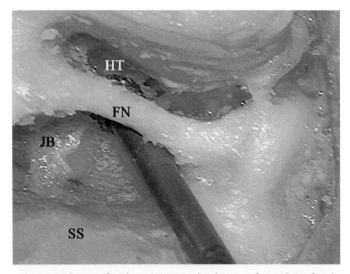

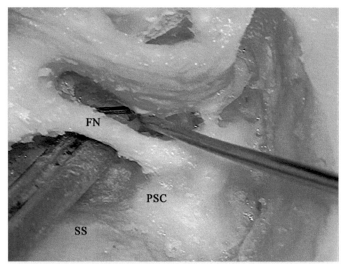

Fig. 3.14 The retrofacial tympanotomy has been performed. FN, facial nerve; HT, hypotympanum; JB, jugular bulb; SS, sigmoid sinus.

Fig. 3.15 The combination of extended tympanotomy and retrofacial tympanotomy provides wider access for management of the hypotympanum. FN, facial nerve; PSC, posterior semicircular canal; SS, sigmoid sinus.

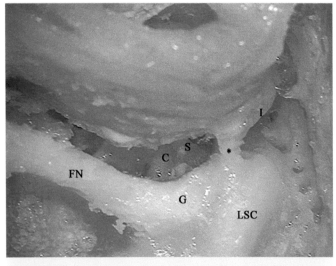

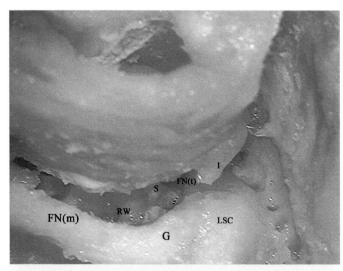

Fig. 3.16 The last step is to remove the strut of bone (*) left to protect the incus (I) using a curette. C, cochlea; FN, facial nerve; G, genu; LSC, lateral semicircular canal; S, stapes.

Fig. 3.17 The bone strut has been removed, and the tympanic segment of the facial nerve (FN[t]) is now under control. FN(m), mastoid segment of the facial nerve; G, genu; I, incus; LSC, lateral semicircular canal; RW, round window; S, stapes.

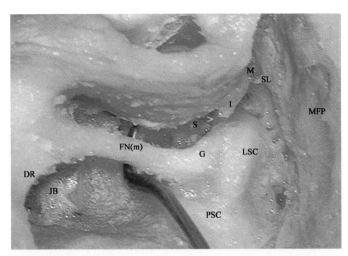

Fig. 3.18 The view after completing the approach. >, tympanic segment of the facial nerve; DR, digastric ridge; FN(m), mastoid segment of the facial nerve; G, genu; I, incus; JB, jugular bulb; LSC, lateral semicircular canal; M, malleus; MFP, middle fossa plate; PSC, posterior semicircular canal; S, stapes; SL, suspensory ligament.

Right Ear

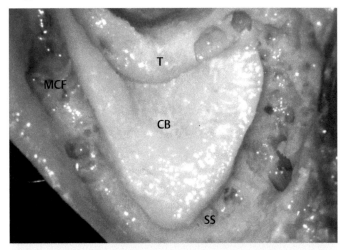

Fig. 3.19 The triangle of attack has been created in a right temporal bone. CB, cortical bone; MCF, level of the middle cranial fossa; SS, expected level of the sigmoid sinus; T, posterior tangent to the external auditory canal.

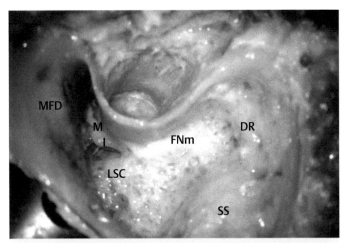

Fig. 3.20 Mastoidectomy and atticotomy have been completed. The incus (I) and the malleus are under view. DR, digastric ridge; FN(m), mastoid segment of the facial nerve; LSC, lateral semicircular canal; MFD, middle fossa dura; SS, sigmoid sinus.

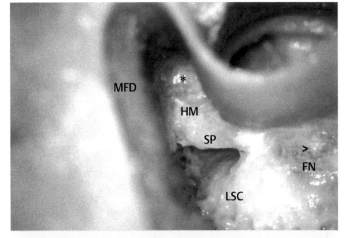

Fig. 3.21 Atticotomy, closer view. Note the articulation between the incus and the malleus and the space between the short process of the incus (SP), the lateral semicircular canal (LSC), and the facial nerve (FN), which is the area for the posterior tympanotomy (>). A thin shell of bone (*) should be further removed to gain access to the anterior epitympanum and supratubal recess. HM, head of the malleus; MFD, middle fossa dura.

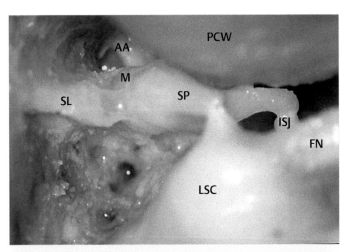

Fig. 3.22 Closer view after posterior tympanotomy. AA, anterior attic; FN, facial nerve; ISJ, incudostapedial joint; LSC, lateral semicircular canal; M, malleus; PCW, posterior canal wall; SL, suspensory ligament; SP, short process of the incus.

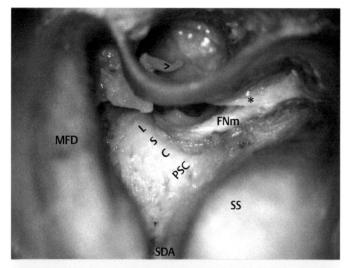

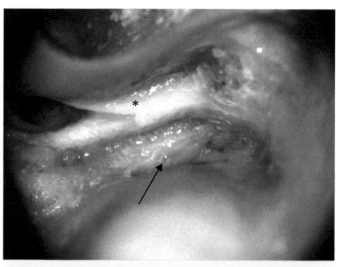

Fig. 3.23 The posterior tympanotomy has been extended inferiorly and the mastoid, genu, and tympanic segment of the facial nerve have been skeletonized. Note the origin of the chorda tympani (*). The mastoid sement of the facial nerve (FN[m]) lies just anteriorly to the ampullary end of the posterior semicircular canal (PSC), which forms an angle of 90 degrees with the lateral semicircular canal (LSC). The tympanic membrane has been removed and the handle of the malleus is visible (>). MFD, middle fossa dure; SDA, sinodural angle; SS, sigmoid sinus.

Fig. 3.24 Closer view of ▶ Fig. 3.23. Note the origin of the chorda tympani (*). Tre retrofacial air cells are started to be dissected to skeletonize the jugular bulb (*arrow*).

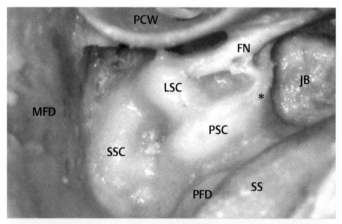

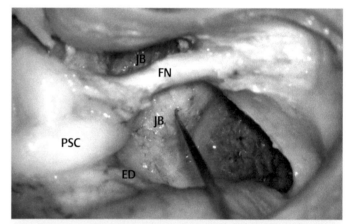

Fig. 3.25 The jugular bulb (JB) has been skeletonized in its retrofacial portion. In this case the jugular bulb is high and reaches the ampullary end of the posterior semicircular canal (*). Note the relation between the facial nerve (FN) and the lateral and posterior canals. The superior semicircular canal (SSC) has been skeletonized too. LSC, lateral semicircular canal; MFD, middle fossa dura; PCW, posterior canal wall; PFD, posterior fossa dura; PSC, posterior semicircular canal; SS, sigmoid sinus.

Fig. 3.26 Retrofacial tympanotomy has been performed. Note the relation of the facial nerve (FN) with the jugular bulb (JB), which is usually located two-thirds posterior and one-third anterior to the nerve. The endolymphatic duct (ED) is visible posterior to the ampulla of the posterior semicircular canal (PSC). The chorda tympani has been cut.

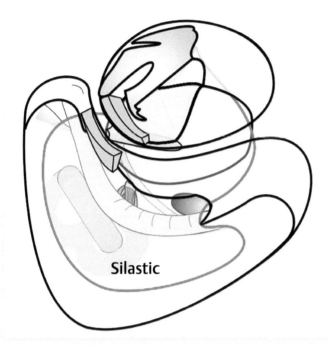

Fig. 3.27 Before closure, inserting a sheet of Silastic into the middle ear and mastoid cavity enhances the growth of healthy mucosa.

3.2 Open Tympanoplasty

3.2.1 Indications

- Cholesteatoma in cases of the following:
  - Contracted mastoid.
  - Large epitympanic erosions.
  - Recurrence after the closed tympanoplasty.
  - Bilateral cholesteatoma.
  - Cleft palate and Down's syndrome.
  - Only hearing ear.
  - Large labyrinthine fistula.
  - Severe sensorineural hearing loss.
- Some benign tumors involving the middle ear.

3.2.2 Surgical Steps

▸ Fig. 3.28, ▸ Fig. 3.29, ▸ Fig. 3.30, ▸ Fig. 3.31, ▸ Fig. 3.32, ▸ Fig. 3.33, ▸ Fig. 3.34, ▸ Fig. 3.35, ▸ Fig. 3.36, ▸ Fig. 3.37, ▸ Fig. 3.38, ▸ Fig. 3.39, ▸ Fig. 3.40, ▸ Fig. 3.41, ▸ Fig. 3.42, ▸ Fig. 3.43, ▸ Fig. 3.44, ▸ Fig. 3.45, ▸ Fig. 3.46, ▸ Fig. 3.47, ▸ Fig. 3.48, ▸ Fig. 3.49, ▸ Fig. 3.50, ▸ Fig. 3.51, ▸ Fig. 3.52, ▸ Fig. 3.53, ▸ Fig. 3.54, ▸ Fig. 3.55, ▸ Fig. 3.56, ▸ Fig. 3.57.

This approach can be performed in two ways: transcortically, carrying out a closed tympanoplasty with atticotomy first, followed by removal of the posterior canal wall either using the drill or the rongeur; or transmeatally, identifying the middle fossa plate at the level of the external auditory canal with initially and following it posteriorly. In the first case, the initial steps are identical to those described for closed tympanoplasty. After the closed tympanoplasty approach has been completed, a large cutting burr is used to drill away the posterior canal wall until the level of the FN is reached, as indicated by the digastric ridge and the

lateral semicircular canal. When the level of the FN is approached, the burr is changed to a diamond burr of the same large size, and drilling is continued parallel to the orientation of the FN with ample suction irrigation. The superior canal wall is then lowered in the same manner, with care being taken not to drill over the ossicular chain, which by now should have been examined and its continuity has been ascertained.

1. If the start was transmeatal, superior canal wall drilling is started in an anterior to posterior manner until the middle fossa plate is identified. This level should be followed posteriorly to the sinodural angle and medially until a thin shell of bone is left covering the ossicles (the facial bridge).

2. The drilling is now shifted to the posterior canal wall, which is gradually lowered using a large cutting burr until the level of the annulus is reached. Further medial drilling in this region would jeopardize the FN, since no landmarks for the nerve have been identified yet.

3. For this reason, drilling is continued posteriorly, and the mastoid antrum and sigmoid sinus are identified. In this way, the mastoid cavity is gradually opened from anterior to posterior. While the drilling is being carried out, the cavity must always be saucerized and gradually deepened, bony overhangs should be removed from the edges, and a round-shaped cavity should be obtained. In live surgery, if bone is removed appropriately, the middle fossa dura is clearly identified through the thinned bone by its pinkish color, and the sigmoid sinus is clearly identified by its bluish color.

4. In addition to identifying the lateral semicircular canal, one of the landmarks for the mastoid segment of the nerve, this step would also lead to widening of the approach, facilitating further drilling.

5. Identification of the other landmark of the mastoid segment of the FN—the digastric ridge, at the anterior border of the lower portion of the sigmoid sinus in the area of the mastoid tip—is carried out next. Drilling is started in a posterior to anterior direction until the whole digastric ridge is developed, and the FN will be found lying anteriorly.

6. Removal and exteriorization of all air cells between the mastoid segment of the facial nerve and the sigmoid sinus is carried out.

7. Before the lowering of the FN ridge is completed, the thin shell of bone left covering the ossicles and the FN bridge is removed with a curette. This provides better visualization of the tympanic segment of the FN, which can be used as a landmark when lowering the facial ridge. The anterior buttress of the bridge is drilled away using a small burr, with care being taken not to touch the ossicular chain lying behind. If there is prominent protrusion in the anterior or inferior wall, canalplasty should be carried out. The anterior meatal skin is cut laterally and detached from the bone toward the annulus. The medially folded meatal skin flap is protected with an aluminum sheet. The anterior or the inferior meatal walls, or both, are drilled to obtain a round-shaped cavity. Care should be taken not to expose the temporomandibular joint beneath the anterior wall.

8. In the last part of the approach, a large diamond burr is used to lower the FN ridge. While this step is being carried out, the direction of the movement of the burr should always be

parallel to the nerve, and drilling should take place with ample suction irrigation to allow early identification of the nerve. The level to which the FN ridge should be lowered is indicated by the pathology. For management of chronic otitis media, the level to which the ridge should be lowered should be sufficient to allow adequate drainage of the mastoid cavity without the ridge hampering it. On the other hand, if the approach is being carried out for an FN tumor, further lowering should be performed. In the poorly pneumatized mastoid frequently seen in patients with chronic otitis media, the level of the ideally drilled facial ridge is almost on the same plane as the drilled mastoid cavity.

9. The final shape of the cavity is a reversed pyramid, with rounded external edges with no bony overhang in the cavity. Drilling to obtain the correct cavity shape should be carried out to this extent.

3.2.3 Hints and Pitfalls

- Do not leave any bony overhangs in the edge of the cavity. The bony edges must be removed and rounded as much as possible in order to obtain a saucerized cavity.
- Thin the middle fossa plate and the sigmoid sinus plate sufficiently, but do not expose them. Open the sinodural angle widely.
- A deep, pneumatized mastoid tip must be lowered and removed.

- A posteroinferiorly based soft tissue flap is used to obliterate the area of the mastoid tip if there is a deep dip left after these procedures.
- The facial ridge must be lowered sufficiently.
- Spaces that may become aerated and deep, especially retrofacial cells, are obliterated with autologous cartilage or bone paste, or both.
- Attention should always be paid to the facial nerve and its anatomical landmarks. An important landmark for lowering the facial ridge at the level of the antrum is the prominence of the lateral semicircular canal. The second genu of the nerve is located inferomedial to the prominence.
- Drilling over the mastoid segment of the facial nerve must be carried out with large burrs, and always with continuous suction irrigation. The burrs should be moved parallel to the nerve.
- The anterior buttress must be removed. Leaving the buttress in place may facilitate ingrowth of skin underneath it.
- Perilabyrinthine cells in the attic must be drilled out. Care should be taken not to damage the superior semicircular canal and the labyrinthine segment of the facial nerve, located medial to the geniculate ganglion.

Right Ear—Transcortical Approach

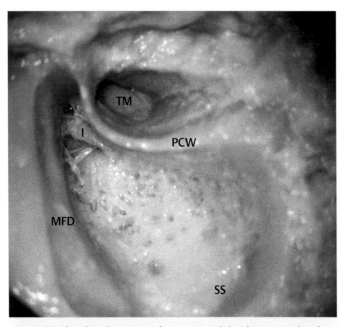

Fig. 3.28 The closed tympanoplasty approach has been completed. I, incus; MFD, middle fossa dura; PCW, posterior canal wall; SS, sigmoid sinus; TM, tympanic membrane.

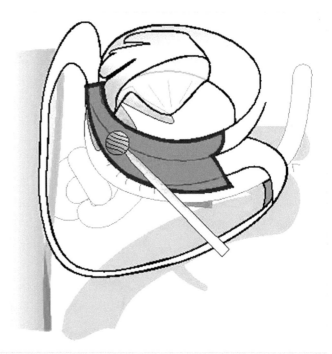

Fig. 3.29 A diagram showing the extent of drilling of the posterior and superior canal walls required to convert a closed tympanoplasty into an open one.

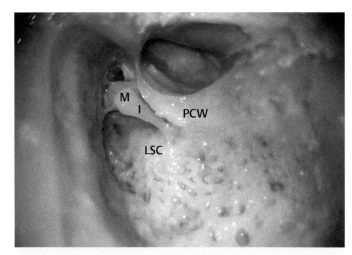

Fig. 3.30 The posterior canal wall (PCW) has been progressively drilled. I, incus; LSC, lateral semicircular canal; M, malleus.

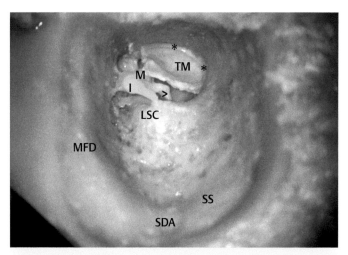

Fig. 3.31 The posterior canal wall (PCW) and the anterior buttress have been completely drilled and the anterior canalplasty is performed. The anterior and inferior part of the annulus (*) as well as incudostapedial joint (>) are visible. I, incus; LSC, lateral semicircular canal; M, malleus; MFD, middle fossa dura; SDA, sinodural angle; SS, sigmoid sinus; TM, tympanic membrane.

Left Ear—Transcortical Approach

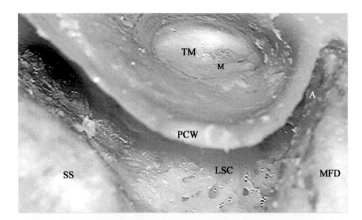

Fig. 3.32 A closed tympanoplasty with atticotomy has already been carried out in a left ear. A, attic; LSC, lateral semicircular canal; M, handle of the malleus; MFD, middle fossa dura; PCW, posterior canal wall; SS, sigmoid sinus; TM, tympanic membrane.

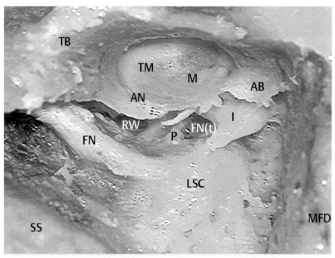

Fig. 3.33 The posterior canal wall has been drilled away, and the facial nerve (FN) has been skeletonized. AB, anterior buttress; AN, annulus; FN(t), tympanic segment of the facial nerve; I, incus; LSC, lateral semicircular canal; M, handle of the malleus; MFD, middle fossa dura; P, pyramidal process; RW, round window; SS, sigmoid sinus; TB, tympanic bone; TM, tympanic membrane.

Right Ear—Transcanal Approach

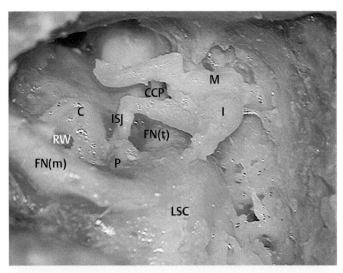

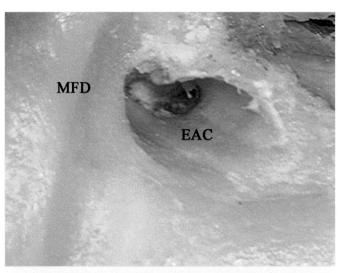

Fig. 3.34 The tympanic membrane, the anterior buttress of bone, and the remnants of the posterior canal wall have been removed, and the approach has been completed. C, cochlea; CCP, tensor tympani tendon passing through the cochleariform process; FN(m), mastoid segment of the facial nerve; FN(t), tympanic segment of the facial nerve; I, incus; ISJ, incudostapedial joint; LSC, lateral semicircular canal; M, malleus; P, pyramidal process; RW, round window.

Fig. 3.35 In this case of open tympanoplasty, the approach was started transmeatally in a right ear. The identification of the middle fossa plate (MFD) was started by drilling the superior wall of the external auditory canal (EAC). Drilling then was continued posteriorly.

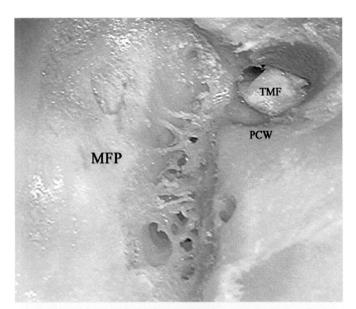

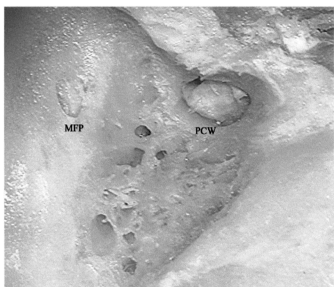

Fig. 3.36 After identification of the middle fossa plate (MFP), drilling has been continued in a medial direction toward the annulus. PCW, posterior canal wall; TMF, tympanomeatal flap.

Fig. 3.37 The posterior canal wall (PCW) has been lowered. MFP, middle fossa plate.

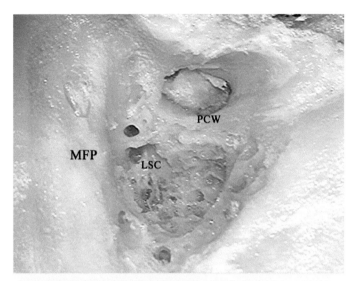

Fig. 3.38 The antrum has been opened, and the lateral semicircular canal (LSC) has been identified. MFP, middle fossa plate; PCW, posterior canal wall.

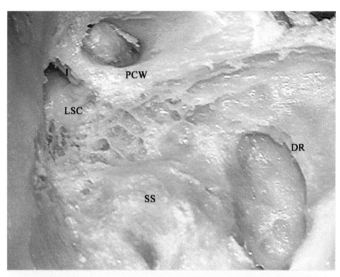

Fig. 3.39 Drilling has been further shifted posteriorly, identifying the sigmoid sinus (SS) and the digastric ridge (DR). I, incus; LSC, lateral semicircular canal; PCW, posterior canal wall.

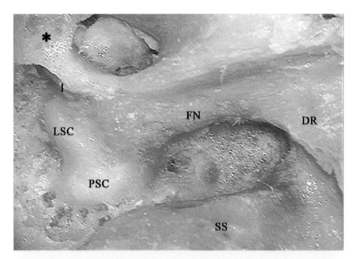

Fig. 3.40 The air cells between the facial nerve (FN) and the sigmoid sinus (SS) have been identified. The thin shell of bone (*) left covering the ossicles in the attic area is to be removed next using a curette. DR, digastric ridge; LSC, lateral semicircular canal; PSC, posterior semicircular canal.

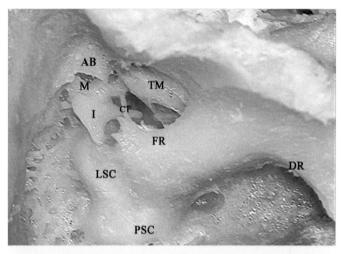

Fig. 3.41 The thin shell of bone covering the attic has been removed. The anterior buttress has yet to be removed. AB, anterior buttress, CT, chorda tympani; DR, digastric ridge; FR, facial ridge; I, incus; LSC, lateral semicircular canal; M, malleus; PSC, posterior semicircular canal; TM, tympanic membrane.

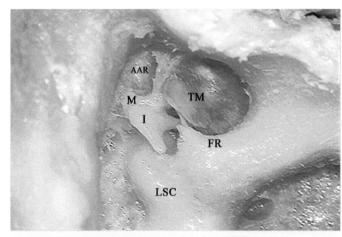

Fig. 3.42 The attic has been adequately opened, and the facial ridge (FR) will next be lowered. AAR, anterior attic recess; I, incus; LSC, lateral semicircular canal; M, head of the malleus; TM, tympanic membrane.

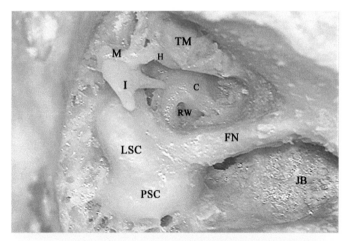

Fig. 3.43 The facial bridge has been adequately lowered, and the tympanic membrane (TM) has been reflected anteriorly. C, basal turn of the cochlea (promontory); FN, facial nerve; H, handle of the malleus; I, incus; JB, jugular bulb; LSC, lateral semicircular canal; M, malleus; PSC, posterior semicircular canal; RW, round window.

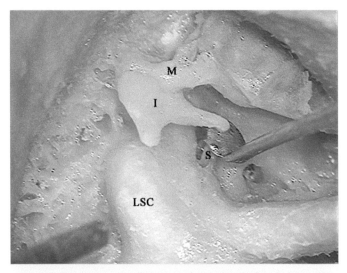

Fig. 3.44 The incudostapedial joint is being disarticulated. I, incus; LSC, lateral semicircular canal; M, malleus; S, stapes.

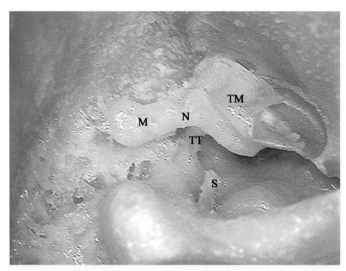

Fig. 3.45 The incus has been removed. The malleus (M) is now to be cut at the level of the neck (N). S, stapes; TM, tympanic membrane; TT, tensor tympani tendon.

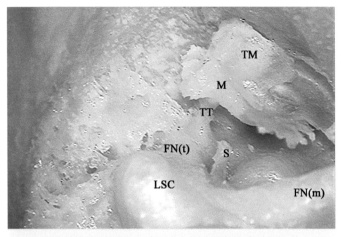

Fig. 3.46 The head of the malleus has been removed. Note the attachment of the tensor tympani (TT) to the medial aspect of the neck of the malleus, preventing anterior reflection of the malleus handle (M) together with the attached tympanic membrane (TM) to examine the anterior part of the mesotympanum. FN(m), mastoid segment of the facial nerve; FN(t), tympanic segment of the facial nerve; LSC, lateral semicircular canal; S, stapes.

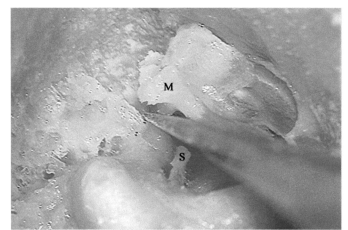

Fig. 3.47 The tensor tympani tendon is being cut. M, malleus; S, stapes.

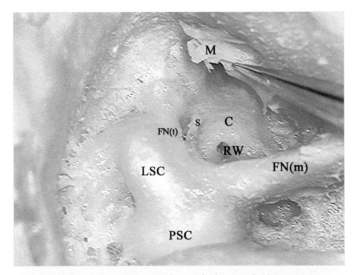

Fig. 3.48 The malleus (M), together with the attached tympanic membrane, can now be reflected anteriorly, and the middle ear cavity can be well visualized. C, basal turn of the cochlea (promontory); FN(m), mastoid segment of the facial nerve; FN(t), tympanic segment of the facial nerve; LSC, lateral semicircular canal; PSC, posterior semicircular canal; RW, round window; S, stapes.

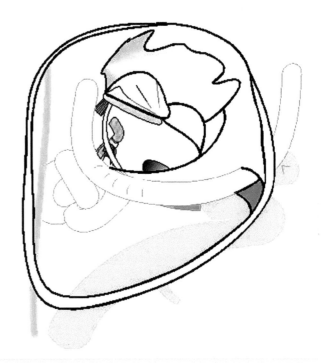

Fig. 3.49 A schematic presentation of the exposure required in an open tympanoplasty.

Left Ear—Transcanal Approach

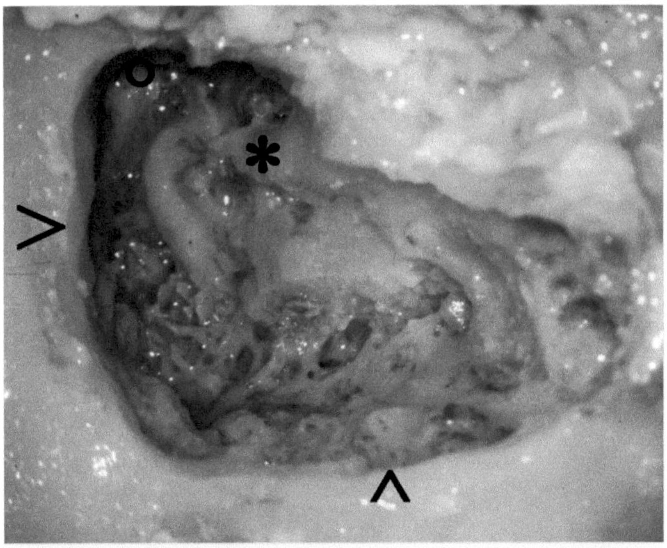

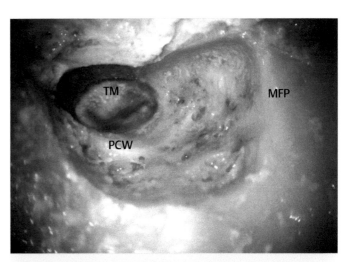

Fig. 3.50 An example of an incorrectly performed open tympanoplasty. The mistakes that can be seen are the edges at the level of both the middle fossa plate (>) and the sigmoid sinus (^) are overhanging and not saucerized, the facial ridge is too high (*), and the anterior attic recess (O) has not been adequately opened.

Fig. 3.51 Left ear. Canal wall down tympanoplasty started transmeatally. The level of the middle fossa plate (MFP) has been identified and the mastoid air cells are starting to be seen. PCW, posterior canal wall; TM, tympanic membrane.

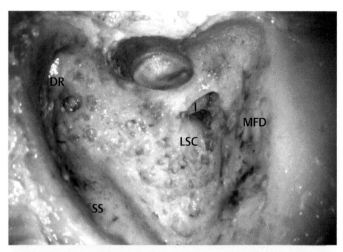

Fig. 3.52 The antrum and the mastoid air cells have been opened. The middle fossa dura (MFD), the sigmoid sinus (SS), the lateral semicircular canal (LSC), and the short process of the incus (I) are under view. DR, digastric ridge.

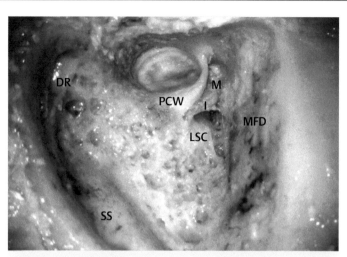

Fig. 3.53 The drilling has been continued anterosuperiorly and all the epitympanic area has been opened with further skeletonization of the middle fossa dura (MFD). The posterior canal wall (PCW) is starting to be thinned. DR, digastric ridge; I, incus; LSC, lateral semicircular canal; M, malleus; SS, sigmoid sinus.

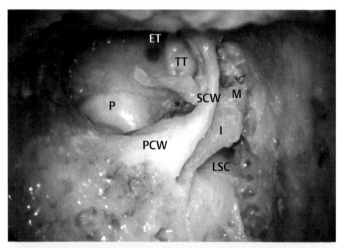

Fig. 3.54 Closer view after removal of the tympanic membrane. *, chorda tympani; ET, eustachian tube; I, incus; LSC, lateral semicircular canal; M, malleus; P, promontory; PCW, posterior canal wall; SCW, superior canal wall; TT, tensor tympani muscle.

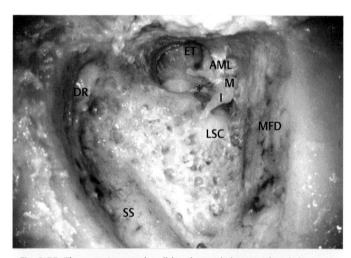

Fig. 3.55 The anterior canal wall has been skeletonized and the posterior canal wall has beed further lowered. The malleus is completely visible. The chorda tympani is under view (*). AML, anterior malleolar ligament; DR, digastric ridge; ET, eustachian tube; I, incus; LSC, lateral semicircular canal; M, malleus; MFD, middle fossa dura; SS sigmoid sinus.

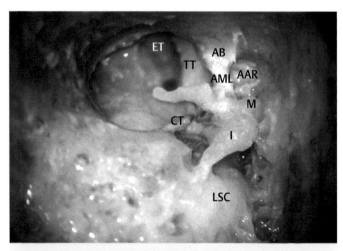

Fig. 3.56 Closer view. AAR, anterior attic recess; AB, anterior buttress; AML, anterior malleolar ligament; CT, chorda tympani; ET, eustachian tube; I, incus; LSC, lateral semicircular canal; M, malleus; TT, tensor tympani muscle.

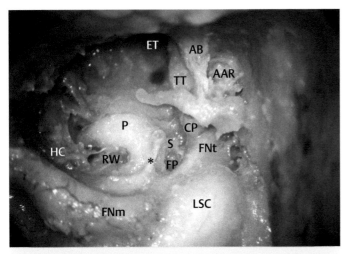

Fig. 3.57 Closer view after removal of the incus, posterior canal wall, and complete skeletonization of the mastoid portion of the facial nerve (FN[m]). Note the relationship between the facial nerve and the lateral semicircular canal (LSC). The anterior buttress (AB) has to be removed to get complete control of the anterior attic recess (AAR). *, tendon of the stapedius muscle; CP, cochleariform process; ET, eustachian tube; FN(t), tympanic portion of the facial nerve; FP, footplate; HC, hypotympanic cells; M, malleus; P, promontory; RW, round window; S, stapes; TT, tensor tympani muscle.

3.3 Modified Bondy's Technique

Some patients with cholesteatoma maintain good or better hearing in the diseased ear, and hearing preservation is of first importance. Closed tympanoplasty may give a chance of maintaining hearing. However, if the ossicular chain is reconstructed during middle ear surgery, preservation of normal or good preoperative hearing is not always possible, and the second operation may carry an additional risk to the hearing. In modified Bondy's technique, the posterior canal wall is removed, but the articulations between the ossicles are not touched. The prerequisite conditions for using this technique are an intact ossicular chain and the tympanic membrane with cholesteatoma located laterally to the chain, usually epitympanic cholesteatoma. A contracted mastoid is preferred. Significant benefits of this technique are constant retention of preoperative hearing, due to the preservation of ossicular articulations, low recurrence, and low rate of residues compared to closed technique, and that it is a one-stage operation that does not necessitate a second intervention. The risk of this procedure is sensorineural hearing loss at the high frequencies due to acoustic trauma, especially when drilling around the chain, since the ossicular chain remains intact throughout the surgery. Drilling around the chain should be conducted correctly and meticulously. With appropriate selection of cases, there are no further disadvantages compared with other open mastoidectomy procedures.

3.3.1 Indications

- Epitympanic cholesteatoma in a normal or good hearing ear with an intact tympanic membrane, ossicular chain, and tympanic cavity (▶ Fig. 3.58).
- Epitympanic cholesteatoma in the better or only hearing ear with slightly injured ossicular chain.
- Some cases of bilateral postinflammatory canal stenosis.

3.3.2 Surgical Steps

See the steps listed below and also refer to ▶ Fig. 3.59, ▶ Fig. 3.60, ▶ Fig. 3.61, ▶ Fig. 3.62, ▶ Fig. 3.63, ▶ Fig. 3.64, ▶ Fig. 3.65, ▶ Fig. 3.66, ▶ Fig. 3.67, ▶ Fig. 3.68, ▶ Fig. 3.69, ▶ Fig. 3.70, ▶ Fig. 3.71, ▶ Fig. 3.72, ▶ Fig. 3.73, ▶ Fig. 3.74, ▶ Fig. 3.75, ▶ Fig. 3.76, ▶ Fig. 3.77, ▶ Fig. 3.78, ▶ Fig. 3.79, ▶ Fig. 3.80, ▶ Fig. 3.81, ▶ Fig. 3.82, ▶ Fig. 3.83, ▶ Fig. 3.84, ▶ Fig. 3.85.

1. A mastoidectomy is completed using one of two techniques described earlier. Sufficient lowering of the facial ridge to the level of the tympanic annulus is of tremendous importance. The drill should be moved parallel to the nerve during this procedure.
2. A highly pneumatized mastoid tip should be amputated as described previously. Extensive pneumatizations in the cavity are filled with cartilage or bone paste. (See the section on Open Tympanoplasty).
3. In transcortical mastoidectomy, posterior epitympanotomy is performed taking care not to touch the intact ossicular chain. The specimen should be tilted away from the surgeon to help identify the chain as soon as possible. The burr should be moved from an area near the ossicles to elsewhere, but never toward the ossicles.
4. If canalplasty is required, the anterior meatal skin is cut and folded medially. The inferior canal wall is widened to give a round cavity. The tympanomeatal flap should be protected with a thin aluminum sheet during the drilling.
5. The facial bridge is removed with a curette, taking special care not to injure the chain. Burrs may be used, but since the ossicular chain remains intact, this might carry more risks. The anterior and the posterior buttresses are also removed in the same way. The anterior epitympanum should be fully opened. The facial ridge is further lowered.
6. In live surgery, cholesteatoma is removed from the attic and the mastoid. The posterosuperior annulus is partially detached from the tympanic sulcus, and the tympanic cavity is carefully inspected to ensure absence of cholesteatoma. Pathologic tissue, such as scar and granulation tissue, if any, is dissected with meticulous care from the ossicular chain. Minor invagination of cholesteatoma matrix behind the body of the incus and the head of the malleus is carefully dissected from the chain. Meatoplasty is performed to obtain sufficiently large access to the cavity postoperatively. The conchal cartilage is harvested for the subsequent reconstruction.
7. A piece of cartilage is placed in the attic, medially to the body of the incus and the head of the malleus. This cartilage prevents retraction of the reconstructed tympanic membrane behind the ossicles. Bone paste should not be used in this area to avoid fixation of the ossicular chain. The eustachian tube and the tympanic cavity are packed with Gelfoam.
8. A longitudinal cut is made in the temporalis fascia. One tongue is placed medial to the body of the incus and the head of the malleus, extending anteriorly under the anterosuperior quadrant of the tympanic membrane. The other tongue is inserted lateral to the long process of the incus and medial to the handle of the malleus making the fascia underlay. In some cases, a thin piece of cartilage may be inserted over the long process of the incus to avoid retraction of the posterosuperior quadrant.
9. As large an exposed bony surface as possible is covered with the posterior extension of the fascia. Another piece of fascia may be

placed to cover exposed bone and materials used for obliteration. The tympanomeatal flap is replaced on the temporal fascia.

10. If the ossicular chain is substantially involved in the cholesteatoma and its dissection is difficult, it is necessary to remove the body of the incus with or without the head of the malleus. This converts the technique to open tympanoplasty. The chain may be reconstructed in the same stage.

3.3.3 Hints and Pitfalls

- The modified Bondy's technique forms a part of the main system of surgery, with which a skilled and experienced surgeon must be familiar.
- The major advantage of this technique over others is that it is a single-stage procedure. This is safer if preservation of hearing is of prime importance.
- When the procedure is carried out correctly in the right patient, a dry and self-cleaning cavity can be obtained in the majority of cases (> 95% of our cases).

- It should always be borne in mind that the entire ossicular chain is intact and directly connected to the inner ear. Do not touch the intact ossicular chain with burrs.
- Drilling of the epitympanic area must be carried out very carefully. The drill is moved from medial to lateral, or away from the ossicular chain, to avoid touching it accidentally.
- The last portion of the superior canal wall (the facial bridge) is removed with a curette, rather than burrs. Do not leave the anterior buttress. This will favor invagination of the skin anterior to the head of the malleus, which is very difficult to manage.
- Insert autologous conchal cartilage beneath the body of the incus and the head of the malleus in order to avoid retraction, which creates deep spaces medial to these structures.
- If protrusion of the anterior canal wall is not too prominent, do not drill it out. This will avoid unnecessary danger not only to the temporomandibular joint but also to the ossicular chain.

Right Ear

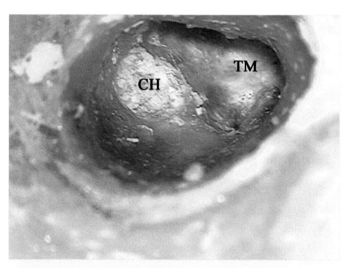

Fig. 3.59 View of the tympanic membrane (TM), with an attic cholesteatoma (CH) in a right ear.

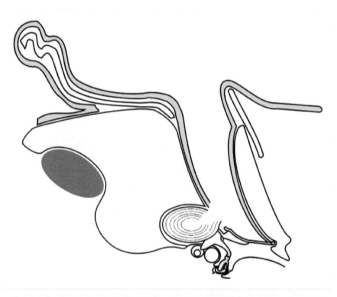

Fig. 3.58 The indication for performing a modified Bondy procedure. Note that the cholesteatoma (C) is invading only the attic lateral to the malleus and incus, so that both the malleus and incus and also the tympanic membrane remain intact.

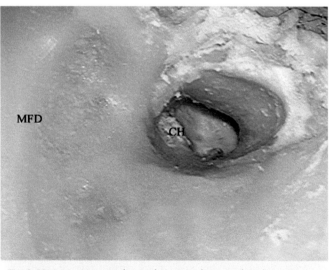

Fig. 3.60 An incision similar to that carried out in closed tympanoplasty is made. The level of the middle fossa dura (MFD) has been delineated here, and drilling has been started from the level of the anterior canal wall. CH, cholesteatoma.

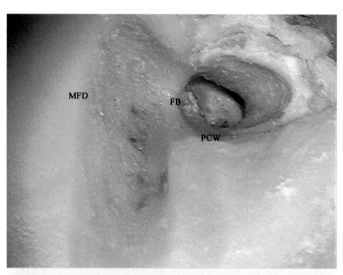

Fig. 3.61 The drilling has been advanced medially, leaving only a thin shell of bone covering the ossicles. FB, facial bridge; MFD, level of the middle fossa dura; PCW, posterior canal wall.

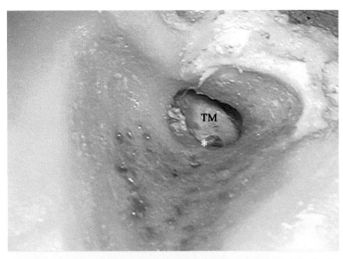

Fig. 3.62 The posterior canal wall has been lowered down to the level of the annulus (*). TM, tympanic membrane.

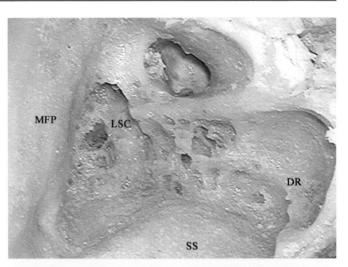

Fig. 3.63 The lateral semicircular canal (LSC), sigmoid sinus (SS), and digastric ridge (DR) have been identified. MFP, middle fossa plate.

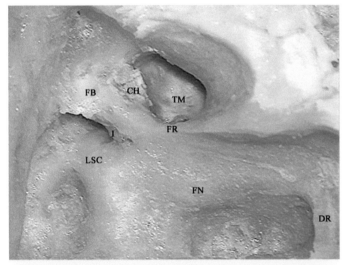

Fig. 3.64 The short process of the incus (I) and the facial nerve (FN) have been identified. CH, cholesteatoma; DR, digastric ridge; FB, facial bridge; FR, facial ridge; LSC, lateral semicircular canal; TM, tympanic membrane.

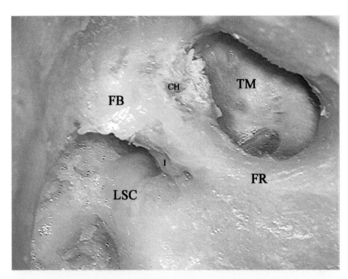

Fig. 3.65 The facial ridge (FR) has been lowered further.
CH, cholesteatoma; FB, facial bridge; I, incus; LSC, lateral semicircular canal; TM, tympanic membrane.

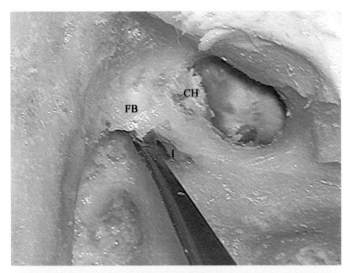

Fig. 3.66 The curette is used to remove the facial bridge (FB) and the last bone covering the ossicles. CH, cholesteatoma; I, incus.

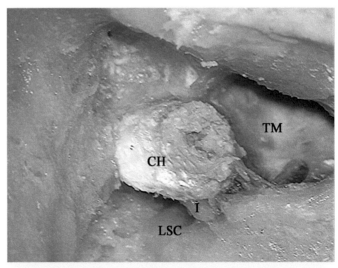

Fig. 3.67 The cholesteatoma (CH) can be seen located lateral to the incus (I) in the attic area. LSC, lateral semicircular canal; TM, tympanic membrane.

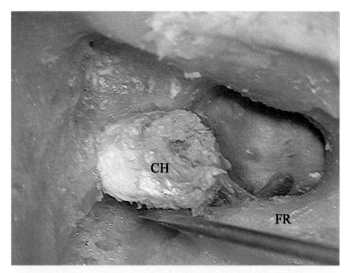

Fig. 3.68 Dissection of the cholesteatoma (CH). FR, facial ridge.

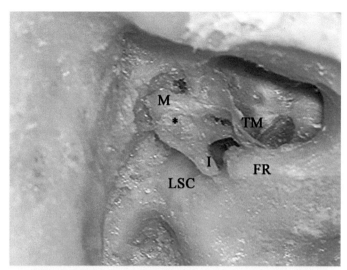

Fig. 3.69 The cholesteatoma has been removed, and the ossicles are seen to be intact, except for mild erosion (*) of the body of the incus (I). FR, facial ridge; LSC, lateral semicircular canal; M, malleus; TM, tympanic membrane.

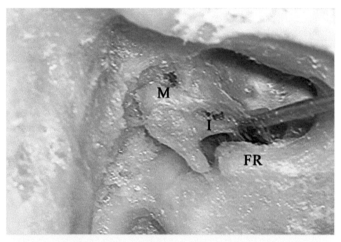

Fig. 3.70 Elevation of the tympanic membrane to examine the mesotympanum. FR, facial ridge; I, incus; M, malleus.

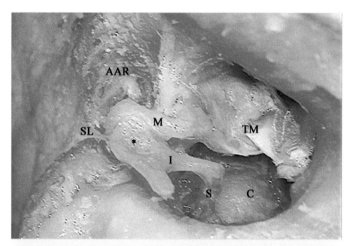

Fig. 3.71 The tympanic membrane (TM) has been reflected anteriorly. The ossicles are intact, and no cholesteatoma is found. *, erosion of the body of the incus; AAR, anterior attic recess; C, basal turn of the cochlea (promontory); I, incus; M, malleus; S, stapes; SL, superior suspensory ligament.

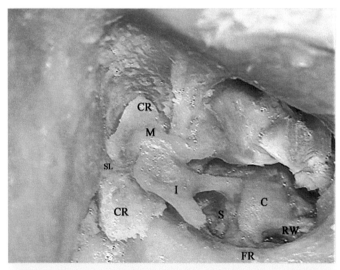

Fig. 3.72 The reconstruction is started by inserting a piece of cartilage (CR) medial to the body of the incus (I) and head of the malleus (M). C, basal turn of the cochlea (promontory); FR, facial ridge; RW, round window; S, stapes; SL, superior suspensory ligament.

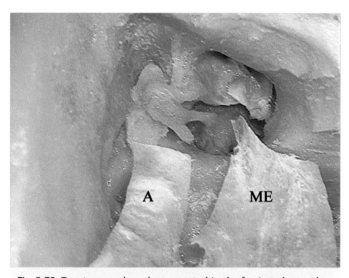

Fig. 3.73 Two tongues have been created in the fascia to be used during construction. The smaller tongue (A) will be inserted into the attic medial to the body of the incus and head of the malleus, and lateral to the cartilage, while the larger tongue (ME) will be inserted between the handle of the malleus and the long process of the incus.

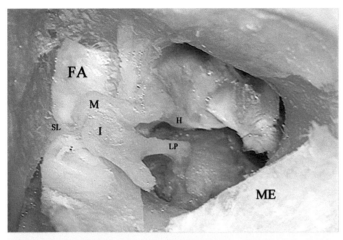

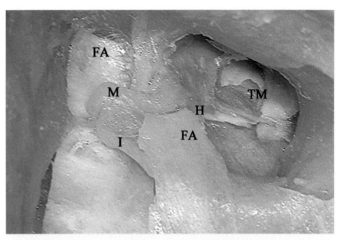

Fig. 3.74 The small tongue of the fascia (FA) is in place. H, handle of the malleus; I, body of the incus; LP, long process of the incus; M, head of the malleus; ME, larger tongue; SL, suspensory ligament.

Fig. 3.75 The large tongue of the fascia (FA, right) is in place. H, handle of the malleus; I, body of the incus; M, head of the malleus; TM, tympanic membrane.

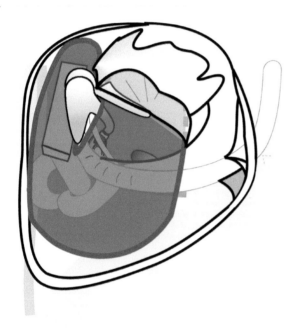

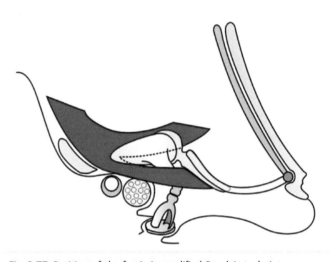

Fig. 3.77 Position of the fascia in modified Bondy's technique.

Fig. 3.76 Diagrams illustrating the relationship of the cartilage and fascia to the ossicles. A piece of cartilage is placed medial to the head of the malleus and the body of the incus and is covered with a tongue of fascia. The rest of the fascia is placed between the handle of the malleus and the long process of the incus.

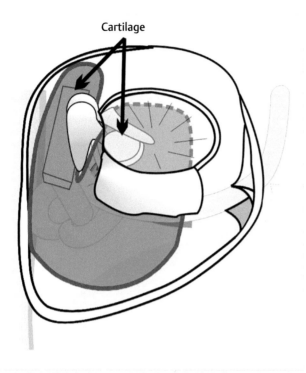

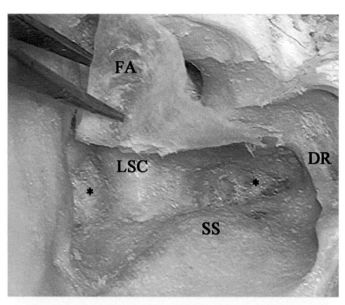

Fig. 3.79 To prevent secretions from collecting, the depression in the mastoid cavity (*) should be obliterated. DR, digastric ridge; FA, fascia; LSC, lateral semicircular canal; SS, sigmoid sinus.

Fig. 3.78 An additional piece of cartilage is placed between the handle of the malleus and the long process of the incus, and the posterior meatal skin flap is reflected backward to cover the fascia.

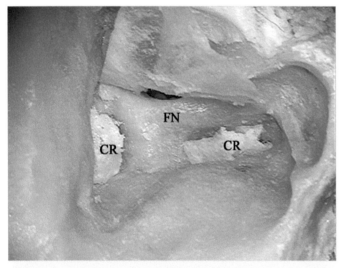

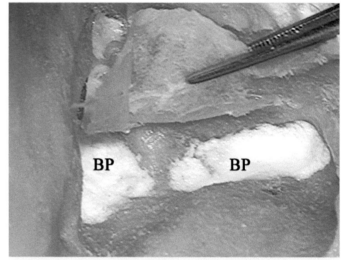

Fig. 3.80 Small pieces of cartilage (CR) are used first. FN, facial nerve.

Fig. 3.81 Bone paste (BP) is added to cover the cartilage.

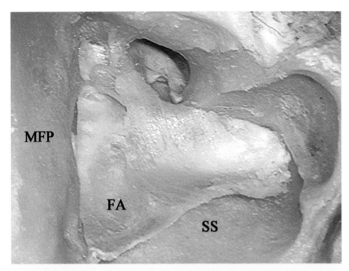

Fig. 3.82 The rest of the fascia (FA) is reflected posteriorly to cover as much of the mastoid cavity as possible. MFP, middle fossa plate; SS, sigmoid sinus.

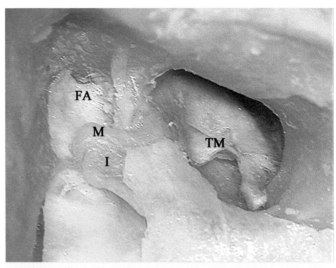

Fig. 3.83 The remnants of the tympanic membrane (TM) are reflected back. FA, fascia; I, body of the incus; M, head of the malleus.

Left Ear

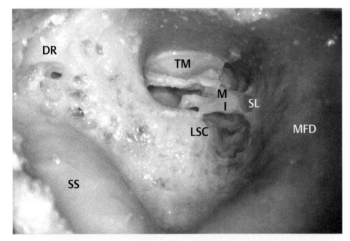

Fig. 3.84 View after completion of a modified Bondy technique tympanoplasty in a left ear. The posterior canal wall has been lowered to the level of the annulus and the ossicles have been left in place. DR, digastric ridge; I, incus; LSC, lateral semicircular canal; M, malleus; MFD, middle fossa dura; SL, superior suspensory ligament; SS, sigmoid sinus; TM, tympanic membrane.

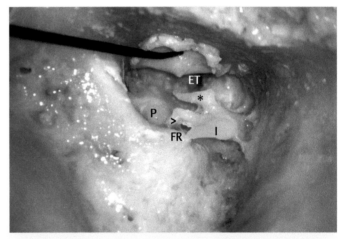

Fig. 3.85 Closer view after elevation of the tympanic membrane. The handle of the malleus (*) is visible as well as the incudostapedial joint (>). ET, eustachian tube; FR, facial ridge; I, incus; P, promontory.

3.4 Radical Mastoidectomy

The difference between this technique and open tympanoplasty is that it involves complete removal of the middle ear, including the sound transmission system (except for the footplate of the stapes), and eradication of the tubal function. This technique is used mainly in elderly patients with a preoperative dead ear or nonserviceable hearing, in whom the only goal of surgery is to obtain a dry and safe ear (▶ Fig. 3.86, ▶ Fig. 3.87). Other indications are as follows:

- Presence of cochlear fistulas.
- Presence of middle ear cholesteatoma in difficult-to-reach areas—for example, deep sinus tympani.
- Cholesteatoma with intracranial complications.
- Benign tumors in the middle ear and the mastoid, with severe sensorineural hearing loss.

Right Ear

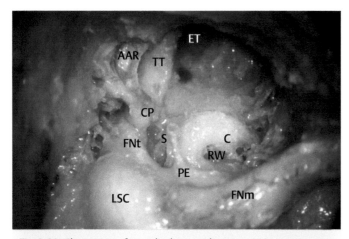

Fig. 3.86 Closer view after radical mastoidectomy. AAR, anterior attic recess; C, basal turn of the cochlea (promontory); CP, cochleariform process; ET, eustachian tube; FN(m), mastoid segment of the facial nerve; FN(t), tympanic segment of the facial nerve; LSC, lateral semicircular canal; PE, pyramidal eminence; RW, round window; S, stapes; TT, tensor tympani muscle.

Left Ear

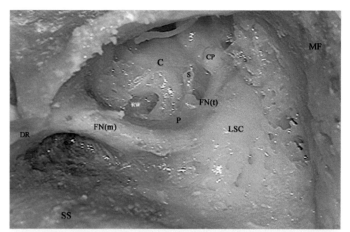

Fig. 3.87 The appearance after radical mastoidectomy. C, basal turn of the cochlea (promontory), CP, cochleariform process; DR, digastric ridge; FN(m), mastoid segment of the facial nerve; FN(t), tympanic segment of the facial nerve; LSC, lateral semicircular canal; MF, middle fossa plate; P, pyramid; RW, round window; S, stapes; SS, sigmoid sinus.

3.5 Subtotal Petrosectomy

In this approach, after radical mastoidectomy has been completed, complete drilling of the air cells of the temporal bone is carried out, leaving only the inner ear. The air cells to be removed include retrofacial, retrolabyrinthine, infralabyrinthine, supralabyrinthine, peritubal, and pericarotid air cells, if present. Blind-sac closure of the external auditory canal can be added to the approach, depending on the indication. Refer to ▸ Fig. 3.88, ▸ Fig. 3.89, ▸ Fig. 3.90, ▸ Fig. 3.91, ▸ Fig. 3.92, ▸ Fig. 3.93, ▸ Fig. 3.94, ▸ Fig. 3.95, ▸ Fig. 3.96, ▸ Fig. 3.97, ▸ Fig. 3.98, ▸ Fig. 3.99, ▸ Fig. 3.100, ▸ Fig. 3.101, ▸ Fig. 3.102, ▸ Fig. 3.103, ▸ Fig. 3.104, ▸ Fig. 3.105, ▸ Fig. 3.106, ▸ Fig. 3.107, ▸ Fig. 3.108.

3.5.1 Indications

- Canal wall–down cavity with intractable inflammation with no serviceable hearing.
- Chronic otitis media with no serviceable hearing with multiple previous surgeries.
- Recurrent cholesteatoma with huge mastoid aeration.
- Sustained CSF leak with either spontaneous, posttraumatic, or surgical origin.
- Large meningoencephalic herniation.
- Extensive exposure of middle fossa dura.
- Cochlear implants in special cases.
- Paragangliomas of class B3.

Right Ear

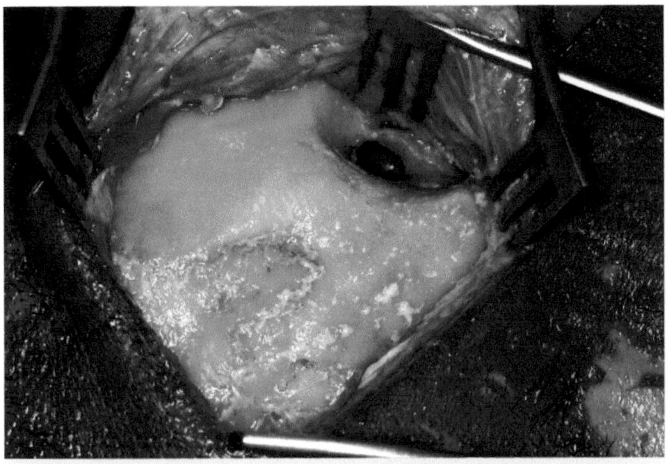

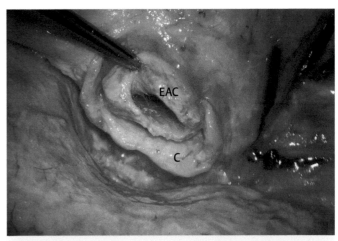

Fig. 3.89 Blind-sac closure of the external auditory canal (EAC) is starting. Meticulous dissection of the skin from the anterior cartilage (C) has to be performed.

Fig. 3.88 Skin incision, transection of the external auditory canal, and creation of the musculoperiosteal flap have been performed in a right ear.

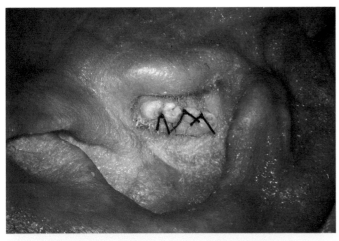

Fig. 3.90 The skin is everted and sutured with silk sutures.

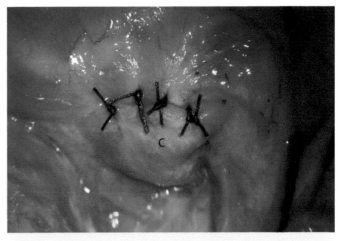

Fig. 3.91 Medially, the anterior cartilage of the external auditory canal (C) is sutured with the soft tissues of the concha. This second layer is of utmost importance in case of CSF leakage.

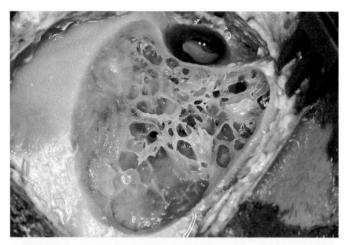

Fig. 3.92 Cortical mastoidectomy has been started.

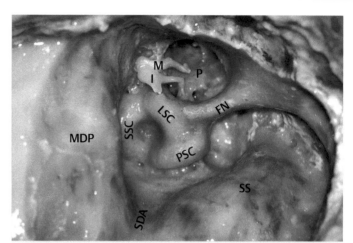

Fig. 3.93 An extended canal wall–down mastoidectomy has been performed. All the perilabyrinthine, retrolabyrinthine, and retrofacial air cells have been removed. FN, facial nerve; I, incus; LSC, lateral semicircular canal; M, malleus; MDP, middle fossa dura plate; P, promontory; PSC, posterior semicircular canal; SDA, sinodural angle; SS, sigmoid sinus; SSC, superior semicircular canal.

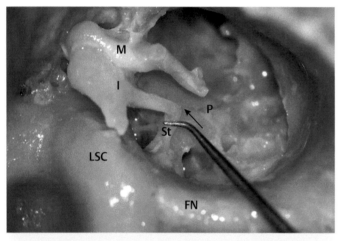

Fig. 3.94 Closer view. The incudostapedial joint is disarticulated. FN, facial nerve; I, incus; LSC, lateral semicircular canal; M, malleus; P, promontory; St, stapes.

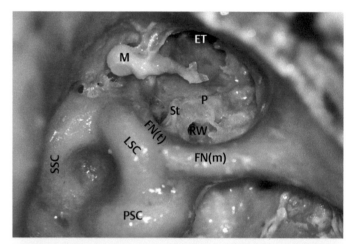

Fig. 3.95 The incus has been removed. ET, eustachian tube; FN(m), mastoid segment of the facial nerve; FN(t), tympanic segment of the facial nerve; I, incus; LSC, lateral semicircular canal; M, malleus; P, promontory; PSC, posterior semicircular canal; RW, round window; SSC, superior semicircular canal; St, stapes.

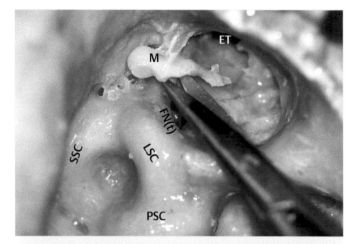

Fig. 3.96 The tendon of the malleus is cut. ET, eustachian tube; FN(t), tympanic segment of the facial nerve; LSC, lateral semicircular canal; M, malleus; PSC, posterior semicircular canal; SSC, superior semicircular canal.

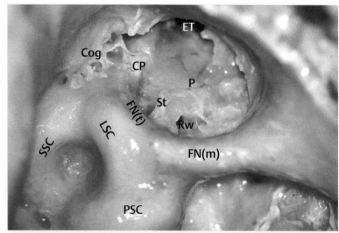

Fig. 3.97 After removal of the malleus, tha anterior attic is under view. The **Cog** is a bony septum which separates the anterior from the posterior epitympanum. CP, cochleariform process; ET, eustachian tube; FN(m), mastoid segment of the facial nerve; FN(t) tympanic segment of the facial nerve; I, incus; LSC, lateral semicircular canal; M, malleus; P, promontory; PSC, posterior semicircular canal; RW, round window; SSC, superior semicircular canal; St, stapes.

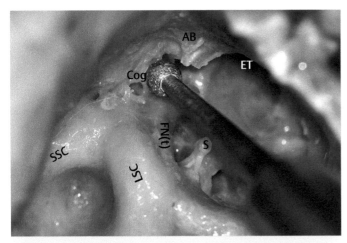

Fig. 3.98 Drilling the **Cog** exposes the anterior attic recess (also known as "supratubal recess"). AB, anterior buttress; ET, eustachian tube; FN(t), tympanic segment of the facial nerve; LSC, lateral semicircular canal; SSC, superior semicircular canal; St, stapes.

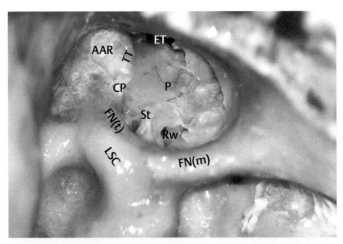

Fig. 3.99 The anterior attic recess (AAR) is under view. CP, cochleariform process; ET, eustachian tube; FN(m), mastoid segment of the facial nerve; FN(t), tympanic segment of the facial nerve; LSC, lateral semicircular canal; P, promontory; RW, round window; St, stapes; TT, tensor tympani muscle.

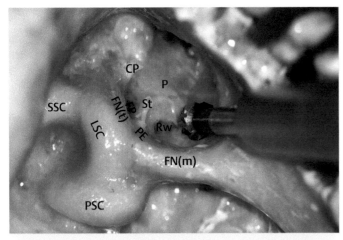

Fig. 3.100 In case of a class B3 paraganglioma, the infralabyrinthine air cells have to be removed (drill). CP, cochleariform process; FP, footplate; FN(m), mastoid segment of the facial nerve; FN(t) tympanic segment of the facial nerve; LSC, lateral semicircular canal; P, promontory; PSC, posterior semicircular canal; PE, pyramidal eminence; RW, round window; SSC, superior semicircular canal; St, stapes.

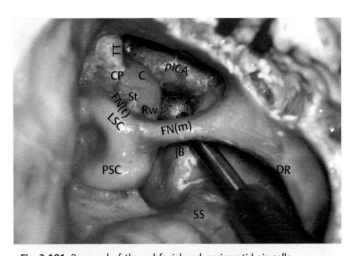

Fig. 3.101 Removal of the subfacial and pericarotid air cells. C, cochlea; CP, cochleariform process; DR, digastric ridge; FN(m), mastoid segment of the facial nerve; FN(t), tympanic segment of the facial nerve; JB, jugular bulb; LSC, lateral semicircular canal; pICA, petrous internal carotid artery; PSC, posterior semicircular canal; RW, round window; SS, sigmoid sinus; St, stapes; TT, tensor tympani muscle.

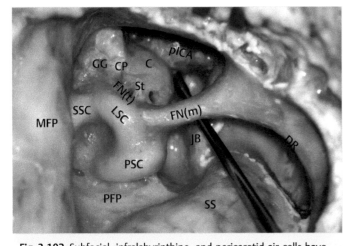

Fig. 3.102 Subfacial, infralabyrinthine, and pericarotid air cells have been removed. C, cochlea; CP, cochleariform process; DR, digastric ridge; FN(m), mastoid segment of the facial nerve; FN(t), tympanic segment of the facial nerve; GG, geniculate ganglion; JB, jugular bulb; LSC, lateral semicircular canal; PFP, posterior fossa plate; pICA, petrous internal carotid artery; PSC, posterior semicircular canal; SS, sigmoid sinus; SSC, superior semicircular canal; St, stapes.

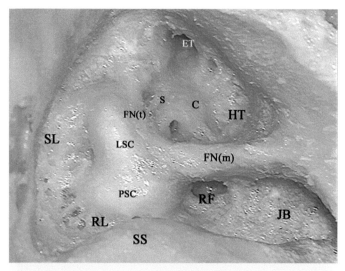

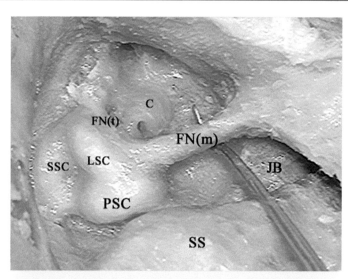

Fig. 3.103 Another case. The groups of air cells that need to be drilled out to achieve a subtotal petrosectomy in a right temporal bone. C, basal turn of the cochlea (promontory); ET, eustachian tube; FN(m), mastoid segment of the facial nerve; FN(t), tympanic segment of the facial nerve; HT, hypotympanic air cells; JB, jugular bulb; LSC, lateral semicircular canal; PSC, posterior semicircular canal; RF, retrofacial air cells; RL, retrolabyrinthine air cells; S, stapes; SL, supralabyrinthine air cells, SS, sigmoid sinus.

Fig. 3.104 The retrofacial and hypotympanic air cells have been drilled, as shown by the passage of the pointer medial to the mastoid segment of the facial nerve (FN[m]). C, basal turn of the cochlea (promontory); FN(t), tympanic segment of the facial nerve; JB, jugular bulb; LSC, lateral semicircular canal; PSC, posterior semicircular canal; SS, sigmoid sinus; SSC, superior semicircular canal.

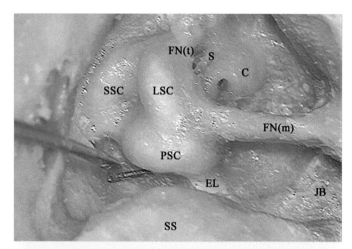

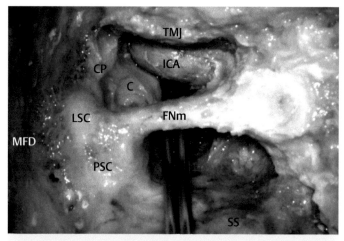

Fig. 3.105 The perilabyrinthine air cells have been drilled away. C, basal turn of the cochlea (promontory); EL, endolymphatic duct; FN(m), mastoid segment of the facial nerve; FN(t), tympanic segment of the facial nerve; JB, jugular bulb; LSC, lateral semicircular canal; PSC, posterior semicircular canal; S, stapes; SS, sigmoid sinus; SSC, superior semicircular canal.

Fig. 3.106 Another case of subtotal petrosectomy in a right ear. In this case hypotympanic, retrofacial, infralabyrinthine cells have been drilled toward the petrous apex (suction tip). The vertical portion and genu of the petrosal internal carotid artery (ICA) have been exposed. C, cochlea; CP, cochleariform process; FN(m), mastoid portion of the facial nerve; LSC, lateral semicircular canal; MFD, middle fossa dura; PSC, posterior semicircular canal; SS, sigmoid sinus; TMJ, temporomandibular joint.

Left Ear

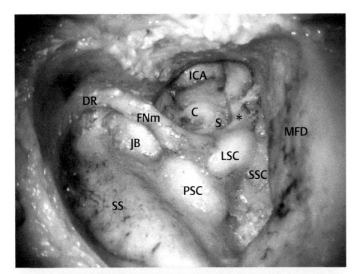

Fig. 3.107 Subtotal petrosectomy in a left ear. The pneumatic cells of the temporal bone have been removed and all the structures are under view. *, tympanic segment of the facial nerve; C, basal turn of the cochlea (promontory); DR, digastric ridge; FN(m), mastoid segment of the facial nerve; JB, jugular bulb; LSC, lateral semicircular canal; PSC, posterior semicircular canal; S, stapes; SS, sigmoid sinus; SSC, superior semicircular canal; MFD, middle fossa dura; ICA, internal carotid artery.

3.6 En Bloc Excision of the External Auditory Canal (Lateral Temporal Bone Resection)

3.6.1 Indication

- Malignant tumors of the external auditory canal (class T1 or T2 tumors, according to the modified Pittsburg staging system for squamous cell carcinoma of the external auditory canal).

3.6.2 Surgical Steps

See the steps listed below and also refer to ▶ Fig. 3.109, ▶ Fig. 3.110, ▶ Fig. 3.111, ▶ Fig. 3.112, ▶ Fig. 3.113, ▶ Fig. 3.114, ▶ Fig. 3.115, ▶ Fig. 3.116, ▶ Fig. 3.117, ▶ Fig. 3.118, ▶ Fig. 3.119, ▶ Fig. 3.120, ▶ Fig. 3.121, ▶ Fig. 3.122, ▶ Fig. 3.123, ▶ Fig. 3.124, ▶ Fig. 3.125, ▶ Fig. 3.126, ▶ Fig. 3.127, ▶ Fig. 3.128, ▶ Fig. 3.129, ▶ Fig. 3.130, ▶ Fig. 3.131, ▶ Fig. 3.132, ▶ Fig. 3.133.

1. A closed mastoidectomy is carried out, as described previously.
2. The posterior tympanotomy is extended inferiorly to expose the hypotympanum.
3. Anteroinferior extension of the tympanotomy is carried out. Drilling is continued using an appropriately sized diamond burr to separate the inferior portion of the tympanic bone from the medial wall of the middle ear in the area of the hypotympanum. The drilling should be extended anteriorly until the temporomandibular joint is reached.
4. The mastoid tip is dissected away, with care being taken not to injure the closely related facial nerve. In case of associated superficial parotidectomy, the extratemporal portion of the facial nerve is dissected.
5. The incudostapedial joint is disarticulated in order to avoid sensorineural hearing loss in live surgery while carrying out the remaining drilling in the attic area.

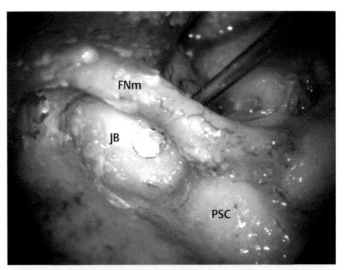

Fig. 3.108 Closer view. The retrofacial cells have been removed and the third portion of the facial nerve skeletonized. Note the space between the facial nerve and the jugular bulb, as shown by the dissector. FN(m), mastoid segment of the facial nerve; JB, jugular bulb; PSC, posterior semicircular canal.

6. The atticotomy is now extended anteriorly until the temporomandibular joint is opened.
7. The tensor tympani tendon attachment to the malleus is sharply cut. This step allows safe removal of the external auditory canal without the risk of leaving behind any residual tumor as a result of the tendon pulling on the malleus and leading to rupture of the tympanic membrane.
8. Using the thumb, gentle anterior pressure on the external auditory canal leads to fracturing of the last attachment at the anterior wall level.
9. Inspection of both the middle ear and the medial aspect of the tympanic membrane removed with the specimen is now carried out to ensure that no remnants are left behind.

3.6.3 Hints and Pitfalls

- When the posterior tympanotomy is being extended anteroinferiorly, the intraparotid facial nerve may be injured. For this reason, in live surgery, identification of the intraparotid facial nerve as far as the bifurcation is carried out before the extension. This step is also useful if the superficial loop of the parotid gland is to be included with the specimen.
- Before the sample is removed, cutting the attachment of the tensor tympani tendon to the malleus prevents the unfortunate occurrence of rupture of the tympanic membrane due to pulling on the handle of the malleus when it is integrated into the membrane layers.
- In cases in which the tumor is small and localized in the posterior wall of the external auditory canal, the anterior wall of the canal (the posterior wall of the temporomandibular joint) can be preserved, thus avoiding any masticatory problems. In these cases, the drilling need not be extended into the joint, and the anteriorly attached soft tissues can be sharply dissected from the bone.
- In cases in which the tumor has infiltrated the temporomandibular joint through the anterior wall of the canal, the articulation (mandibular head and disk) should be included with the specimen.

Right Ear

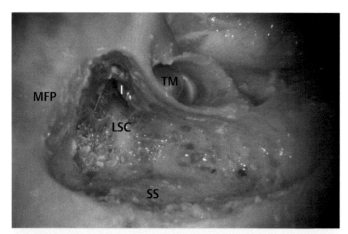

Fig. 3.109 Closed mastoidectomy has been carried out. I, incus; LSC, lateral semicircular canal; MFP, middle fossa plate; SS, sigmoid sinus; TM, tympanic membrane.

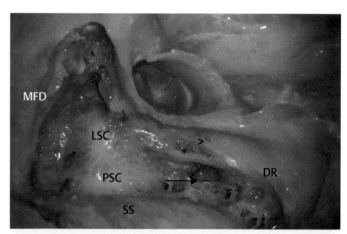

Fig. 3.110 The digastric ridge (DR), the mastoid portion of the facial nerve (*), and the chorda tympani (>) are under view. The retrofacial air cells are starting to be drilled toward the jugular bulb (*arrow*). LSC, lateral semicircular canal; MFD, middle fossa dura; PSC, posterior semicircular canal.

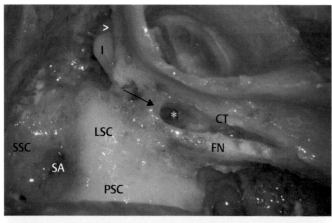

Fig. 3.111 Posterior tympanotomy is starting (*arrow*). The area of the round window is visible (*). The division between the mastoid portion of the facial nerve (FN[m]) and the chorda tympani (CT) has been maintained. The atticotomy has been further extended anteriorly and the head of the malleus can be seen (>). I, incus; LSC, lateral semicircular canal; PSC, posterior semicircular canal; SA, subarcuate artery; SSC, superior semicircular canal.

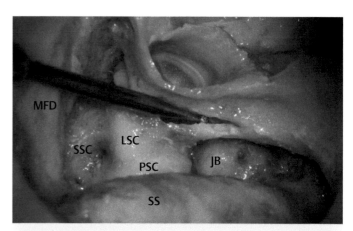

Fig. 3.112 The retrofacial air cells have been drilled and the jugular bulb (JB) is visible. The posterior tympanotomy is extended inferiorly, still maintaining the division between the mastoid portion of the facial nerve and the chorda tympani. LSC, lateral semicircular canal; MFD, middle fossa dura; PSC, posterior semicircular canal; SS, sigmoid sinus; SSC, superior semicircular canal.

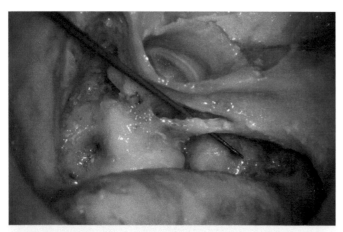

Fig. 3.113 Subfacial recess tympanotomy has been completed (hook).

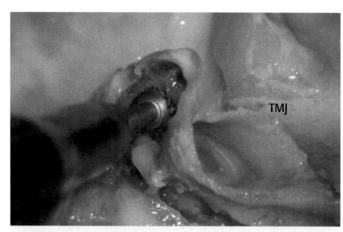

Fig. 3.114 The atticotomy is further extended anteriorly toward the temporomandibular joint (TMJ).

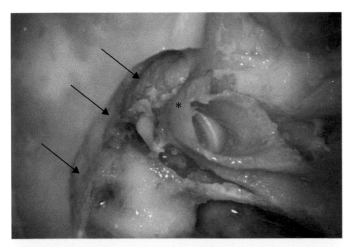

Fig. 3.115 Wider view. The dura of the middle fossa has been followed from the mastoid to the middle ear (*arrows*). This is of utmost importance in case of a T1- or T2-stage tumor of the external auditory canal, in which a lateral temporal bone resection is required, to get clear bony margins in the superior portion of the specimen (*).

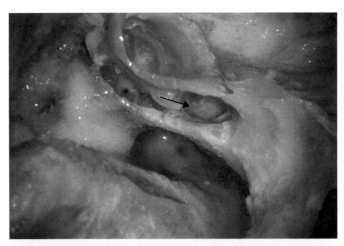

Fig. 3.116 Posterior tympanotomy has been extended inferiorly (*arrow*). The chorda tympani has been cut. *, round window niche.

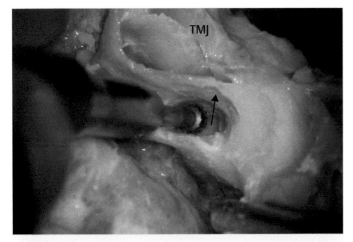

Fig. 3.117 The posterior tympanotomy is further extended anteroin-feriorly (*arrow*) to separate the inferior portion of the tympanic bone from the medial wall of the middle ear in the area of the hypotympanum. The drillling has to be extended to the area of the temporomandibular joint (TMJ).

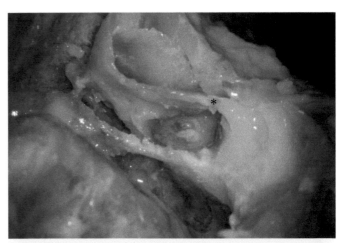

Fig. 3.118 View after completion of the anteroinferior tympanotomy. The last shell of bone (*) has to be removed to free the inferior portion of the specimen. In this step care should be taken not to injure the extratemporal portion of the facial nerve in the area of the stylomastoid foramen. For this reason, in live surgery some authors advocate routine identification of the extratemporal portion of the facial nerve in the parotid before completing this step.

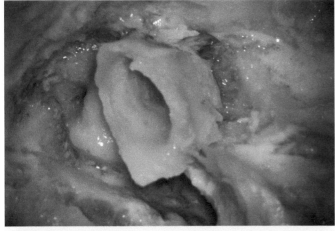

Fig. 3.119 With a gentle pressure the specimen is detached at the level of anterior and inferior walls. The incudostapedial joint has already been disarticulated.

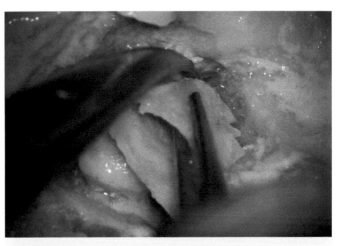

Fig. 3.120 The tensor tympani tendon attachment to the malleus is sharply cut.

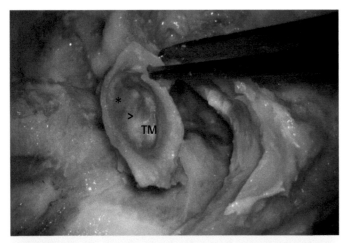

Fig. 3.121 Specimen with intact tympanic membrane (TM), malleus (>), and incus (*).

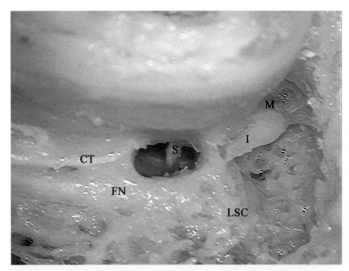

Fig. 3.122 View after en block excision of the external auditory canal. *, stapes; C, basal turn of the cochlea (promontory); ET, eustachian tube; FN, facial nerve; LSC, lateral semicircular canal; MFD, middle fossa dura; PSC, posterior semicircular canal; SSC, superior semicircular canal; SS, sigmoid sinus; TT, tensor tympani muscle.

Left Ear

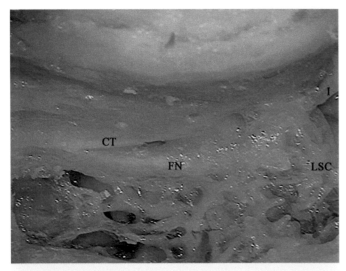

Fig. 3.123 Mastoidectomy has been carried out, and the facial nerve (FN) has been identified. CT, chorda tympani; I, incus; LSC, lateral semicircular canal.

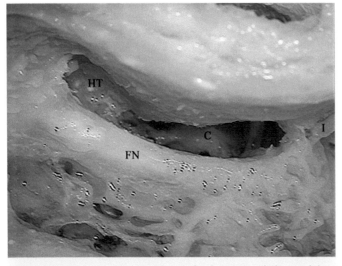

Fig. 3.125 The posterior tympanotomy has been extended toward the hypotympanum (HT). C, basal turn of the cochlea (promontory); FN, facial nerve; I, incus.

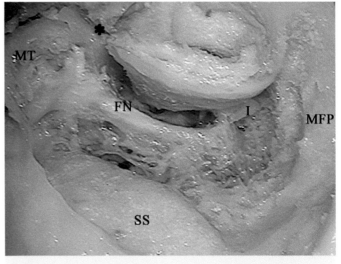

Fig. 3.124 Posterior tympanotomy has been started. CT, chorda tympani; FN, facial nerve; I, incus; LSC, lateral semicircular canal; M, malleus; S, stapes.

Fig. 3.126 Anteroinferior extension of the tympanotomy (*) has separated the inferior portion of the tympanic bone from the medial wall of the middle ear in the area of the hypotympanum. FN, facial nerve, I, incus; MFP, middle fossa plate; MT, mastoid tip; SS, sigmoid sinus.

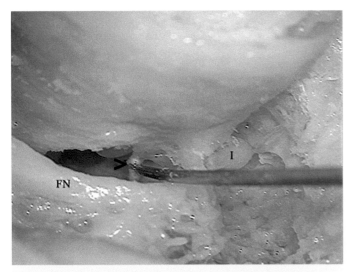

Fig. 3.127 The incudostapedial joint (>) has been disarticulated. FN, facial nerve; I, incus.

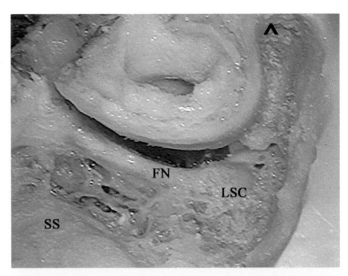

Fig. 3.128 Atticotomy has been carried out. The arrow (^) shows the last piece of bone to be removed in order to reach the temporomandibular joint. FN, facial nerve; LSC, lateral semicircular canal; SS, sigmoid sinus.

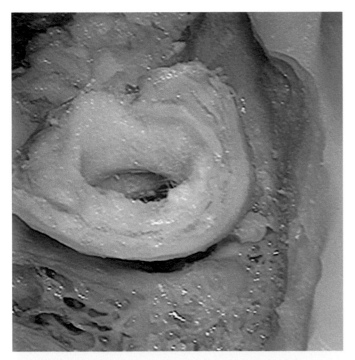

Fig. 3.129 The atticotomy is now extended anteriorly until the temporomandibular joint is opened.

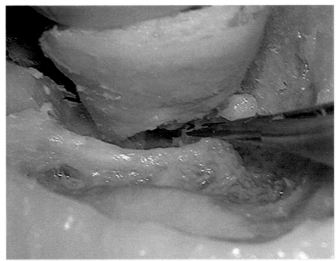

Fig. 3.130 The tensor tympani tendon (>) attachment to the malleus is sharply cut.

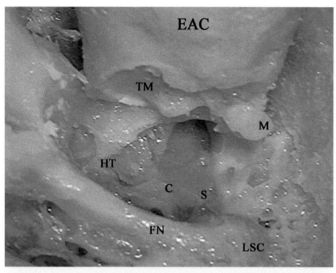

Fig. 3.131 Gentle anterior pressure on the external auditory canal (EAC) leads to fracturing of the last attachment at the level of the anterior wall. C, basal turn of the cochlea (promontory); FN, facial nerve; HT, hypotympanum; LSC, lateral semicircular canal; M, malleus; S, stapes; TM, tympanic membrane.

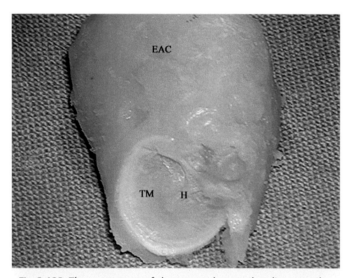

Fig. 3.133 The appearance of the removed external auditory canal (EAC) together with the intact tympanic membrane (TM). H, handle of the malleus.

3.7 Endolymphatic Sac Decompression

3.7.1 Surgical Anatomy

The endolymphatic sac is a blind sac connected to the membranous labyrinth through the endolymphatic duct. Both the endolymphatic duct and the proximal part of the sac lie within a bony canal, the vestibular aqueduct, which runs medial to the posterior semicircular canal to enter the vestibule. The terminal part of the sac lies between the two layers of the posterior fossa dura, inferior to a line extending through the lateral semicircular canal (Donaldson's line).

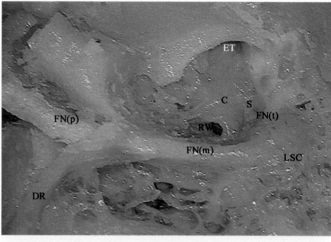

Fig. 3.132 The appearance after the procedure has been completed. C, basal turn of the cochlea (promontory); DR, digastric ridge; ET, eustachian tube; FN(m), mastoid segment of the facial nerve; FN(p), extratemporal facial nerve; FN(t), tympanic segment of the facial nerve; LSC, lateral semicircular canal; RW, round window; S, stapes.

3.7.2 Indication

• Intractable Ménière's disease with serviceable hearing.

3.7.3 Surgical Steps

See steps listed below and also refer to ▶ Fig. 3.134, ▶ Fig. 3.135, ▶ Fig. 3.136, ▶ Fig. 3.137, ▶ Fig. 3.138, ▶ Fig. 3.139, ▶ Fig. 3.140, ▶ Fig. 3.141, ▶ Fig. 3.142, ▶ Fig. 3.143, ▶ Fig. 3.144, ▶ Fig. 3.145, ▶ Fig. 3.146.

1. Complete cortical mastoidectomy.
2. Bone over the sigmoid sinus is removed using a large diamond burr until a very thin shell of bone remains over the sinus. The jugular bulb is identified and skeletonized. The posterior semicircular canal is identified, but not blue-lined.
3. With the suction irrigator, the sigmoid sinus is gently depressed, and the posterior fossa dura in front of the sinus is carefully detached from the overlying bone. Bone between the sigmoid sinus and posterior semicircular canal can now be removed safely without injuring the dura. The posterior fossa dura should be widely exposed.
4. The exposed dura is gently depressed with a septal dissector, thus identifying the point at which the sac enters the vestibular aqueduct. If a double-curved raspatory is moved along the plane of the posterior fossa dura from superior to inferior, it fails to pass freely, since it is obstructed by the sac from entering the vestibular aqueduct. Another identifying characteristic of the sac is that it is relatively whiter in comparison with the surrounding bluish posterior fossa dura.
5. The sac is sharply opened, and the lateral wall of the sac is removed. A Silastic tube is then inserted into the lumen.

3.7.4 Hints and Pitfalls

• Bone removal and exposure of the posterior fossa dura should be as wide as possible, and not only restricted to the expected sac location. Failure to remove the bone in the retrofacial cells would lead to an inability to locate the sac.

- In some cases, the sac may be intimately related to the jugular bulb. Care should be taken in these cases not to injure the bulb while opening the sac.
- Since the position of the endolymphatic sac is quite variable, the various methods of identifying the sac described in the literature are of little significance in live surgery.

Right Ear

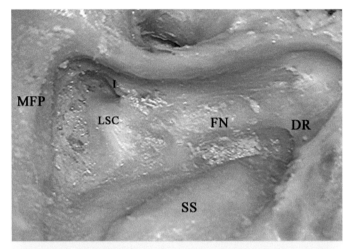

Fig. 3.134 An extended mastoidectomy has been carried out in a right temporal bone. Note that the bone thinning of has been extended over the sigmoid sinus (SS), while the middle fossa plate (MFP) has only been identified. DR, digastric ridge; FN, facial nerve; I, iIncus; LSC, lateral semicircular canal.

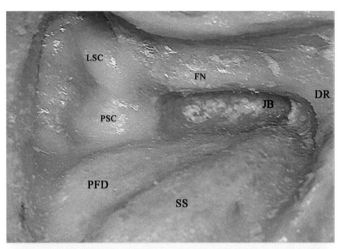

Fig. 3.135 The posterior semicircular canal (PSC) has been identified, and the bone overlying the sigmoid sinus (SS) and the posterior fossa dura (PFD) anterior to it has been thinned. DR, digastric ridge; FN, facial nerve; JB, jugular bulb; LSC, lateral semicircular canal.

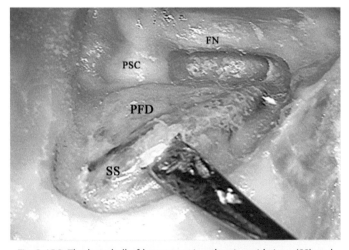

Fig. 3.136 The last shell of bone covering the sigmoid sinus (SS) and the posterior fossa dura (PFD) is being removed. FN, facial nerve; PSC, posterior semicircular canal.

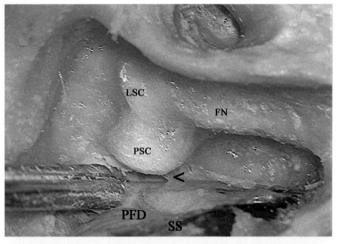

Fig. 3.137 After the sigmoid sinus (SS) and the posterior fossa dura (PFD) have been uncovered, retraction of the dura posteriorly reveals the endolymphatic duct (<) exiting medial to the posterior semicircular canal (PSC). FN, facial nerve; LSC, lateral semicircular canal.

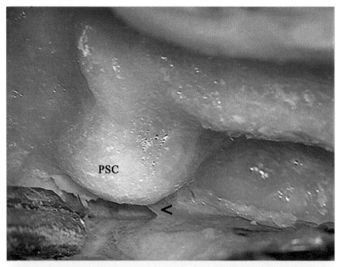

Fig. 3.138 At higher magnification, the relationship between the endolymphatic duct (<) and the posterior semicircular canal (PSC) can be better appreciated.

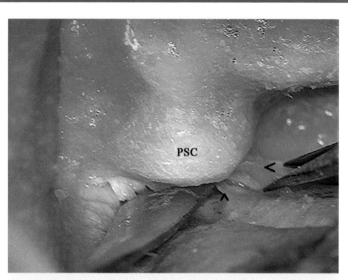

Fig. 3.139 Using microscissors, the lateral wall of the endolymphatic sac (<) is separated from its medial wall (^). PSC, posterior semicircular canal.

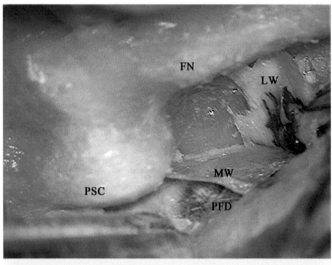

Fig. 3.140 The lateral wall of the endolymphatic sac (LW) has been dissected from the medial wall (MW). FN, facial nerve; PFD, posterior fossa dura; PSC, posterior semicircular canal.

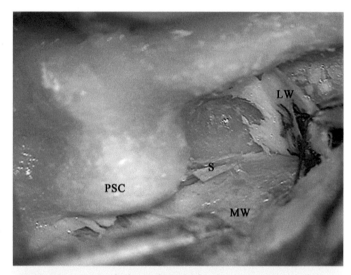

Fig. 3.141 A piece of Silastic sheet (S) has been inserted into the endolymphatic duct as it emerges from behind the posterior semicircular canal (PSC). LW, lateral wall of the endolymphatic sac; MW, medial wall of the endolymphatic sac.

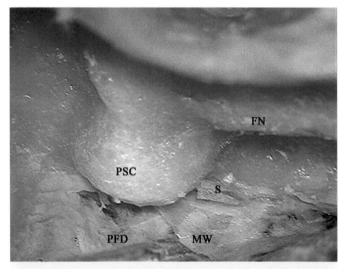

Fig. 3.142 The lateral wall of the endolymphatic sac has been excised in order to avoid closure of the drain by scar tissue. FN, facial nerve; MW, medial wall of the endolymphatic sac; PFD, posterior fossa dura; PSC, posterior semicircular canal; S, Silastic.

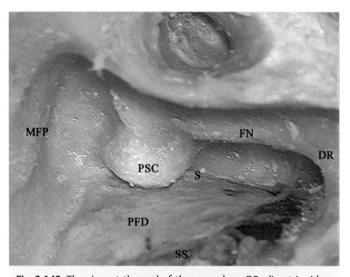

Fig. 3.143 The view at the end of the procedure. DR, digastric ridge; FN, facial nerve; MFP, middle fossa plate; PFD, posterior fossa dura; PSC, posterior semicircular canal; S, Silastic; SS, sigmoid sinus.

Left Ear

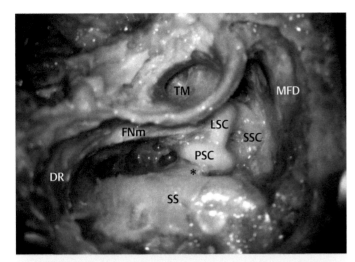

Fig. 3.144 Extended mastoidectomy has been carried out and the sigmoid sinus has been completely skeletonized. Even the bone over the posterior fossa dura has been removed and the endolymphatic duct (*), exiting medial to the posterior semicircular canal (PSC), is visible. DR, digastric ridge; FN(m), mastoid portion of the facial nerve; LSC, lateral semicircular canal; MFD, middle fossa dura; SS, sigmoid sinus; SSC, superior semicircular canal; TM, tympanic membrane.

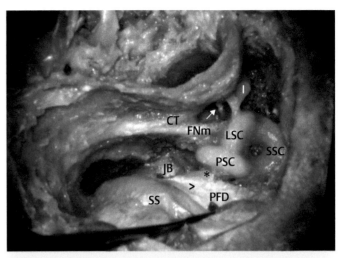

Fig. 3.145 Closer view. The posterior fossa dura (PFD) is gently retracted with a dissector. The course of the endolymphatic duct (*) is visible, from the posterior surface of the posterior semicircular canal (PSC) to the endolymphatic sac (>). Arrow, incudostapedial joint; CT, chorda tympani; FN(m), mastoid portion of the facial nerve; I, incus; LSC, lateral semicircular canal; JB, jugular bulb; SS sigmoid sinus, SSC superior semicircular canal.

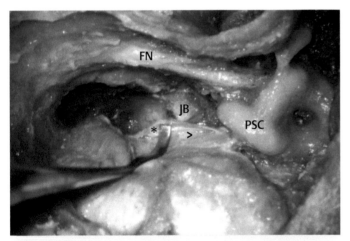

Fig. 3.146 The lateral wall of the endolymphatic sac (*) has been dissected and cut from the medial wall (>). FN, facial nerve; JB, jugular bulb; PSC, posterior semicircular canal.

3.8 Cochlear Implantation

3.8.1 Indication

- Profound bilateral sensorineural hearing loss, prelingual or postlingual.

3.8.2 Surgical Steps

See the steps listed below and also refer to ▶ Fig. 3.147, ▶ Fig. 3.148, ▶ Fig. 3.149, ▶ Fig. 3.150, ▶ Fig. 3.151, ▶ Fig. 3.152, ▶ Fig. 3.153, ▶ Fig. 3.154, ▶ Fig. 3.155, ▶ Fig. 3.156, ▶ Fig. 3.157, ▶ Fig. 3.158, ▶ Fig. 3.159, ▶ Fig. 3.160, ▶ Fig. 3.161, ▶ Fig. 3.162, ▶ Fig. 3.163, ▶ Fig. 3.164, ▶ Fig. 3.165, ▶ Fig. 3.166, ▶ Fig. 3.167, ▶ Fig. 3.168, ▶ Fig. 3.169, ▶ Fig. 3.170, ▶ Fig. 3.171, ▶ Fig. 3.172, ▶ Fig. 3.173, ▶ Fig. 3.174, ▶ Fig. 3.175, ▶ Fig. 3.176.

1. After the incision has been completed and the flaps have been elevated, a limited canal wall–up mastoidectomy is drilled. Since the aim of the mastoidectomy in cases of cochlear implantation is only to provide access to the facial recess, the size of the mastoidectomy cavity should be as small as possible. After the mastoidectomy has been completed in live surgery, the FN monitor is turned on.

2. The identification of the landmarks for the mastoid segment of the FN is started. Drilling between the lateral semicircular canal and the digastric ridge is started using an appropriately sized drill. To avoid injury to the nerve, drilling should be parallel to the direction of the nerve and should be carried out with ample suction irrigation in order to reduce heat injury and allow maximum visualization. As drilling advances closer to the nerve, a diamond drill should be used.

3. Once the FN has been identified, the size of the burr used is reduced and a posterior tympanotomy is started. As in cholesteatoma surgery, the extent of drilling is limited initially by four landmarks: the facial nerve medially, the annulus laterally, the bar of bone to the left covering the short process of the incus superiorly, and finally the chorda tympani inferiorly.

4. After completion of the drilling, access to the round window is assessed. If the lower rim of the round window can be visualized through the posterior tympanotomy, the approach is sufficient. Otherwise, the chorda tympani is sacrificed and the posterior tympanotomy is extended inferiorly until the whole round window niche can be seen.

5. Using a water-resistant colored pen, the model provided with the implant is used to mark the extent of drilling needed to create the bed for the receiver–stimulator complex of the cochlear implant. The location of the bed lies posterior and slightly superior to the mastoid cavity created. A large cutting burr is used initially; when the depth is sufficient as

checked by the implant, a diamond burr is used to smooth out the edges.

6. Two tunnels are drilled in the bone at the side of the bed, and a thick silk suture is passed into both tunnels to form a cross over the bed.

7. Attention is now paid to the round window. The superior overhang of the round window niche is drilled out. For this purpose, a small diamond burr of adequate length is used.

8. The round window membrane is identified, and drilling is continued anterolaterally to create an opening in the scala tympani adequate for insertion of the implant array. A piece of fibrous tissue is used to obliterate the opening created.

9. The receiver–stimulator complex of the implant is fitted into the bed and fixed in place by tightening the suture.

10. After the complex has been fixed in place, the surgeon is now able to use both hands to insert the array. The fibrous tissue is removed from the round window, the array is held gently with a nontoothed, straight forceps (this prevents damage to the expensive array by the forceps' teeth, unlike the microear forceps which are generally used to allow easy manipulation). To allow optimal positioning of the electrodes, the direction of the stylet should always be kept pointing inferiorly—that is, to the right of the surgeon when operating on a right ear, and vice versa.

11. In live surgery, after the insertion of the array, the audiologist is given time to check the impedance of the electrodes and thus examine whether the positioning is correct. After correct positioning has been confirmed, the leading wire is withdrawn. Care should be taken to avoid accidental withdrawal of the wire before confirmation is obtained, because of the difficulty of reinserting it, which can lead to damage to the electrodes.

12. After withdrawal of the wire, pieces of fibrous tissue are used to seal the round window. The seal is reinforced by the addition of tissue glue if the need is felt. This step helps reinforce the fixation of the array, reducing the risk of CSF leakage and meningitis and reducing the incidence of postoperative vertigo. Another piece of fibrous tissue is used to separate the array and the facial nerve, to reduce the chances of FN stimulation by the electrical impulse. The adequacy of the insulation can be checked by asking the audiologist to apply some stimulation to the implant while the FN monitor is on.

13. Cases of ossified cochlea are occasionally encountered after meningitis-induced deafness. In the majority of these cases, the ossification is limited to the basal turn of the cochlea. In these cases, a small-diamond burr with a long shaft is used, and drilling in the area of round window and neo-ossification is carried out in an anteromedial direction, creating a tunnel in the supposed area of the basal turn. While this step is being carried out, care must be taken not to injure the FN, and the site of drilling is checked frequently to confirm the correct direction of drilling, as assessed by changes in the color and consistency of the exposed bone. Drilling is stopped whenever the opening of the scala tympani is identified, the red color of the carotid artery is encountered, or the depth of drilling exceeds 8 mm within the bone. The reason for this is that after this distance, the cochlea starts to turn superomedially, making further drilling not only dangerous to the carotid artery but also useless, since electrodes inserted afterward will be lying away from the modiolus.

14. In cases of total ossification of the cochlea, complete identification of all the cochlear turns, using a subtotal petrosectomy, is the method of choice.

3.8.3 Hints and Pitfalls

- The reason for creating a small mastoidectomy during the cochlear implant procedure is to reduce surgical trauma as much as possible and to preserve the surrounding bone to serve as a bed for the implant.
- While the posterior tympanotomy is being created, preservation of the chorda tympani should be attempted only if the access created allows adequate visualization of the round window niche; otherwise, the tympanotomy is extended inferiorly, sacrificing the chorda in order to obtain an adequate and safe approach.
- While the posterior tympanotomy is being carried out, care should be taken not to advance drilling too far anteriorly in an attempt to avoid the FN, thus leading to injury to the annulus and the tympanic membrane. The best way of avoiding such a mishap is to drill using the appropriate burr size after actively identifying the FN by visualizing it through the canal.
- While the round window niche is being drilled through the posterior tympanotomy, extreme care must be taken to avoid contact between the rotating shaft of the drill and the thinned FN canal. Inadvertent contact of this type can lead to injury to the nerve due to either heat or direct physical trauma.
- Cochlear implants in an ossified cochlea and revision implantation are surgically demanding procedures and should be carried out by the most experienced surgeon in the team.

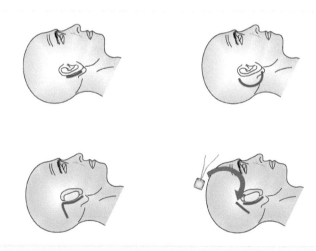

Fig. 3.147 Types of incision for cochlear implantation.

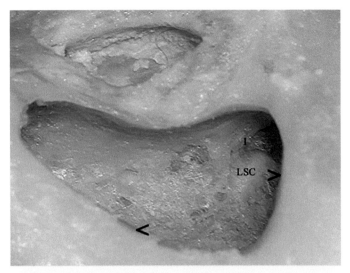

Fig. 3.148 A simple canal wall–up mastoidectomy has been carried out in a left temporal bone. Note that the superior (>) and posterior (<) limits of the cavity are not beveled and that the underlying structures have not been reached. I, incus; LSC, lateral semicircular canal.

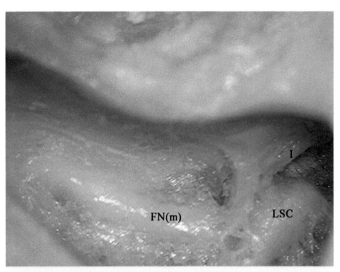

Fig. 3.149 The mastoid segment of the facial nerve (FN[m]) has been identified. I, incus; LSC, lateral semicircular canal.

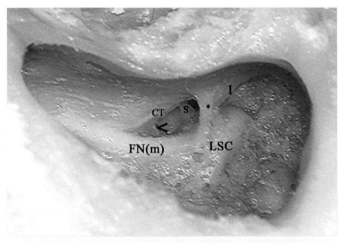

Fig. 3.150 The posterior tympanotomy has been started. Note that the lower angle (<) between the chorda tympani (CT) and the facial nerve (FN[m]) still has some bone, which should be removed. *, strut of bone to protect the ossicles; I, incus; LSC, lateral semicircular canal; S, stapes.

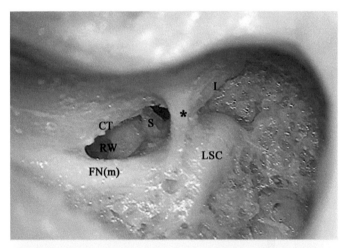

Fig. 3.151 The tympanotomy has been completed, preserving the chorda tympani (CT). Note that the round window (RW) is not yet under adequate control, so that the posterior tympanotomy needs to be further extended inferiorly, with the chorda tympani having to be sacrificed. *, strut of bone to protect the ossicles; FN(m), mastoid segment of the facial nerve; I, incus; LSC, lateral semicircular canal; S, stapes.

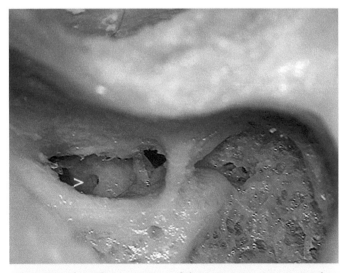

Fig. 3.152 After inferior extension of the posterior tympanotomy, the lower limit of the round window (>) can be clearly seen.

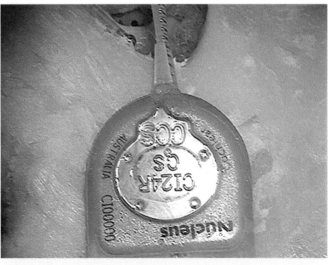

Fig. 3.153 The model provided with the implant is used to mark the implant bed.

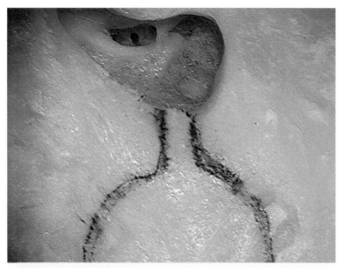

Fig. 3.154 Water-resistant ink is used to mark the area to be drilled.

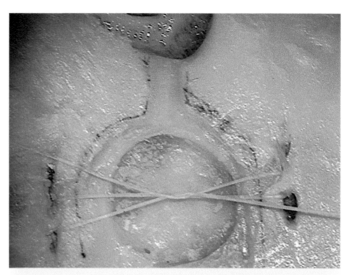

Fig. 3.155 The bed and the two tunnels at its side have been drilled, and the surgical thread used to fix the implant's receiver–stimulator complex in place has been inserted.

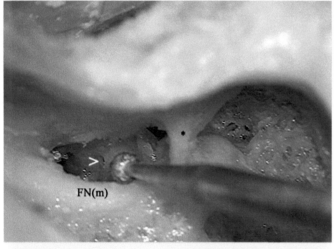

Fig. 3.156 A small-diamond burr of adequate length is used to drill the round window niche overhang (>). *, strut of bone; FN(m), mastoid segment of the facial nerve.

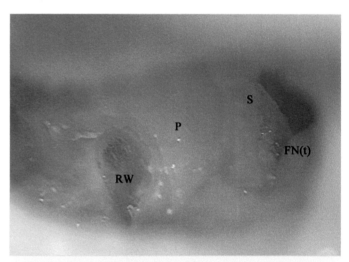

Fig. 3.157 The overhang has been drilled, and the round window membrane (RW) can clearly be seen. FN(t), tympanic segment of the facial nerve; P, promontory; S, stapes.

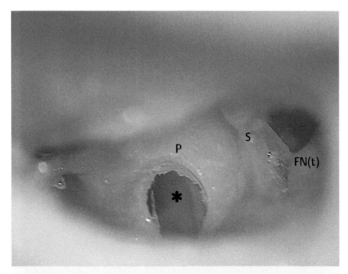

Fig. 3.158 The oval window and the scala tympani (*) have been adequately opened. FN(t), tympanic segment of the facial nerve; P, promontory; S, stapes.

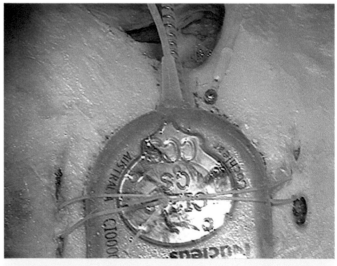

Fig. 3.159 The receiver–stimulator complex of the cochlear implant has been fixed in its bed.

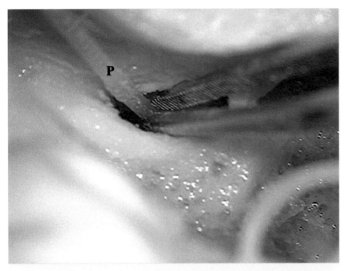

Fig. 3.160 A nontoothed forceps is used to insert the array (P) into the scala tympani.

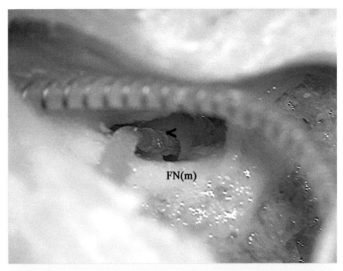

Fig. 3.161 Adequate insertion, as seen by contact between the middle ring on the array (<) and the edge of the cochleostomy, has been achieved. FN(m), mastoid segment of the facial nerve.

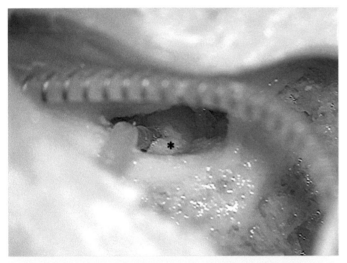

Fig. 3.162 A piece of fascia (*) is used to obliterate the space surrounding the array.

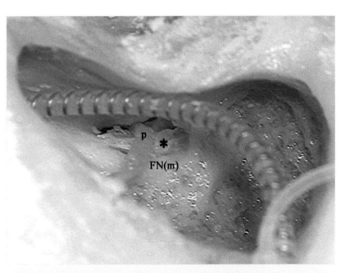

Fig. 3.163 Another piece of fascia (*) is inserted between the array (P) and the mastoid segment of the facial nerve (FN[m]).

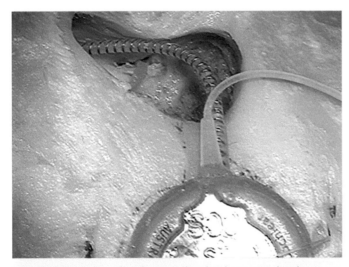

Fig. 3.164 The view after the procedure has been completed.

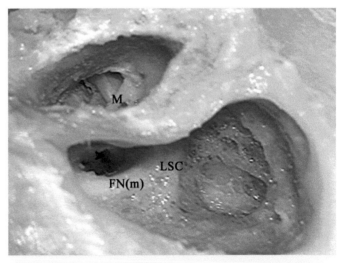

Fig. 3.165 In cases of ossified cochlea, the combined approach can be used to identify the cochlea turns. >, the round window seen through the posterior tympanotomy; FN(m), mastoid segment of the facial nerve; LSC, lateral semicircular canal; M, handle of the malleus.

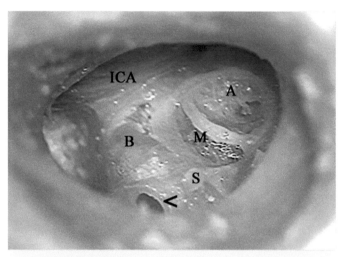

Fig. 3.166 The membranous part of the basal (B), middle (M), and apical (A) turns of the cochlea can be seen after the cortical bony covering has been drilled away. <, the edge of the cochleostomy; ICA, internal carotid artery; S, stapes.

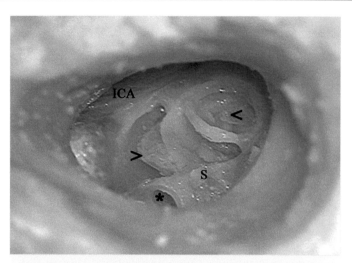

Fig. 3.167 The membranous part of the cochlea has been removed, and the bony spiral lamina (>) and the apex of the modiolus (<) can both be seen. Note that the basal turn of the cochlea starts to curve superiorly near the internal carotid artery (ICA), after a short distance from the level of the round window (*). S, stapes.

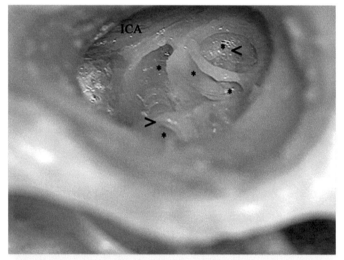

Fig. 3.168 The probe of the cochlear implant has been inserted. Note the course of the probe (***) as it spirals round, hugging the modiolus and reaching as far as the apical turn (<). >, the edge of the cochleostomy; ICA, internal carotid artery.

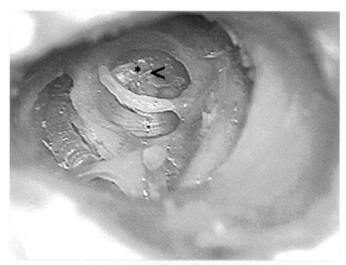

Fig. 3.169 Another, clearer view of this relationship. *, tip of the array; <, tip of the modiolus.

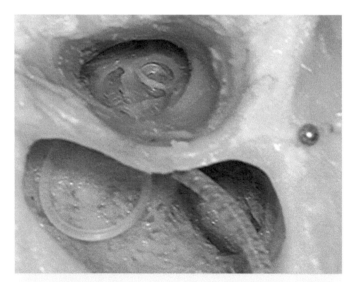

Fig. 3.170 The overall view after the procedure has been completed.

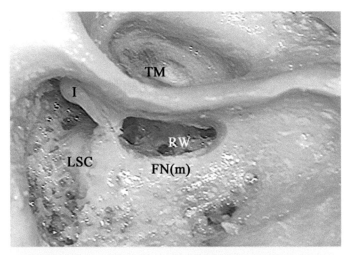

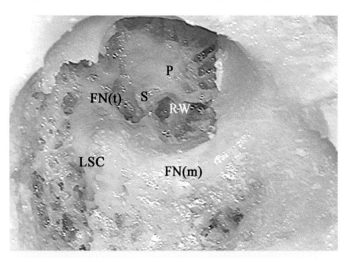

Fig. 3.171 Another option for dealing with the implantation of an ossified cochlea is to identify the cochlear turns through a subtotal petrosectomy. A canal wall–up mastoidectomy and posterior tympanotomy have been carried out in this right temporal bone just for dissection purposes. FN(m) mastoid segment of the facial nerve; I, incus; LSC, lateral semicircular canal; RW, round window; TM, tympanic membrane.

Fig. 3.172 The posterior and superior canal walls, tympanic membrane, malleus, and incus have all been removed. FN(m), mastoid segment of the facial nerve; FN(t), tympanic segment of the facial nerve; LSC, lateral semicircular canal; P, promontory; RW, round window; S, stapes.

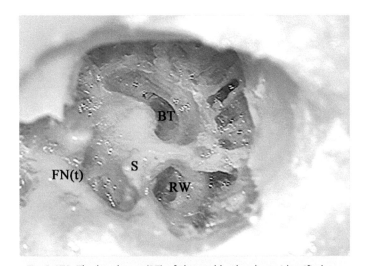

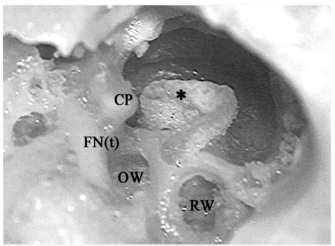

Fig. 3.173 The basal turn (BT) of the cochlea has been identified. FN(t), tympanic segment of the facial nerve; RW, round window; S, stapes.

Fig. 3.174 The whole length of the cochlea turns has been identified. *, modiolus; CP, cochleariform process; FN(t), tympanic segment of the facial nerve; OW, oval window; RW, round window.

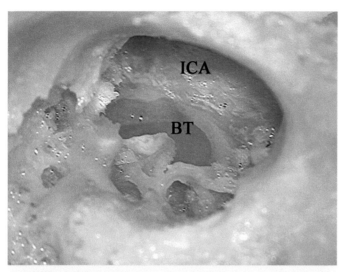

Fig. 3.175 Note that the basal turn of the cochlea (BT) starts to curve superiorly near the internal carotid artery (ICA), a short distance from the level of the round window.

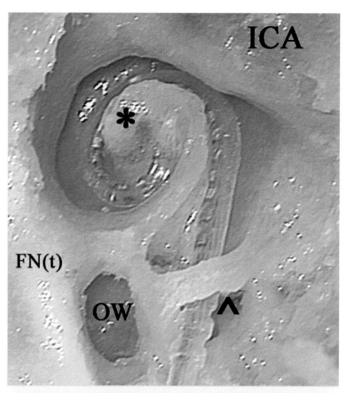

Fig. 3.176 The anterior wall of the external auditory canal and the cochleariform process, along with the tensor tympani muscle, have been removed here to show the relationship between the array and the modiolus (*) and between the array and the tympanic segment of the facial nerve (FN[t]). ^, edge of the round window; ICA, internal carotid artery; OW, oval window.

4 Translabyrinthine Approaches

Abstract

The rationale of this approach is to gain lateral access to the internal auditory canal (IAC) and cerebellopontine angle, allowing removal of cerebellopontine angle lesions with no cerebellar retraction. The enlarged form of the approach provides excellent exposure of the neurovascular structures present in the cerebellopontine angle, and permits removal of all acoustic neurinomas, irrespective of the size. The transapical extension of the approach permits control of the IAC for 320 or 360 degrees of its circumference. Management of cases with high jugular bulb will be provided.

Keywords: translabyrinthine approach, transapical extension, high jugular bulb

4.1 Basic Translabyrinthine Approach

4.1.1 Indications

- Removal of cerebellopontine angle lesions, when hearing preservation is not a concern, is as follows:
  a) Acoustic neurinoma:
    - With unserviceable preoperative hearing, whatever the size of the tumor is. It should be noted that giant tumors can be safely removed through this approach.
    - Acoustic neurinoma more than 1.5 cm in the extrameatal diameter irrespective of the preoperative hearing.
    - Cases with neurofibromatosis type 2 (NF2), in which preservation of the cochlear nerve and a concomitant cochlear implant (CI) can be attempted. Furthermore, an auditory brainstem implant (ABI) can be placed through this approach even if the cochlear nerve is not preserved.
  b) Meningiomas, posterior to or centered on the IAC, with unserviceable hearing. Cases that lie anterior to the canal require a transapical extension, whereas large petroclival tumors need a modified transcochlear approach.
  c) Other cerebellopontine angle tumors with unserviceable hearing, such as epidermoids, dermoids, etc.
- Vertigo surgery:
  - Labyrinthectomy
  - Vestibular neurectomy

4.1.2 Surgical Steps

See ▸ Fig. 4.1, ▸ Fig. 4.2, ▸ Fig. 4.3, ▸ Fig. 4.4, ▸ Fig. 4.5, ▸ Fig. 4.6, ▸ Fig. 4.7, ▸ Fig. 4.8, ▸ Fig. 4.9, ▸ Fig. 4.10, ▸ Fig. 4.11, ▸ Fig. 4.12, ▸ Fig. 4.13, ▸ Fig. 4.14, ▸ Fig. 4.15, ▸ Fig. 4.16, ▸ Fig. 4.17, ▸ Fig. 4.18, ▸ Fig. 4.19, ▸ Fig. 4.20, ▸ Fig. 4.21, ▸ Fig. 4.22, ▸ Fig. 4.23, ▸ Fig. 4.24, ▸ Fig. 4.25, ▸ Fig. 4.26, ▸ Fig. 4.27, ▸ Fig. 4.28, ▸ Fig. 4.29, ▸ Fig. 4.30, ▸ Fig. 4.31, ▸ Fig. 4.32, ▸ Fig. 4.33, ▸ Fig. 4.34, ▸ Fig. 4.35, ▸ Fig. 4.36, ▸ Fig. 4.37, ▸ Fig. 4.38, ▸ Fig. 4.39, ▸ Fig. 4.40, ▸ Fig. 4.41, ▸ Fig. 4.42, ▸ Fig. 4.43, ▸ Fig. 4.44, ▸ Fig. 4.45, ▸ Fig. 4.46, ▸ Fig. 4.47, ▸ Fig. 4.48, ▸ Fig. 4.49, ▸ Fig. 4.50, ▸ Fig. 4.51, ▸ Fig. 4.52, ▸ Fig. 4.53, ▸ Fig. 4.54, ▸ Fig. 4.55, ▸ Fig. 4.56, ▸ Fig. 4.57, ▸ Fig. 4.58, ▸ Fig. 4.59, ▸ Fig. 4.60, ▸ Fig. 4.61, ▸ Fig. 4.62, ▸ Fig. 4.63, ▸ Fig. 4.64, ▸ Fig. 4.65, ▸ Fig. 4.66, ▸ Fig. 4.67, ▸ Fig. 4.68, ▸ Fig. 4.69, ▸ Fig. 4.70, ▸ Fig. 4.71, ▸ Fig. 4.72, ▸ Fig. 4.73, ▸ Fig. 4.74, ▸ Fig. 4.75, ▸ Fig. 4.76, ▸ Fig. 4.77, ▸ Fig. 4.78.

1. An extended mastoidectomy is performed. The middle fossa dura and the sigmoid sinus are identified, leaving a thin shell of bone over them. Bone 2 to 3 cm posterior to the sinus is drilled using a large cutting burr. The middle fossa dura is beveled. The sinodural angle is widely opened.
2. The mastoid air cells are exenterated, and the antrum is widely opened.
3. The digastric ridge is identified at its anterior border. The ridge points directly to the mastoid segment of facial nerve at the area of the stylomastoid foramen. The facial nerve is only skeletonized, and not uncovered.
4. Once the facial nerve has been identified, retrofacial air cells can be safely drilled, and the sigmoid sinus is followed to the jugular bulb.
5. Using a large diamond burr, the last shell of bone covering the sigmoid sinus and the dura posterior to the sigmoid sinus is removed. The sigmoid sinus is gently depressed using the suction irrigation tube, and the posterior fossa dura in front of the sinus is separated from the overlying bone using a large septal dissector. Bone is then drilled using a large cutting burr.
6. When the level of the posterior semicircular canal is reached, the endolymphatic sac is seen passing from its position medial to the sac to enter between the layers of the dura. The duct maintains the posterior fossa dura attached to the labyrinth. Using a Beaver knife with the sharp edge directed against the bone, the duct is cut away, enabling further retraction of the posterior fossa dura.
7. Bone over the middle fossa dura is also removed using a rongeur after it has been separated from the dura. Care is taken to leave a thin shell of bone adjacent to the labyrinth in order to protect the posterior and middle fossa dura while carrying out the labyrinthectomy.
8. The labyrinthectomy starts by opening the lateral semicircular canal (LSC) using a medium-sized cutting burr. The posterior semicircular canal is next opened, followed by the opening of the superior semicircular canal. The labyrinthectomy continues by drilling off the three semicircular canals.

9. Care is taken to leave the anterior lateral part of the LSC, in order to protect the part of facial nerve lying within the concavity of the canal. The medial wall of the ampullae of the superior and LSCs is also left, to protect the labyrinthine segment of the facial nerve and to serve as a landmark for the superior ampullary nerve as well as the upper limit of the IAC.

10. The vestibule is now widely opened. It is important to avoid drilling the floor of the vestibule, in order to avoid entering the fundus of the IAC. The facial nerve runs immediately lateral to the vestibule, and overzealous drilling of the roof of the vestibule would therefore injure the nerve. Drilling in this area should be from superior to inferior or vice versa, and never from medial to lateral, in order to prevent injury to the fundus or the facial nerve.

11. After completion of the labyrinthectomy, the bone left over the posterior and middle fossa dura is successively reduced. Using a large septal dissector, the dura is separated from the bone which is then removed using a rongeur. Following the posterior fossa dura leads to identification of the IAC porus.

12. Identification of the inferior and superior borders of the IAC begins. During this process, drilling should be carried out parallel to the canal and in a medial to lateral direction. The ampulla of the superior semicircular canal serves as a landmark for the superior border of the IAC.

13. The inferior border of the canal is identified by drilling the retrofacial air cells between the jugular bulb inferiorly and the presumed level of the canal superiorly. At this level, drilling identifies the cochlear aqueduct. This is an important landmark for the glossopharyngeal nerve, which lies immediately inferior and medial to it. In live surgery, opening the cochlear aqueduct leads to cerebrospinal fluid (CSF) leakage, thereby reducing intradural tension.

14. Bone between the middle fossa dura and the superior border of the IAC is further drilled. Care is taken while doing this to avoid injury to the facial nerve (FN) or dura.

15. Bone at the level of the porus is further reduced by careful drilling in semicircles starting superior to the IAC, coursing posteriorly and ending inferior to it. Once this bone has been thinned out, it can be separated from the underlying IAC dura using a dissector.

16. The dura of the IAC is now completely exposed. Two troughs have been created superiorly and inferiorly to the IAC, and the canal is exposed over 270 degrees of its circumference.

17. The posterior aspect of the internal auditory canal at the level of the fundus is drilled inferiorly. This exposes the inferior vestibular nerve. Further drilling at a more superior level identifies the transverse crest, which separates the inferior from the superior vestibular nerve. The superior vestibular nerve is followed laterally where it leaves the fundus of the IAC and enters a tiny canal that carries the nerve, which is now called the superior ampullary nerve, to the ampulla of the LSC.

18. The inferior ampullary nerve is detached from the fundus using a hook. With the tip of the hook facing inferiorly, the superior ampullary nerve is detached from its canal. While this step is being carried out, Bill's bar lies anterior to the superior ampullary nerve, protecting the anteriorly lying FN from injury during this maneuver. With the help of a Brackmann suction tip, the hook is used to continue detaching the superior vestibular nerve, separating it from the FN and reflecting it medially. The FN can now be clearly seen entering the intralabyrinthine canal, and the extent of its involvement by the tumor can be assessed.

19. In live surgery, the lines of incision undergo bipolar coagulation before the posterior fossa dura is opened, in order to avoid bleeding.

20. The superior dural incision runs parallel and inferior to the superior petrosal sinus up to the limits of bony drilling. The inferior incision starts just in front of the distal part of the sigmoid sinus and follows the sinus and jugular bulb course to the porus, where it joins the superior incision. The dura of the IAC is next opened. The canal dura at the level of the porus is incised using scissors.

21. At the end of the approach, a double-curved hook is used to remove the incus through the aditus. The middle ear is then packed with periosteum to prevent CSF leakage.

4.1.3 Hints and Pitfalls

- Extensive removal of bone over the middle fossa dura and posterior to the sigmoid sinus, uncovering the posterior fossa dura, is a fundamental step for obtaining a wide approach adequate for tumor removal, in comparison with the classic translabyrinthine approach.
- The sigmoid sinus has to be completely uncovered. Leaving an island of bone over the sigmoid sinus (Bill's island) limits the degree of sinus retraction. The edges of the bone island may injure the sinus wall during retraction.
- Bone between the terminal part of the sigmoid sinus and the jugular bulb should be removed to allow optimal visualization of the lower portion of the cerebellopontine angle. Removing the bone here is a tedious job, and it should be done with care to avoid injuring the fragile jugular bulb.
- The attachment of the endolymphatic sac to the posterior fossa dura impedes posterior retraction of the latter. For this reason, a blade is used to incise the proximal part of the sac, with the tip directed against the bone.
- The facial nerve lies immediately lateral to the vestibule. The utmost care should be taken to avoid injuring the nerve during drilling to open the vestibule. At this level, drilling should be posterior and never medial to the nerve.
- The IAC should be uncovered over 270 degrees rather than only 180 degrees of its circumference.

- A thin shell of bone left covering the IAC until all the drilling around has been completed helps prevent injury to the contents of the canal from the rotating drill in case it slips.
- The original technique described by House for identifying the facial nerve at the fundus depends on identification of the vertical crest (Bill's bar). This is a constant landmark that separates the facial nerve, located anterosuperiorly, from the superior vestibular nerve, located posteriorly. The only disadvantage of this technique is that it carries a potential risk of injury to the facial nerve, particularly in inexperienced hands. In our practice, we use the horizontal crest and the superior ampullary nerve to identify the facial nerve (as described above), and we no longer use House's method, except in the very rare cases when there is doubt regarding the position of the facial nerve.

- Care should be taken while removing the incus to avoid fracturing the footplate, since this can create a communication between the cerebellopontine angle and the middle ear, with subsequent postoperative CSF leakage. The footplate can be protected by placing a small right-angled pick medial to the long process of the incus and distracting in a posterolateral direction.
- Use periosteum rather than fat for the closure of the attic. Periosteum is easier to manipulate, and provides a better seal.
- Do not displace the jugular bulb inferiorly if it was the only bulb or the predominant sinus. The angiomagnetic resonance image should be examined first in order to be sure of the adequacy of the contralateral circulation.

Translabyrinthine approaches

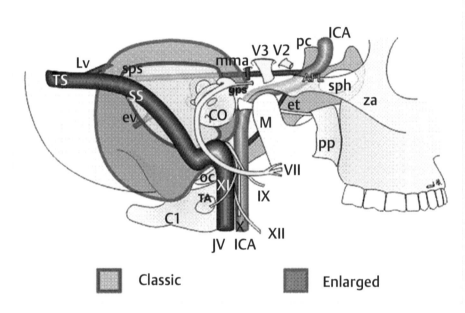

Classic   Enlarged

Fig. 4.1 The structures controlled by the translabyrinthine approach. The shaded area within the red line signifies the extent of exposure achieved by the classical translabyrinthine approach, while the green line shows the extent of exposure achieved by the enlarged translabyrinthine approach. VII, facial nerve; IX, glossopharyngeal nerve; X, vagus nerve; XI, accessory nerve; XII, hypoglossal nerve; AFL, anterior foramen lacerum; C1, atlas; CO, cochlea; et, eustachian tube; ev, emissary vein; gps, greater superficial petrosal nerve; ICA, internal carotid artery; JV, jugular vein; Lv, Labbé's vein; M, mandible; mma, middle meningeal artery; oc, occipital condyle; pc, posterior clinoid; pp, pterygoid process; sph, sphenoid sinus; sps, superior petrosal sinus; SS, sigmoid sinus; TA, lateral process of the atlas; TS, transverse sinus; V2, second division of the trigeminal nerve; V3, third division of the trigeminal nerve; za, zygomatic arch.

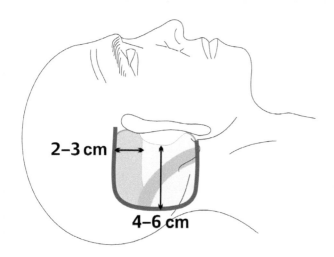

Fig. 4.2 Postauricular skin incision for the enlarged translabyrinthine approach.

Left Ear

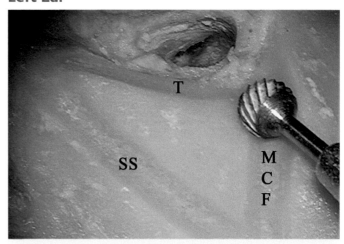

Fig. 4.3 In a left temporal bone, the triangle of attack is created. MCF, level of the middle cranial fossa; SS, level of the sigmoid sinus; T, tangent to the posterior canal wall.

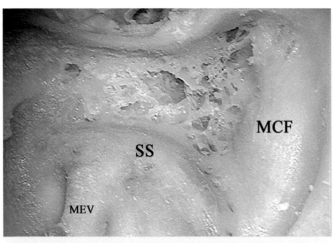

Fig. 4.4 The extended mastoidectomy has been performed. MCF, middle cranial fossa; MEV, mastoid emissary vein; SS, sigmoid sinus.

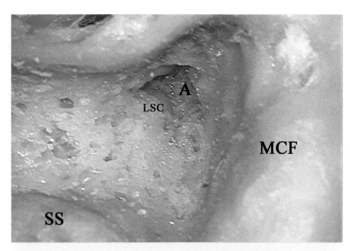

Fig. 4.5 The antrum (A) has been opened. The short process of the incus (*) and the lateral semicircular canal (LSC) are the landmarks for the genu of the facial nerve. MCF, middle cranial fossa; SS, sigmoid sinus.

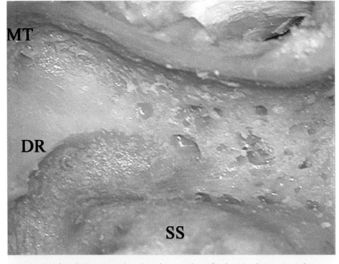

Fig. 4.6 The digastric ridge has been identified. DR, digastric ridge; MT, mastoid tip; SS, sigmoid sinus.

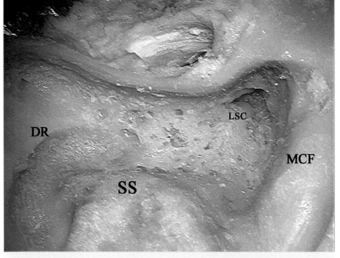

Fig. 4.7 The mastoid segment of the facial nerve between the lateral semicircular canal (LSC) and the digastric ridge (DR) is to be skeletonized. MCF, middle cranial fossa; SS, sigmoid sinus.

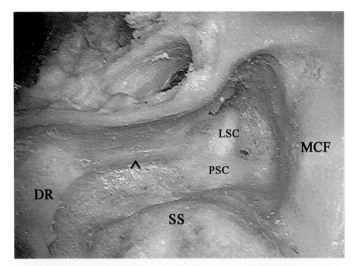

Fig. 4.8 The mastoid segment of the facial nerve (^) has been well skeletonized. *, short process of the incus; DR, digastric ridge; LSC, lateral semicircular canal; MCF, middle cranial fossa; PSC, posterior semicircular canal; SS, sigmoid sinus.

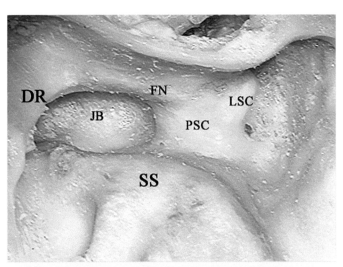

Fig. 4.9 The jugular bulb (JB) has been identified medial to the mastoid segment of the facial nerve (FN). DR, digastric ridge; LSC, lateral semicircular canal; PSC, posterior semicircular canal; SS, sigmoid sinus.

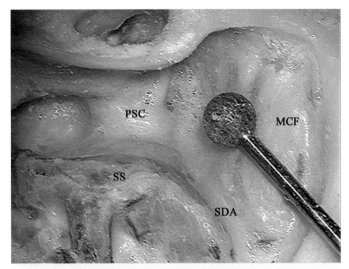

Fig. 4.10 A large diamond burr is used to thin down the bone overlying the sigmoid sinus and the dura into a thin shell. MCF, middle cranial fossa; PSC, posterior semicircular canal; SDA, sinodural angle; SS, sigmoid sinus.

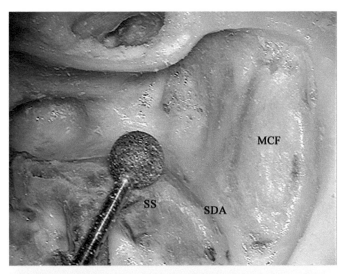

Fig. 4.11 The direction of movement of the burr should be parallel to the structures being skeletonized—the sigmoid sinus (SS) here. MCF, middle cranial fossa; SDA, sinodural angle.

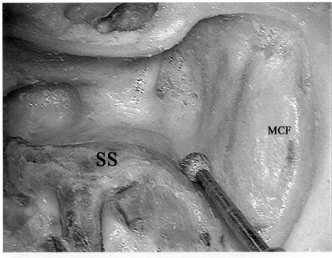

Fig. 4.12 A small diamond burr should be moved from medial to lateral while thinning the bone in the sinodural angle. MCF, middle cranial fossa; **SS,** sigmoid sinus.

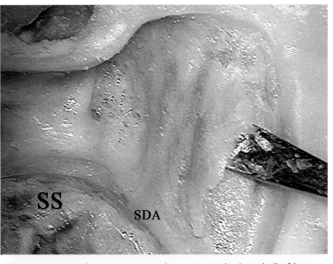

Fig. 4.13 A septal raspatory is used to remove the last shell of bone. SDA, sinodural angle; SS, sigmoid sinus.

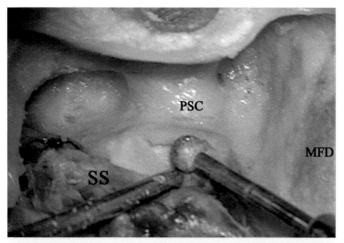

Fig. 4.14 The suction tip is used to retract the dura and sigmoid sinus (SS), while a diamond burr is used the remove the remaining bone. MFD, middle fossa dura; PSC, posterior semicircular canal.

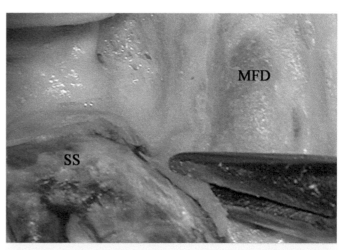

Fig. 4.15 Using a rongeur, the bone at the sinodural angle is removed. MFD, middle fossa dura; SS, sigmoid sinus.

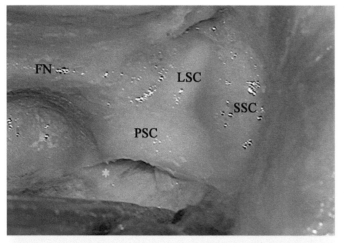

Fig. 4.16 The endolymphatic duct (*) can be seen extending from a position medial to the posterior semicircular canal (PSC) to the posterior fossa dura, preventing adequate retraction. FN, facial nerve; LSC, lateral semicircular canal; SSC, superior semicircular canal.

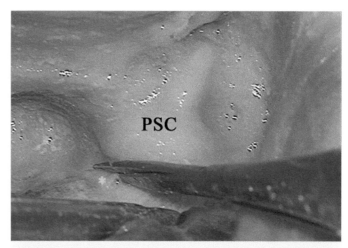

Fig. 4.17 The endolymphatic duct (*) is sharply cut. PSC, posterior semicircular canal.

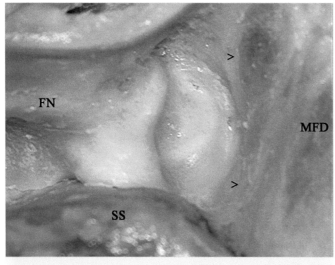

Fig. 4.18 The arrows point to the bone left to protect the dura while labyrinthectomy is being performed. FN, facial nerve; MFD, middle fossa dura; SS, sigmoid sinus.

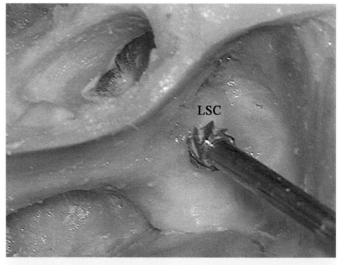

Fig. 4.19 A cutting burr is used to open the labyrinth, starting with the lateral semicircular canal (LSC).

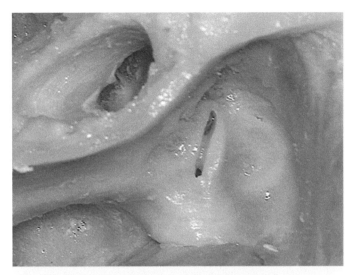

Fig. 4.20 The lateral semicircular canal has been opened.

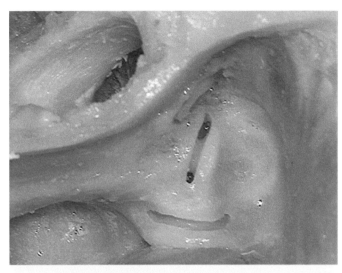

Fig. 4.21 The posterior canal is opened.

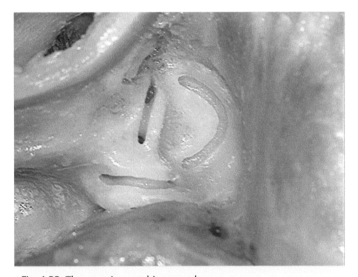

Fig. 4.22 The superior canal is opened.

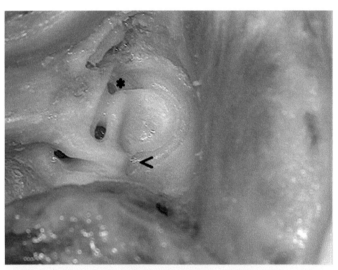

Fig. 4.23 The openings of the canals into the vestibule. <, common crus; *, the joint lateral and superior ampullae.

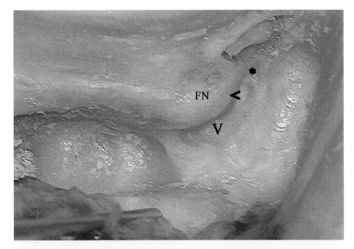

Fig. 4.24 The canals have been drilled away, and the vestibule (V) has been opened. Note the thin amount of bone (<) separating the genu of the facial nerve (FN) from the vestibule. *, the part of the superior canal ampulla left as a landmark to the superior edge of the internal auditory canal.

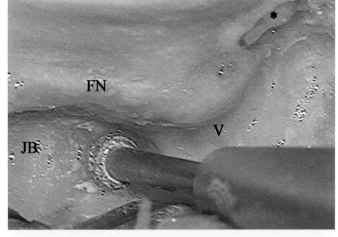

Fig. 4.25 Identification of the lower edge of the internal auditory canal starts by drilling the bone between the jugular bulb (JB) and the expected position of the canal. *, incus; FN, facial nerve; V, vestibule.

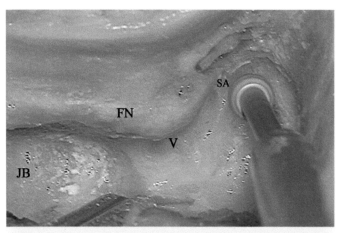

Fig. 4.26 The ampulla of the superior canal (SA) serves as a landmark to the superior edge of the internal auditory canal. The drill should be moved from medial to lateral. FN, facial nerve; JB, jugular bulb; V, vestibule.

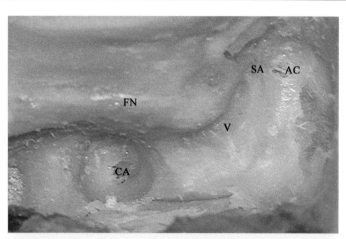

Fig. 4.27 Note the bone (>, <) left to protect the dura from the drill. AC, supralabyrinthine air cells; CA, cochlear aqueduct; FN, facial nerve; SA, ampulla of the superior canal; V, vestibule.

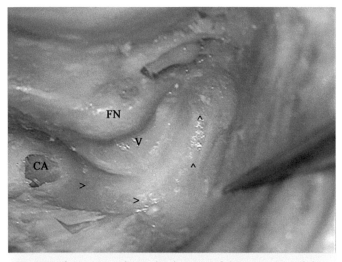

Fig. 4.28 The arrows indicate the direction of the movement of the drill when looking for the internal auditory canal, in a semicircular fashion. *, superior ampulla; CA, cochlear aqueduct; FN, facial nerve; V, vestibule.

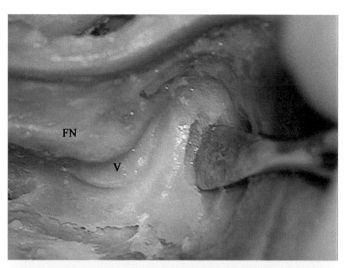

Fig. 4.29 Separating the dura from the drilled bone helps avoid injury to it and leads to early identification of the meatus of the internal auditory canal. FN, facial nerve; V, vestibule.

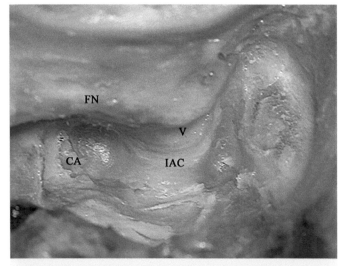

Fig. 4.30 The internal auditory canal (IAC) has been identified, but the overlying bone needs to be thinned further. CA, cochlear aqueduct; FN, facial nerve; V, vestibule.

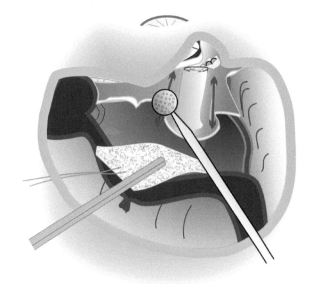

Fig. 4.31 The correct way of using the drill to identify the internal auditory canal is shown. This process is supported by gently pushing the posterior dura and the sigmoid sinus away from the surgical field using a suction irrigator on a surgical patty.

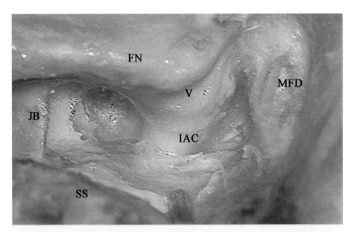

Fig. 4.32 The internal auditory canal (IAC) has been adequately skeletonized. FN, facial nerve; JB, jugular bulb; MFD, middle fossa dura; SS, sigmoid sinus; V, vestibule.

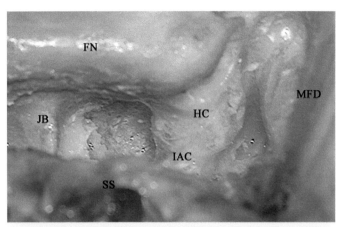

Fig. 4.33 The last shell of bone covering the internal auditory canal (IAC) has been removed using a hook. Note that the sigmoid sinus (SS) lies anteriorly, covering the view of the canal, and should be retracted posteriorly by the suction tube. FN, facial nerve; HC, horizontal crest; JB, jugular bulb; MFD, middle fossa dura.

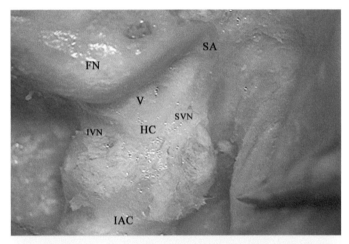

Fig. 4.34 The view of the fully exposed internal auditory canal (IAC). FN, facial nerve; HC, horizontal crest; IVN, inferior vestibular nerve; SA, superior ampulla; SVN, superior vestibular nerve; V, vestibule.

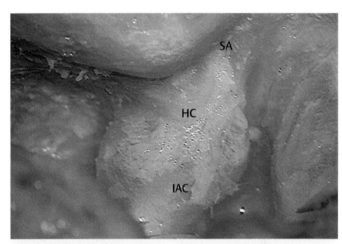

Fig. 4.35 The superior ampullary nerve canal (SA) has been identified. HC, horizontal crest; IAC, internal auditory canal.

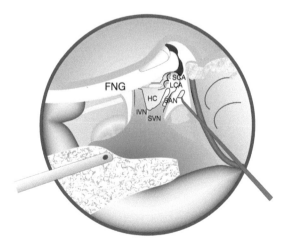

Fig. 4.36 The superior vestibular nerve (SVN) has been followed laterally into the superior ampullary nerve (SAN) canal where the superior ampullary nerve supplies the lateral canal ampulla. FNG, facial nerve genu; HC, horizontal crest; IVN, inferior vestibular nerve; LCA, ampulla of the lateral semicircular canal; SCA, ampulla of the superior semicircular canal.

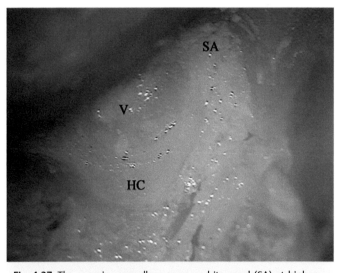

Fig. 4.37 The superior ampullary nerve and its canal (SA) at higher magnification. HC, horizontal crest; V, vestibule.

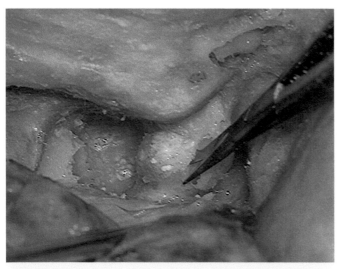

Fig. 4.38 The dura of the internal auditory canal is being opened.

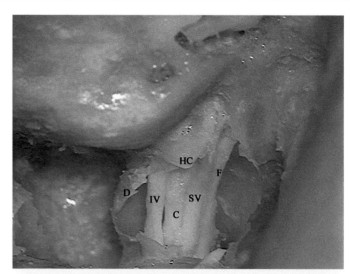

Fig. 4.39 The contents of the canal can be seen. C, cochlear nerve; D, dura of the canal; F, facial nerve; HC, horizontal crest; IV, inferior vestibular nerve; SV, superior vestibular nerve.

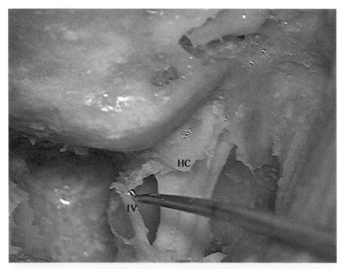

Fig. 4.40 The inferior vestibular nerve (IV) has been detached. HC, horizontal crest.

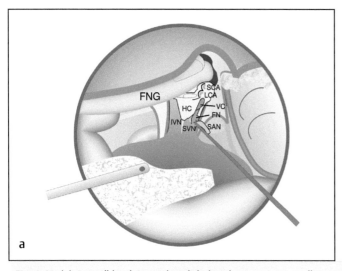

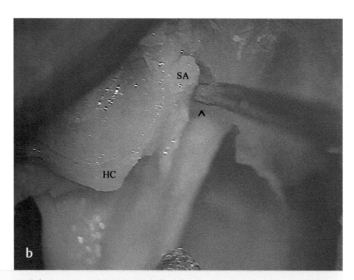

Fig. 4.41 (a) A small hook is used to dislodge the superior ampullary nerve (SA) from its canal (SAC). FNG, facial nerve genu; HC, horizontal crest; IVN, inferior vestibular nerve; LCA, ampulla of the lateral semicircular canal; SCA, ampulla of the superior semicircular canal; SVN, superior vestibular nerve; VC, vertical crest (Bill's bar). (b) Bill's bar (^) can be seen lying anterior to the hook, protecting the labyrinthine segment of the facial nerve. HC, horizontal crest; SA, superior ampullary nerve.

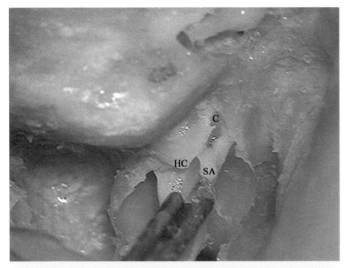

Fig. 4.42 The superior ampullary nerve (SA) has been completely detached from its canal (C). HC, horizontal crest.

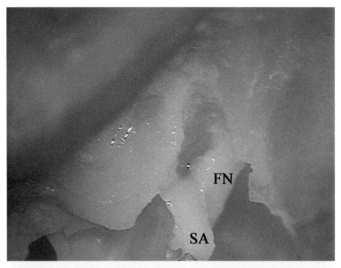

Fig. 4.43 At higher magnification, the relationship between the facial nerve (FN) and the superior ampullary nerve (SA) can be better appreciated.

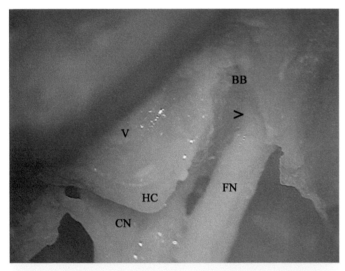

Fig. 4.44 The view of the fundus after removal of the vestibular nerve. >, the beginning of the labyrinthine segment of the facial nerve; BB, Bill's bar; CN, cochlear nerve; FN, facial nerve in the internal auditory canal; HC, horizontal crest; V, vestibule.

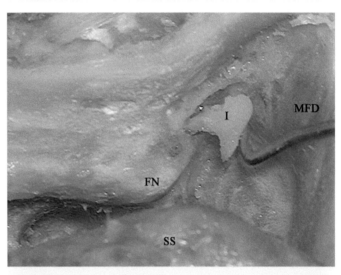

Fig. 4.45 At the end of the approach, the incus (I) is removed through the antrum. FN, facial nerve; MFD, middle fossa dura; SS, sigmoid sinus.

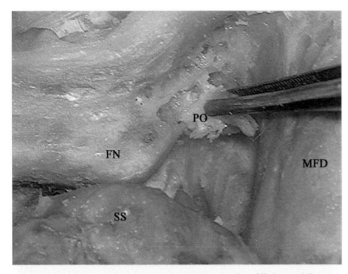

Fig. 4.46 In live surgery, periosteum (PO) is used to fill the middle ear cleft, to prevent cerebrospinal fluid leakage. FN, facial nerve; MFD, middle fossa dura; SS, sigmoid sinus.

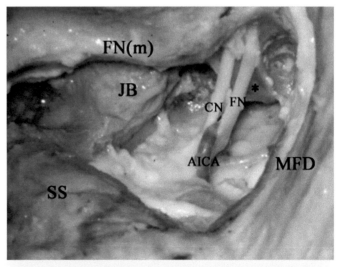

Fig. 4.47 A left-sided cadaveric dissection to show the intracranial structures. *, anterior wall of the internal auditory canal; AICA, anterior inferior cerebellar artery; CN, cochlear nerve; FN, facial nerve; FN(m), mastoid segment of the intracranial nerve; JB, jugular bulb; MFD, middle fossa dura; SS, sigmoid sinus.

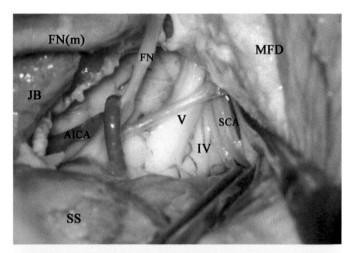

Fig. 4.48 This case shows the benefit of uncovering the dura. The uncovered middle fossa dura (MFD) can be retracted superiorly here to demonstrate the routes of the trigeminal nerve (V), trochlear nerve (IV), and superior cerebellar artery (SCA). AICA, anterior inferior cerebellar artery; FN, facial nerve; FN(m), mastoid segment of the facial nerve; JB, jugular bulb; SS, sigmoid sinus.

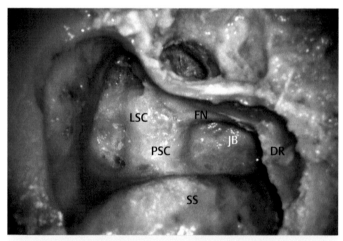

Fig. 4.49 This image shows the benefit of uncovering the sigmoid sinus, the dura posterior to it, and of adequate removal of the bone between the sigmoid sinus and jugular bulb. After these steps have been carried out, the posterior inferior cerebellar artery (PICA), vertebral artery (VA), glossopharyngeal nerve (IX), vagus nerve (X), and accessory nerve (XI) can all be controlled in the lower part of the approach. CBL, cerebellum.

Right Ear

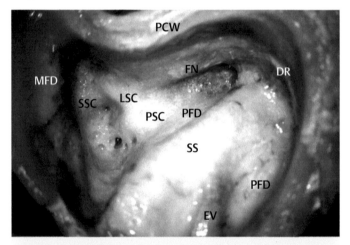

Fig. 4.50 Extended mastoidectomy has been performed. MFD, middle fossa dura; SS, sigmoid sinus; EV, emissary vein; FN, facial nerve; DR, digastric ridge; LSC, lateral semicircular canal; PSC, posterior semicircular canal; SSC, superior semicircular canal; PCW, posterior canal wall; PFD, posterior fossa dura.

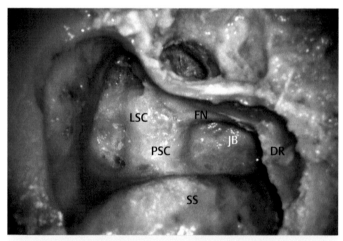

Fig. 4.51 The jugular bulb (JB) has been identified medial to the mastoid segment of the facial nerve. DR, digastric ridge; FN, facial nerve; LSC, lateral semicircular canal; PSC, posterior semicircular canal.

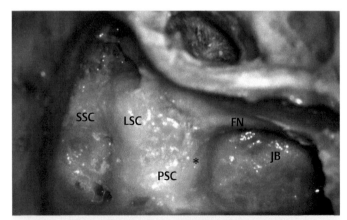

Fig. 4.52 Bigger magnification. Note the relationship between the mastoid portion of the facial nerve (FN), the jugular bulb (JB), and the posterior semicircular canal (PSC). *, ampullary end; I, incus (short process); LSC, lateral semicircular canal; SSC, superior semicircular canal.

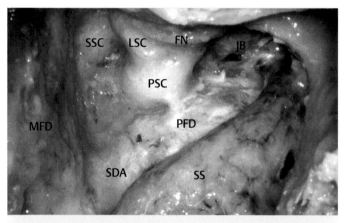

Fig. 4.53 The posterior fossa dura (PFD) has been almost completely skeletonized. A thin shell of bone is still covering the sinodural angle (SDA). FN, facial nerve; JB, jugular bulb; LSC, lateral semicircular canal; MFD, middle fossa dura; PSC, posterior semicircular canal; SS, sigmoid sinus; SSC, superior semicircular canal.

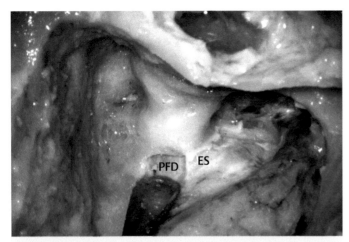

Fig. 4.54 The posterior fossa dura (PFD) is detached from the bone using a raspatory. The endolymphatic sac (ES) is under view.

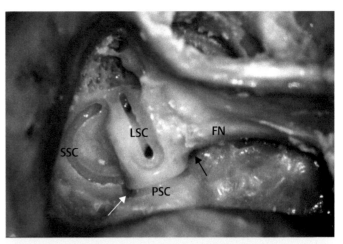

Fig. 4.55 Labirynthectomy has been accomplished and all the three canals opened. Note the relationship between the ampulla of the posterior semicircular canal (*black arrow*) and the facial nerve (FN). White arrow, common crus; LSC, lateral semicircular canal; PSC, posterior semicircular canal; SSC, superior semicircular canal.

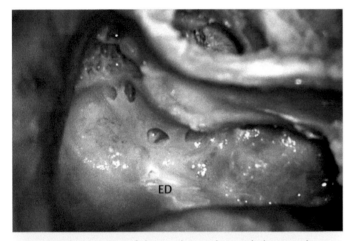

Fig. 4.56 The openings of the canals into the vestibule. Note the endolymphatic duct (ED) running medial to the area of the posterior semicircular canal.

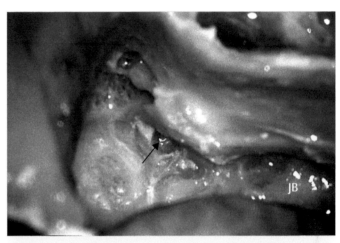

Fig. 4.57 The canals have been drilled away, and the vestibule (*arrow*) has been opened.

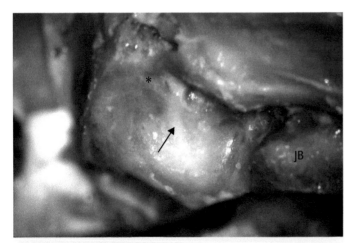

Fig. 4.58 The internal auditory canal is starting to be seen. The ampulla of the superior semicircular canal (*) serves as a landmark for the superior edge of the internal auditory canal and superior vestibular nerve (*arrow*). JB, jugular bulb.

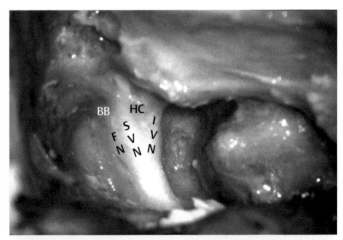

Fig. 4.59 All the internal auditory canal has been identified. BB, Bill's bar; FN, facial nerve, HC, horizontal crest; IFN, inferior vestibular nerve; SVN, superior vestibular nerve.

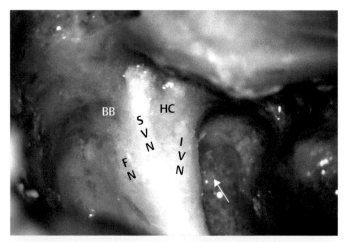

Fig. 4.60 Bigger magnification. The cochlear aqueduct (*arrow*) has been opened. BB, Bill's bar; FN, facial nerve, HC, horizontal crest; IVN, inferior vestibular nerve; SVN, superior vestibular nerve.

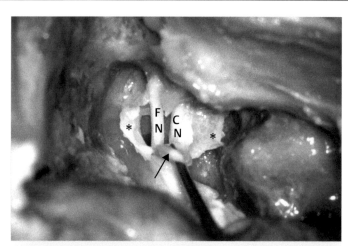

Fig. 4.61 The dura of the internal auditory canal (*) has been opened and the vestibular nerves reflected inferiorly (*arrow*). CA, cochlear nerve; FN, facial nerve.

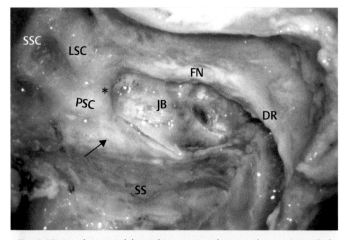

Fig. 4.62 Another translabyrinthine approach in a right ear. Extended mastoidectomy has been performed. The sigmoid sinus (SS) and the jugular bulb (JB) are under view, as well as semicircular canals, facial nerve (FN) and digastric ridge (DR). As in the previous case the jugular bulb is high, reaching the ampulla of the posterior semicircular canal (*). The posterior fossa dura in the area of the endolymphatic sac has been partially uncovered from bone (*arrow*). LSC, lateral semicircular canal; PSC, posterior semicircular canal; SSC, superior semicircular canal.

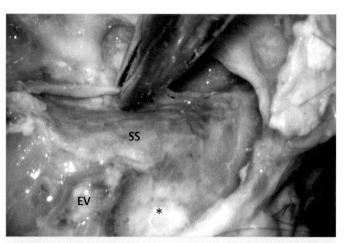

Fig. 4.63 The posterior fossa dura anterior and posterior to the sigmoid sinus (SS) has to be uncovered. Note the uncovered retrosigmoid dura (*). The last shell of bone covering the dura anterior to the sigmoid sinus is removed using a rongeur. EV, emissary vein.

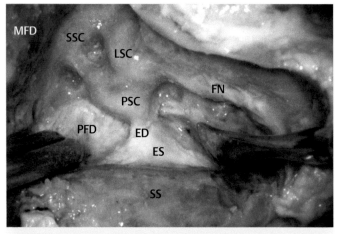

Fig. 4.64 All the posterior fossa dura anterior to the sigmoid sinus has been uncovered and retracted posteriorly. Note the position of the endolymphatic duct (ED) joining the endolymphatic sac (ES). FN, facial nerve; LSC, lateral semicircular canal; MFD, middle fossa dura; PFD, posterior fossa dura; PSC, posterior semicircular canal; SS, sigmoid sinus; SSC superior semicircular canal.

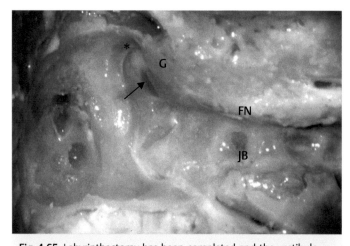

Fig. 4.65 Labyrinthectomy has been completed and the vestibule opened (*arrow*). The ampulla of the superior semicircular canal (*) has been left as a landmark for the superior ampullary nerve. FN, facial nerve (mastoid segment); G, genu of the facial nerve; JB, jugular bulb.

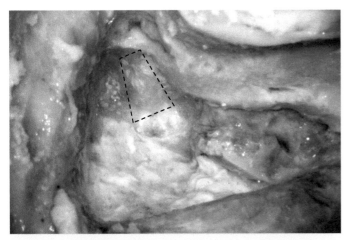

Fig. 4.66 The internal auditory canal is starting to be seen (*dashed lines*).

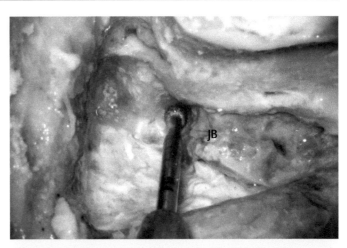

Fig. 4.67 Identification of the lower edge of the internal auditory canal starts by drilling the bone between the jugular bulb (JB) and the expected position of the canal.

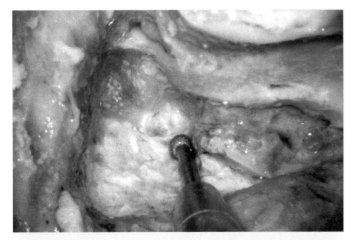

Fig. 4.68 Drilling proceeds posteriorly for the decompression of the high jugular bulb.

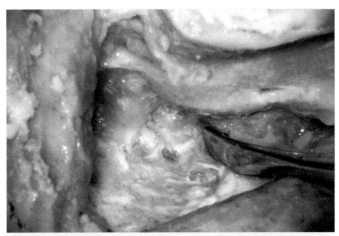

Fig. 4.69 The jugular bulb is pushed downward. In live surgery, Surgicel and bone wax can be used to maintain the jugular bulb displaced inferiorly (see Chapter 4.2 for details).

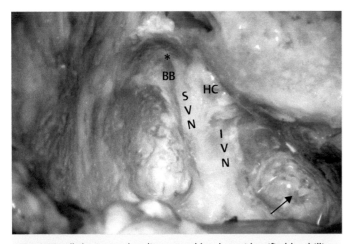

Fig. 4.70 All the internal auditory canal has been identified by drilling the bone between the middle fossa dura and the roof of the canal superiorly and between the floor of the canal and the jugular bulb inferiorly. Superiorly the drill should always be moved from medial to lateral. The cochlear aqueduct has been opened inferiorly (*arrow*). The superior ampullary nerve is visible (*) and serves as a landmark for the superior vestibular nerve (SVN). BB, Bill's bar; HC, horizontal crest; IVN, inferior vestibular nerve.

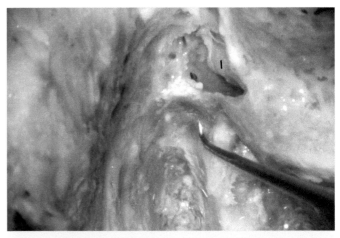

Fig. 4.71 The superior ampullary nerve is detached from its canal using a hook. I, incus.

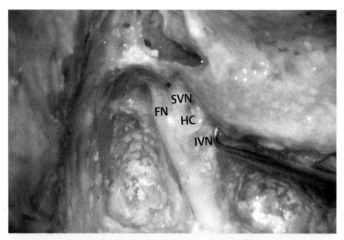

Fig. 4.72 The inferior vestibular nerve (IVN) is starting to be detached using a hook. The superior vestibular nerve (SVN) is then displaced inferiorly. The facial nerve (FN) is under view. *, Bill's bar; HC, horizontal crest.

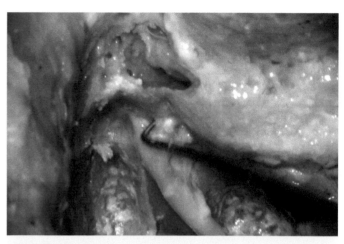

Fig. 4.73 The vestibular nerves are removed and reflected inferiorly with a hook.

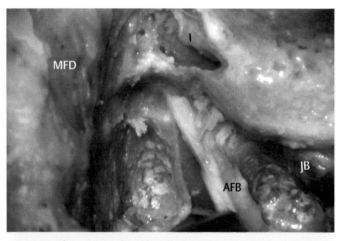

Fig. 4.74 The acousticofacial bundle (AFB) is under view. I, incus; JB, jugular bulb; MFD, middle fossa dura.

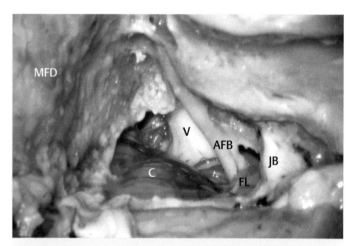

Fig. 4.75 View after opening the posterior fossa dura. AFB, acousticofacial bundle; C, cerebellum; FL, flocculus; JB, jugular bulb; MFD, middle fossa dura; V, trigeminal nerve.

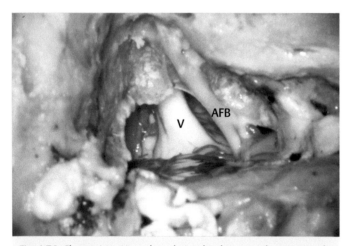

Fig. 4.76 Closer view. Note the relationship between the trigeminal nerve (V) and the acousticofacial bundle (AFB).

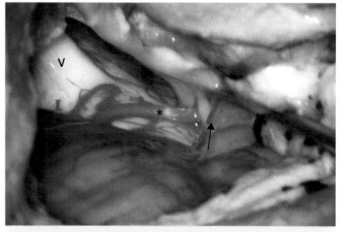

Fig. 4.77 The acousticofacial bundle is displaced inferiorly and a loop of the AICA is clearly seen (*). The flocculus is partially covering the origin of the facial nerve at the pons (*arrow*). V, trigeminal nerve.

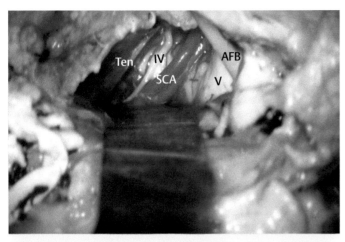

Fig. 4.78 The surgical view is moved superiorly and the cerebellum retracted posteriorly. Note the trochlear nerve (IV), the tentorium (Ten), and the superior cerebellar artery (SCA). AFB, acousticofacial bundle; V, trigeminal nerve.

4.2 Management of High Jugular Bulb

A high jugular bulb is present in about 25% of cases. Particularly in medium-sized or large tumors, a high bulb may obstruct the required view of the area of the lower cranial nerves. In these cases, the high jugular bulb is managed as follows.

4.2.1 Surgical Steps

See ▸ Fig. 4.79, ▸ Fig. 4.80, ▸ Fig. 4.81, ▸ Fig. 4.82, ▸ Fig. 4.83, ▸ Fig. 4.84, ▸ Fig. 4.85, ▸ Fig. 4.86, ▸ Fig. 4.87, ▸ Fig. 4.88, ▸ Fig. 4.89, ▸ Fig. 4.90, ▸ Fig. 4.91.

1. Using a septal elevator, the bulb, together with the surrounding periosteal layer, is dissected from its wall. This should be done very carefully to avoid injury to the thin bulb wall.
2. After adequate dissection has been carried out, the jugular bulb is pressed downward using a large piece of Surgicel over its dome. Surgicel helps control the bleeding that may occur during this step.
3. A piece of bone wax is then placed over the Surgicel to keep the bulb in place. Note that a thin layer of bone must be left around the jugular bulb to support the Surgicel and bone wax.
4. In some cases when there is a high jugular bulb, complete uncovering of the bulb dome (particularly anteriorly) may be difficult to achieve. In this case, the bulb lies anterior to the plane of the facial nerve, and the vertical distance between the bulb and the nerve is very small. In such cases, a large septal dissector cannot be used to dissect the bulb from its walls. Alternatively, a double-curved raspatory can be used. The bulb is managed as described previously.
5. With adequate inferior displacement of the jugular bulb, sufficient bone removal can be safely carried out, creating a bony trough inferior to the IAC.

Right Ear

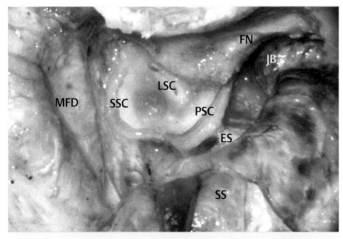

Fig. 4.79 Right ear. Example of a far-advanced sigmoid sinus (SS) combined with a high jugular bulb (JB). Labirynthectomy has been started but decompression of the sigmoid sinus is necessary to gain space. ES, endolymphatic sac; FN, facial nerve; LSC, lateral semicircular canal; PSC, posterior semicircular canal; SSC, superior semicircular canal.

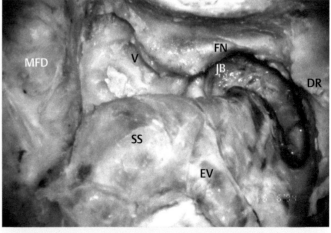

Fig. 4.80 Note the reduction of space without decompression of the sigmoid sinus. DR, digastric ridge; EV, emissary vein; FN, facial nerve; V, vestibule.

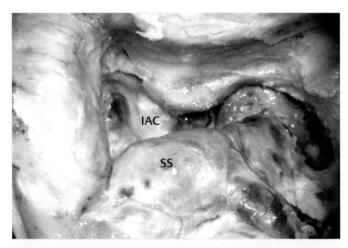

Fig. 4.81 The posterior third of the internal auditory canal (IAC) is covered by the sigmoid sinus (SS).

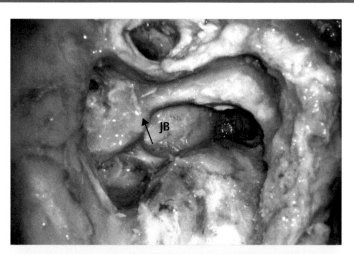

Fig. 4.82 Another example of high jugular bulb (JB) in a right translabyrinthine approach. The dome of the jugular bulb is under the ampulla of the posterior semicircular canal (*arrow*).

Left Ear

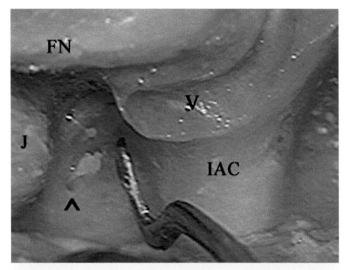

Fig. 4.83 Labyrinthectomy and skeletonization of the internal auditory canal (IAC) have been carried out. Note the narrow distance available between the high jugular bulb (J) and the IAC. ^, cochlear aqueduct; FN, facial nerve; V, vestibule.

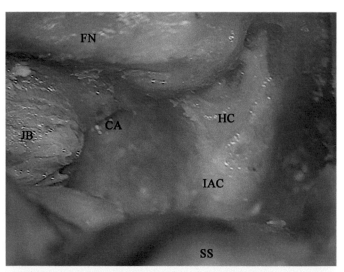

Fig. 4.84 The last shell of bone over the internal auditory canal (IAC) has been removed. CA, cochlear aqueduct; FN, facial nerve; HC, horizontal crest; JB, jugular bulb; SS, sigmoid sinus.

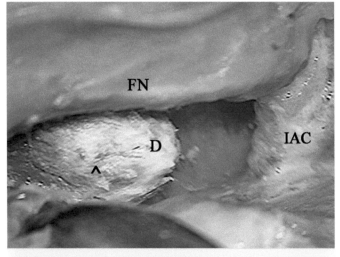

Fig. 4.85 The dome of the jugular bulb (D) has been exposed by carefully removing the overlying bone to the level of the arrow (^). FN, facial nerve; IAC, internal auditory canal.

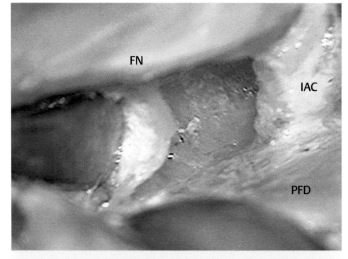

Fig. 4.86 A septal raspatory is carefully used to dissect the jugular bulb from the anteriorly lying bone. FN, facial nerve; IAC, internal auditory canal; PFD, posterior fossa dura.

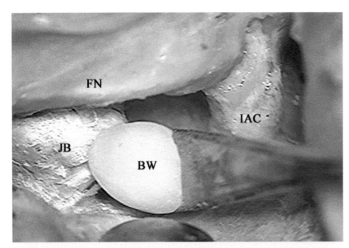

Fig. 4.87 Bone wax (BW) is used to fix the jugular bulb (JB) in its lowered position. FN, facial nerve; IAC, internal auditory canal.

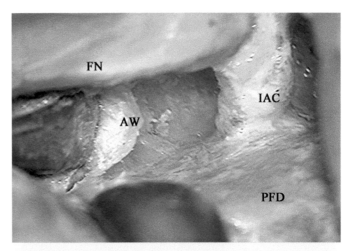

Fig. 4.88 The septal raspatory is used to further push down the bone wax to secure it in place. The extent of lowering should not lead to closure of the bulb. FN, facial nerve; IAC, internal auditory canal; PFD, posterior fossa dura.

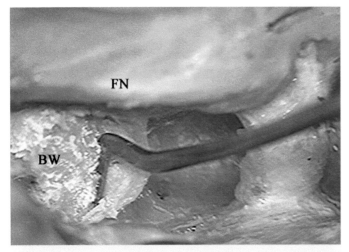

Fig. 4.89 The bone wax (BW) can be seen fixing the bulb in its lowered position. FN, facial nerve.

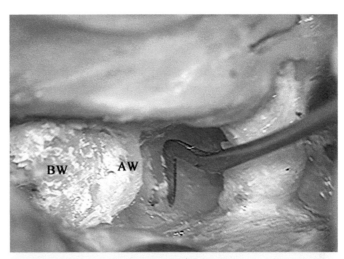

Fig. 4.90 The anterior wall (AW) of the jugular bulb should now be drilled away to widen the surgical field. BW, bone wax.

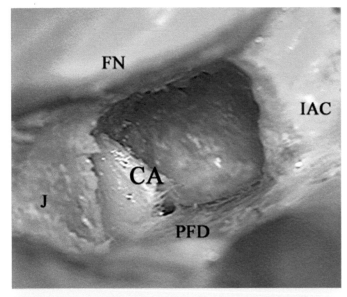

Fig. 4.91 The view after the procedure has been completed. The space gained is less than 1 cm, but this space is considered to be extremely useful in skull base surgery. CA, cochlear aqueduct; FN, facial nerve; IAC, internal auditory canal; J, jugular bulb; PFD, posterior fossa dura.

4.3 The Enlarged Translabyrinthine Approach with Transapical Extension Types (I and II)

4.3.1 Rationale

This approach is an anterior extension of the enlarged translabyrinthine approach, in which the internal auditory canal is drilled for 320 or 360 degrees of its circumference (types I and II, respectively).

4.3.2 Indications

The approach indicated for large cerebellopontine angle tumors, in which hearing preservation is not intended, is as follows:
- Large and giant acoustic neurinomas with anterior extension into the prepontine cisterns (type I approach).
- Large meningioma of the posterior surface of the temporal bone centered on the IAC with significant anterior extension (type II approach).
- Small tumors with marked anterior extension.
- Cases of contracted mastoid.

4.3.3 Surgical Steps

See ► Fig. 4.92, ► Fig. 4.93, ► Fig. 4.94, ► Fig. 4.95, ► Fig. 4.96, ► Fig. 4.97, ► Fig. 4.98, ► Fig. 4.99, ► Fig. 4.100, ► Fig. 4.101, ► Fig. 4.102, ► Fig. 4.103, ► Fig. 4.104, ► Fig. 4.105, ► Fig. 4.106, ► Fig. 4.107, ► Fig. 4.108, ► Fig. 4.109, ► Fig. 4.110, ► Fig. 4.111.
1. The extended mastoidectomy is performed as previously described. Wide bone removal is carried out, exposing approximately 3 cm of the middle fossa dura and the retrosigmoid posterior fossa dura. The sigmoid sinus is completely uncovered.
2. Labyrinthectomy is performed.
3. The IAC is identified and uncovered. Bone is removed for 270 degrees around the canal, as previously described.
4. Bone is further removed inferior to and superior to the IAC, toward the petrous apex. The whole contents of the IAC are pushed inferiorly to allow drilling of the anterior wall of the canal.
5. At the end of the procedure, 360 degrees of the IAC circumference is exposed (type II approach). In the type I approach, it is only necessary to remove 320 degrees of the circumference of the canal.

4.3.4 Hints and Pitfalls

- Transapical drilling should be done with a diamond burr, with extreme care being taken not to injure the facial nerve. A useful trick is to place the suction irrigation tube between the drill and the nerve to provide protection.
- Care should be taken while drilling the petrous apex superior to the IAC so as not to injure the superior petrosal sinus.
- In giant tumors causing high intracranial pressure, the dura usually bulges, hindering access. In such cases, the dura can be opened first to allow drainage of CSF, with a resultant release of pressure and shrinkage of the dura. The drilling can then be continued.
- Particularly in tumors that lie in a far anterior position, the facial nerve is markedly displaced anteriorly. The transapical extension allows much better visualization of the nerve where it starts to curve.
- This approach also allows better control of the trigeminal nerve up to Meckel's cave, and of the abducent nerve, prepontine cistern, and basilar artery.
- Using this approach, we have abandoned the transotic approach for anteriorly located tumors and limit its use only to cases of concomitant cochlear invasion or vertical IAC involvement.

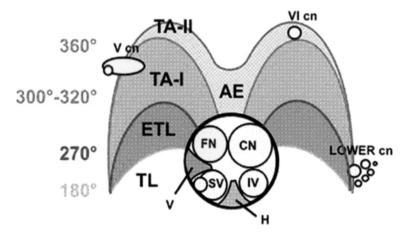

TL   = translabyrinthine
ETL = extended translabyrinthine
TA-I = Transapical type I
TA-II = transapical type II

Fig. 4.92 The extent of drilling around the internal auditory canal needed to achieve the extensions of the translabyrinthine approach. AE, anterior wall of the internal auditory canal; CN, cranial nerve; FN, facial nerve; H, horizontal crest; IV, inferior vestibular nerve; Lower cn, lower cranial nerve; SV, superior vestibular nerve; V, vertical crest; V cn, fifth cranial nerve (trigeminal nerve); VI cn, sixth cranial nerve (abducent nerve).

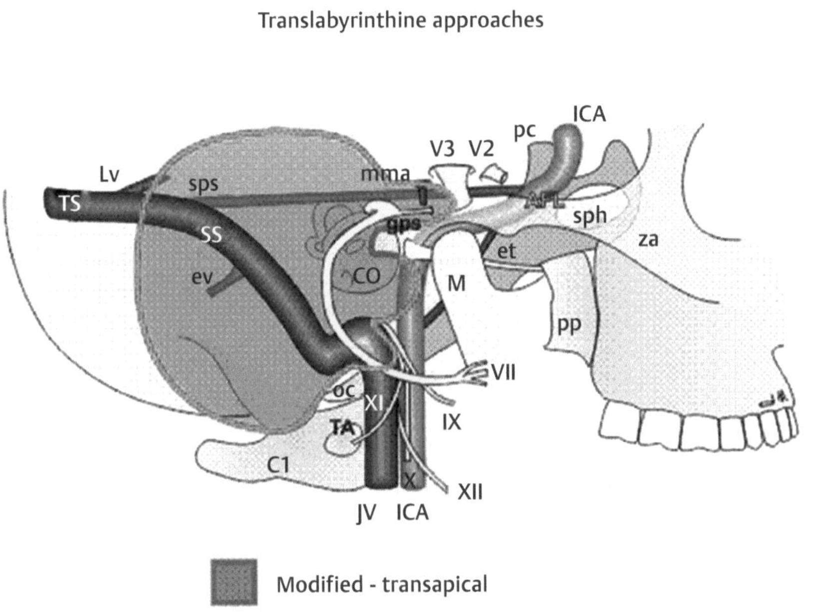

Translabyrinthine approaches

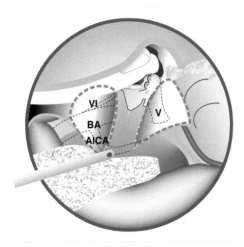

Fig. 4.93 The structures exposed by the trans-labyrinthine–transapical approach. The gray-shaded area indicates the extent of bone removal. Note the transapical extension. See ▶ Fig. 4.1, for key to abbreviation.

Modified - transapical

Right Ear

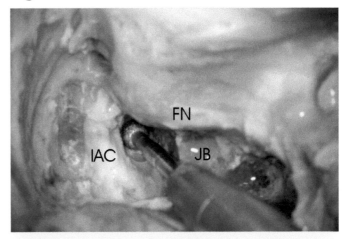

Fig. 4.94 (*Left ear*) Difference between the conventional 180-degree translabyrinthine approach and the 320-degree transapical extension in the surgical view. The dashed line demonstrates the working area for extended bone removal. After this bone work is completed, the important structures can be controlled. AICA, anterior inferior cerebellar artery; BA, basilar artery; V, trigeminal nerve; VI, abducent nerve.

Fig. 4.95 Drilling is being carried out inferior to the internal auditory canal (IAC). FN, facial nerve; JB, jugular bulb.

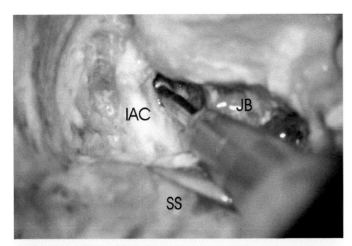

Fig. 4.96 Further extensive drilling is added inferior to the internal auditory canal (IAC) toward the petrous apex. JB, jugular bulb; SS, sigmoid sinus.

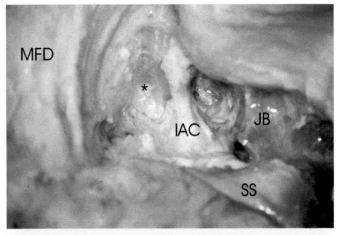

Fig. 4.97 Extensive bone removal inferior and superior to the internal auditory canal (IAC) have been achieved. Bone superior to the canal (*) is still to be removed. JB, jugular bulb; MFD, middle fossa dura; SS, sigmoid sinus.

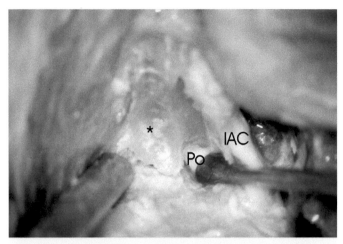

Fig. 4.98 The contents of the internal auditory canal are pushed inferiorly to allow for removal of the remaining bone (*) superior to the internal auditory canal (IAC). Po, porus of the internal auditory canal.

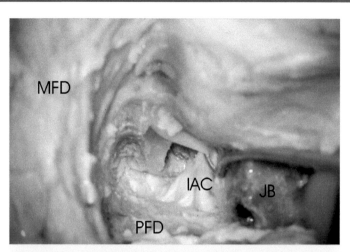

Fig. 4.99 The contents of the internal auditory canal (IAC) are displaced inferiorly to show the extent of bone removal. The anterior wall of the IAC can be further drilled if needed. JB, jugular bulb; MFD, middle fossa dura; PFD, posterior fossa dura.

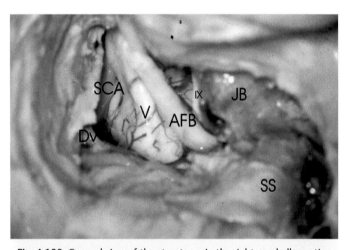

Fig. 4.100 General view of the structures in the right cerebellopontine angle (CPA) after opening the dura. Note the enhanced exposure of the superior CPA and the excellent exposure of the trigeminal nerve (V) and the superior cerebellar artery (SCA). AFB, acousticofacial bundle; Dv, Dandy's vein; JB, jugular bulb; SS, sigmoid sinus; IX, glossopharyngeal nerve.

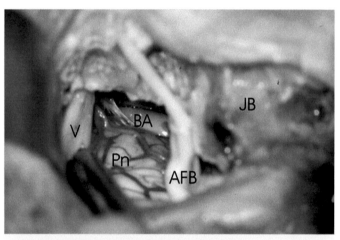

Fig. 4.101 The trigeminal nerve (V) is pushed superiorly. The basilar artery (BA) in the prepontine cistern is clearly visible. AFB, acousticofacial bundle; JB, jugular bulb; Pn, pons.

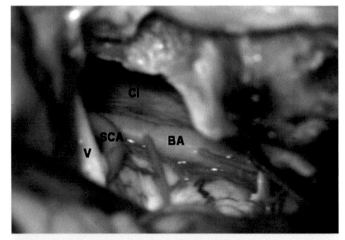

Fig. 4.102 Tilting the microscope anterosuperiorly shows that the superior cerebellar artery (SCA) branches off the basilar artery (BA). The clivus (Cl) can also be visualized. V, trigeminal nerve.

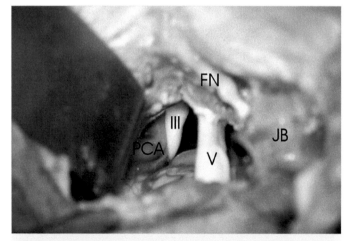

Fig. 4.103 With gentle retraction of the tentorium, the oculomotor nerve (III) is seen between the posterior cerebral artery (PCA) superiorly and the superior cerebellar artery (not labelled) inferiorly. FN, facial nerve; JB, jugular bulb; V, trigeminal nerve.

Left Ear

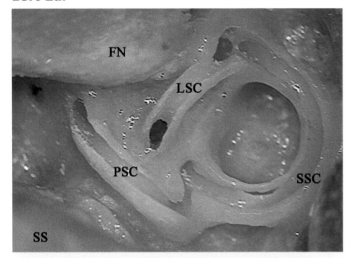

Fig. 4.104 The lateral (LSC), posterior (PSC), and superior (SSC) semicircular canals have been opened in a left temporal bone. FN, facial nerve; SS, sigmoid sinus.

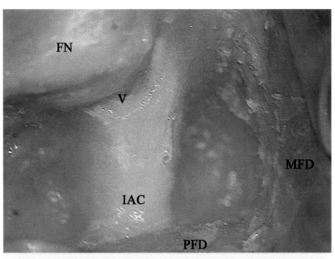

Fig. 4.105 The internal auditory canal (IAC) has been skeletonized over 270 degrees. FN, facial nerve; MFD, middle fossa dura; PFD, posterior fossa dura; V, vestibule.

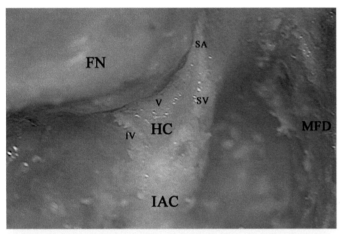

Fig. 4.106 The last shell of bone covering the internal auditory canal (IAC) has been removed. FN, facial nerve; HC, horizontal crest; IV, inferior vestibular nerve; MFD, middle fossa dura; SA, superior ampullary nerve; SV, superior vestibular nerve; V, vestibule.

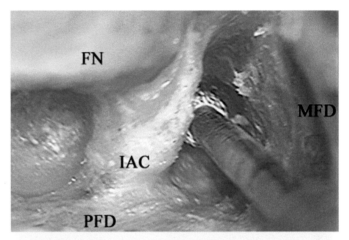

Fig. 4.107 To achieve a type I transapical extension, 320 degrees of the bone surrounding the internal auditory canal (IAC) should be removed. The superior part of the bone removal has been carried out here, as can be seen from the part of the burr head covered by the canal. FN, facial nerve; MFD, middle fossa dura; PFD, posterior fossa dura.

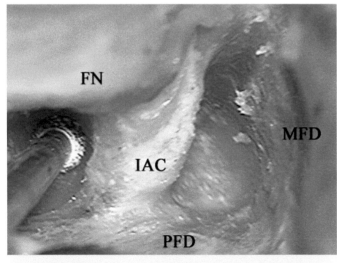

Fig. 4.108 Drilling is now being carried out inferior to the internal auditory canal (IAC) to achieve a type I transapical extension (320 degrees). FN, facial nerve; MFD, middle fossa dura; PFD, posterior fossa dura.

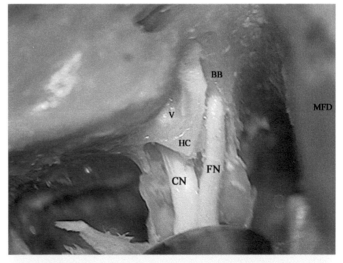

Fig. 4.109 The internal auditory canal has been opened and the vestibular nerves have been removed. BB, Bill's bar; CN, cochlear nerve; FN, facial nerve; HC, horizontal crest; MFD, middle fossa dura; V, vestibule.

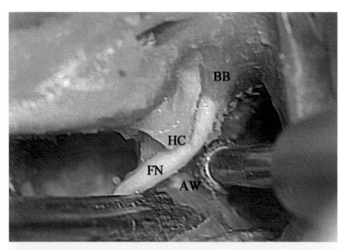

Fig. 4.110 The type II transapical extension involves drilling of all the bone surrounding the internal auditory canal (360 degrees). To achieve this, the contents of the canal should be gently retracted using the suction tip, and the anterior wall of the internal auditory canal (AW) should be carefully drilled using a diamond burr. BB, Bill's bar; FN, facial nerve; HC, horizontal crest.

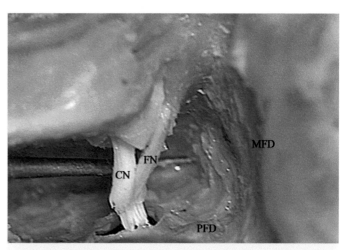

Fig. 4.111 A type II transapical extension has been completed. CN, cochlear nerve; FN, facial nerve; MFD, middle fossa dura; PFD, posterior fossa dura.

5 Facial Nerve Decompression

Abstract

The facial nerve (FN) could be freed from the fallopian canal through different surgical approaches. Transmastoid and translabyrinthine techniques for FN decompression will be described in this chapter.

Keywords: facial nerve decompression, translabyrinthine approach

5.1 Transmastoid Facial Nerve Decompression

Transmastoid FN decompression can be carried out via either closed or open tympanoplasty. In patients with normal hearing, closed tympanoplasty allows the pathology to be managed while preserving the patient's hearing. By contrast, open tympanoplasty is used in patients whose hearing has already been lost.

5.1.1 Indications

- In the past, the procedure was indicated in case of a longitudinal temporal bone fracture with concomitant FN paralysis in which the fracture line is parallel to the tympanic or mastoid segment of the facial nerve without involving a more proximal segment. Nowadays, there is no reliable benefit of this technique for the improvement of facial nerve fuction, so, it has no longer been indicated.
- Facial nerve tumors localized to the mastoid or tympanic segments of the facial nerve.

5.1.2 Surgical Techniques

Closed Tympanoplasty Facial Nerve Decompression

See ▶ Fig. 5.1, ▶ Fig. 5.2, ▶ Fig. 5.3, ▶ Fig. 5.4, ▶ Fig. 5.5, ▶ Fig. 5.6, ▶ Fig. 5.7, ▶ Fig. 5.8, ▶ Fig. 5.9, ▶ Fig. 5.10, ▶ Fig. 5.11, ▶ Fig. 5.12, ▶ Fig. 5.13.

1. A closed tympanoplasty with an extended posterior tympanotomy, as described in Chapter 3, is performed.
2. The bone covering the FN is thinned down to eggshell consistency using a large diamond burr under ample suction irrigation. The mastoid segment of the facial nerve should be skeletonized to a total of 270 degrees of its circumference.
3. Skeletonization of the facial nerve genu is mainly carried out on the anterior and lateral surfaces. The lateral semicircular canal lies immediately posterior to the genu, and care must be taken not to open it. Care also must be taken not to touch the short process of the incus, which lies in close proximity to the lateral surface of the genu. The level of exposure that can be achieved here is only 180 degrees. A small diamond burr is used. The drill should be rotated at a low speed and away from the incus. The bone covering the anterior and lateral surfaces of the genu is thinned out.

4. Attention is now directed to the narrowest part of the approach—the tympanic segment of the FN. This segment has to be approached through the space available between the body of the incus laterally and the anterior part of the lateral semicircular canal, the ampullae of the lateral and superior semicircular canals medially, and the middle fossa dural plate superiorly. A small diamond burr is mounted on a curved handpiece to allow maximal utilization of the narrow visual field available. The length of the burr should also be adjusted so that the handpiece will not interrupt the vision. The speed of the drill is adjusted to a low level, and the drill is rotated away from the ossicular chain. In the middle part of this segment, care also must be taken not to open the ampullated ends of the lateral and superior semicircular canals lying superior to the nerve. Drilling is advanced cautiously anteriorly until the geniculate ganglion (GG) is uncovered.
5. The last shell of thin bone covering the nerve is removed using a double-curved hook, thus uncovering the full length of the FN from the geniculate ganglion to the stylomastoid foramen.
6. At this point, the suction irrigation tube is changed to a smaller Brackmann's suction tube.
7. Using a new Beaver knife with the sharp border facing away from the nerve, the perineural sheath of the nerve is incised, thereby completing the decompression.

Open Tympanoplasty Facial Nerve Decompression

See ▶ Fig. 5.14, ▶ Fig. 5.15.

An open tympanoplasty approach for FN decompression makes the procedure much easier, both because of the ambient space provided and because this approach is usually indicated in patients in whom hearing is not to be preserved or has already been lost.

1. An open tympanoplasty is performed as previously described.
2. After the completion of the approach, a large diamond burr is used to thin down the bony covering of the mastoid segment to a very thin transparent shell of bone. The level of exposure here should be 270 degrees. The exposure involves the posterior, lateral, and anterior surfaces.
3. When drilling reaches the genu, the size of the drill is reduced to avoid unnecessary opening of the lateral canal, even if hearing is not to be conserved, in order to prevent postoperative vertigo.
4. Drilling is then advanced toward the tympanic segment and the geniculate ganglion, with care being not to injure the superiorly lying lateral canal and ampullae of the lateral and superior canal. If needed, the size of the burr can be further reduced.
5. The last shell of bone is removed in the usual manner using the double-curved hook, and the perineural sheath is incised as in closed tympanoplasty decompression.

5.1.3 Hints and Pitfalls

- In the lower part of its mastoid portion, the FN should be skeletonized up to 270 degrees in order to facilitate surgical manipulation. However, this degree of exposure is not feasible in the area of the second genu and the tympanic segment, because of the close relationship to the canals and the ossicular chain.
- At the level of the genu, the short process of the incus lies in close proximity to the lateral surface of the facial nerve, and the lateral semicircular canal forms its posterior relationship. The working space is thus very limited, allowing only 180 degrees of skeletonization. Any slippage of the drill can lead to sensorineural hearing loss.
- In the fortunate occurrence of a dehiscent tympanic segment or a very thin fallopian canal in this area, drilling can be avoided and the thin shell of bone can be removed using a double-curved hook, which should also be used with extreme care. If the bony canal is thick, using a hook is dangerous due to the high chance of slippage, leading to injury to the ossicular chain or the middle fossa dura.
- During skeletonization of the tympanic segment of the facial nerve, extreme attention should be paid not only to the burr head but also to the shaft, which can also lead to sensorineural hearing loss if it touches the ossicles while rotating.
- After the nerve has been completely uncovered, the suction tube is exchanged for a Brackmann suction tube. This tube has side holes that prevent direct suction on delicate structures, thus avoiding unnecessary trauma to the FN.

Left Ear

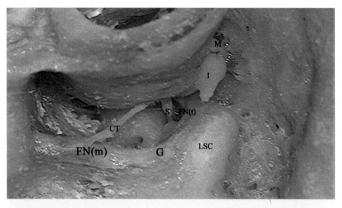

Fig. 5.1 A transmastoid decompression of the mastoid (FN[m]) and tympanic (FN[t]) segments of the facial nerve in a left temporal bone. A closed tympanoplasty with an extended facial recess has been carried out. Note that the mastoid genu (G) and tympanic segments of the facial nerve are controlled. CT, chorda tympani; I, incus; LSC, lateral semicircular canal; M, malleus; S, stapes.

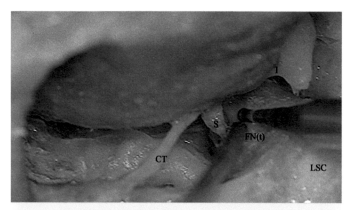

Fig. 5.2 After decompression of the mastoid segment of the nerve, attention now shifts to the tympanic segment (FN[t]). Note that a small diamond burr is being used; note also that marked attention is being paid to both the burr's head and shaft, neither of which is brought into contact with the intact ossicular chain. CT, chorda tympani; I, incus; LSC, lateral semicircular canal; S, stapes.

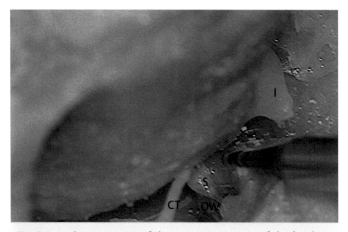

Fig. 5.3 As decompression of the tympanic segment of the facial nerve advances more anteriorly, the working angle becomes more difficult. The surgeon may have to ask for the bed to be tilted anteriorly with the head downward. Extreme attention must be given to the head and shaft of the burr. *, long process of the incus; CT, chorda tympani; I, incus; OW, oval window; S, stapes.

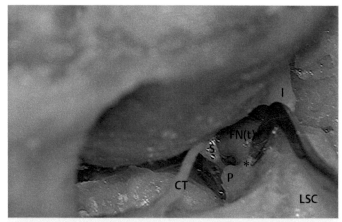

Fig. 5.4 A double-curved hook is used to remove the last shell of bone (*). Care must be taken to prevent it from slipping and injuring either the nerve or the ossicles. CT, chorda tympani; FN(t), tympanic segment of the facial nerve; I, incus; LSC, lateral semicircular canal; P, pyramidal process; S, stapes.

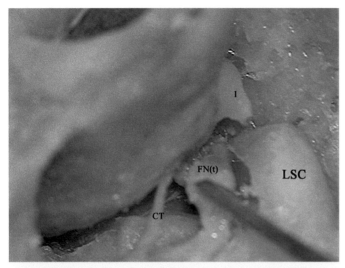

Fig. 5.5 After complete removal of the overlying bone, the nerve can now be dislocated from the fallopian canal. CT, chorda tympani; FN(t), tympanic segment of the facial nerve; I, incus; LSC, lateral semicircular canal.

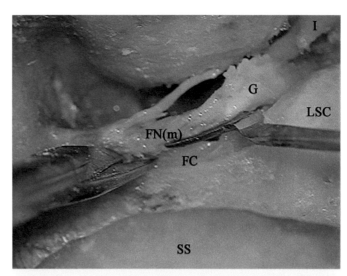

Fig. 5.6 The adhesions between the medial surface of the mastoid segment of the facial nerve (FN[m]) and the fallopian canal (FC) have to be sharply cut. G, genu of the facial nerve; I, incus; LSC, lateral semicircular canal; SS, sigmoid sinus.

Right Ear

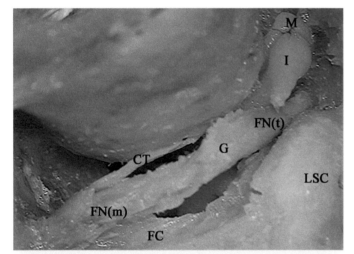

Fig. 5.7 The mastoid segment (FN[m]), genu (G), and tympanic segment (FN[t]) of the facial nerve have now been freed from the fallopian canal (FC), completing the decompression. CT, chorda tympani; I, incus; LSC, lateral semicircular canal; M, malleus.

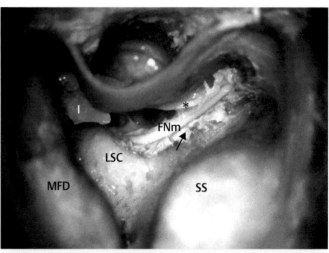

Fig. 5.8 A closed mastoidectomy with posterior tympanotomy has been completed in a right ear. The perineural sheath (*arrow*) of the mastoid segment of the facial nerve (FN[m]) has been opened. I, incus; LSC, lateral semicircular canal; MFD, middle fossa dura; SS, sigmoid sinus.

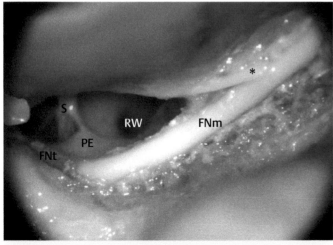

Fig. 5.9 Closer view. Note the origin of the chorda tympani (*). The round window niche (RW), the pyramidal eminence (PE), the stapes (S), and the second portion of the facial nerve (FN[t]) are visible. FN(m), mastoid portion of the facial nerve.

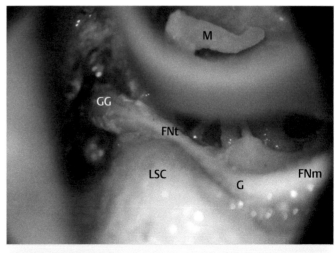

Fig. 5.10 Bone over the second portion of the facial nerve (FN[t]) has been removed. The area of the geniculate ganglion (GG) is under view. FN(m), mastoid portion of the facial nerve; G, genu of the facial nerve; LSC, lateral semicircular canal; M, malleus.

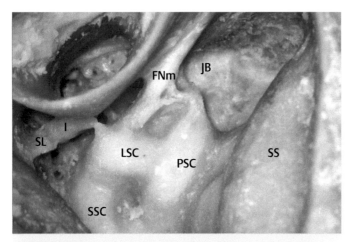

Fig. 5.11 Right ear. Decompression of the mastoid portion of the facial nerve with a close tympanoplasty. Posterior tympanotomy has been accomplished and the retrofacial air cells have been drilled. FN(m), mastoid portion of the facial nerve; JB, jugular bulb; I, incus; LSC, lateral semicircular canal; PSC, posterior semicircular canal; SL, suspensory ligament; SSC, superior semicircular canal; SS, sigmoid sinus.

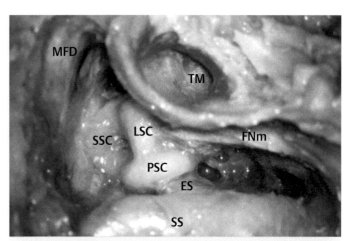

Fig. 5.12 Right ear. Another closed tympanoplasty with decompression of the mastoid portion of the facial nerve. The labyrinth has been completely skeletonized. ES, endolymphatic sac; FN(m), mastoid portion of the facial nerve; JB, jugular bulb; LSC, lateral semicircular canal; MFD, middle fossa dura; PSC, posterior semicircular canal; SSC, superior semicircular canal; SS, sigmoid sinus; TM, tympanic membrane.

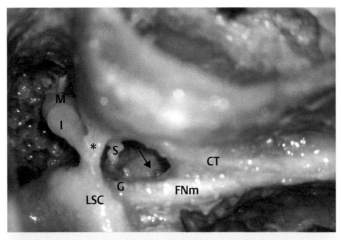

Fig. 5.13 Posterior tympanotomy. The chorda tympani (CT) is visible as well as the area of the oval window (*arrow*). Note the relationship between the genu of the facial nerve (G), the lateral semicircular canal (LSC), and the incus (I), which is still protected by a bony bridge (*). FN(m), mastoid portion of the facial nerve; I, incus; M, malleus; S, stapes.

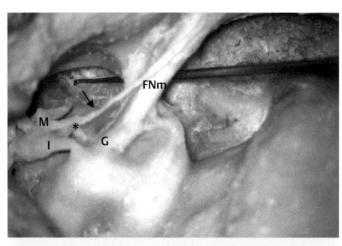

Fig. 5.14 The posterior canal wall has been removed and subfacial tympanotomy perfomed (hook). The chorda tympani (*arrow*) is under view. *, stapes; FN(m), mastoid portion of the facial nerve; G, genu of the facial nerve; I, incus; M, malleus.

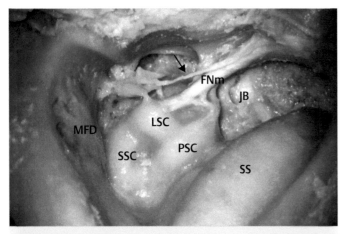

Fig. 5.15 Wider view. Arrow, chorda tympani; FN(m), mastoid portion of the facial nerve; JB, jugular bulb; LSC, lateral semicircular canal; MFD, middle fossa dura; PSC, posterior semicircular canal; SS, sigmoid sinus; SSC, superior semicircular canal.

5.2 Translabyrinthine Facial Nerve Decompression

See ▶ Fig. 5.16, ▶ Fig. 5.17, ▶ Fig. 5.18, ▶ Fig. 5.19, ▶ Fig. 5.20.

Facial nerve decompression via the translabyrinthine approach is carried out whenever decompression of the full length of the facial nerve is required in the absence of useful hearing. The procedure is practically a combination of closed tympanoplasty with the translabyrinthine approach. Decompression of the mastoid, tympanic segments, and the geniculate ganglion parts of the facial nerve is achieved through the closed tympanoplasty. Labyrinthectomy and exposure of the internal auditory canal allows decompression of the tympanic and internal auditory canal parts of the nerve.

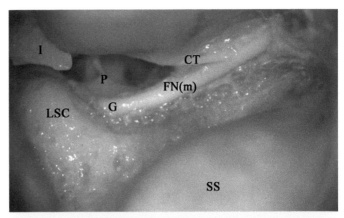

Fig. 5.16 A closed tympanoplasty and extended posterior tympanotomy have been carried out in a right temporal bone. The mastoid segment of the facial nerve (FN[m]) has been well skeletonized. CT, chorda tympani; G, genu; I, incus; LSC, lateral semicircular canal; P, pyramidal process; SS, sigmoid sinus.

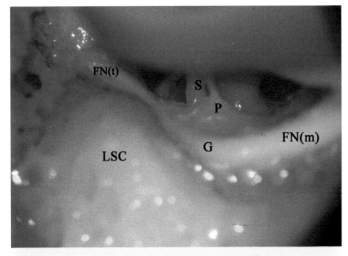

Fig. 5.17 Through the atticotomy, decompression of the tympanic segment of the facial nerve (FN[t]) is carried out. FN(m), mastoid segment of the facial nerve; G, genu; LSC, lateral semicircular canal; P, pyramidal process; S, stapes.

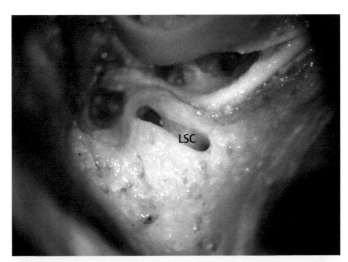

Fig. 5.18 Labyrinthectomy starts with opening of the lateral semicircular canal (LSC).

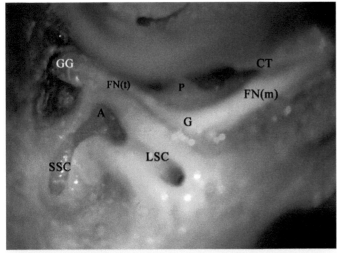

Fig. 5.19 Labyrinthectomy proceeds. The joint ampulla (A) of the lateral (LSC) and superior (SSC) semicircular canals can be seen, closely related to the tympanic segment of the facial nerve (FN[t]). CT, chorda tympani; FN(m), mastoid segment of the facial nerve; G, genu; GG, geniculate ganglion; P, pyramidal process.

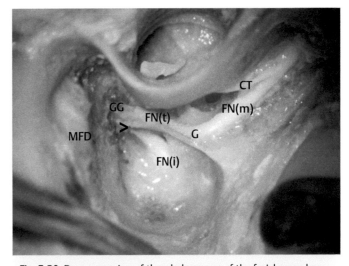

Fig. 5.20 Decompression of the whole course of the facial nerve has been achieved. >, labyrinthine segment of the facial nerve; CT, chorda tympani; FN(i), internal auditory canal segment of the facial nerve; FN(m), mastoid segment of the facial nerve; FN(t), tympanic segment of the facial nerve; G, genu; GG, geniculate ganglion; MFD, middle fossa dura.

6 Middle Cranial Fossa Approaches

Abstract

The middle fossa approaches are classified into the following:
- Middle fossa approach to the internal auditory canal (IAC); The enlarged middle fossa approach, with exposure of the IAC and surrounding bone, increasing the access to the cerebello-pontine angle (CPA);
- The middle fossa transpetrous approach, with removal of the petrous apex. This approach is designed basically for the anterior CPA, ventral surface of the pons, and the upper clivus.
- With the middle cranial fossa (MCF) approach, it is possible to remove lesions involving the CPA preserving the hearing function.
- The MCF can be combined with a transmastoid approach to achieve adequate exposure of the full length of the intratemporal facial nerve without compromising preoperatively preserved hearing.

Keywords: enlarged middle cranial fossa approach, facial nerve tumor, middle cranial fossa–transpetrous approach, transmastoid–middle cranial fossa approach

6.1 Enlarged Middle Cranial Fossa Approach

6.1.1 Indications

The enlarged middle fossa approach allows a complete exposure of the IAC, but a limited exposure of the CPA through the superior surface of the temporal bone. The enlarged approach (▶ Fig. 6.2) differs from the classic middle fossa approach (▶ Fig. 6.1), in which wider bone removal is carried out anterior and posterior to the IAC. This approach allows hearing preservation as well as complete exposure of the full length of the internal auditory canal from the porus to the fundus.

The following pathologies are indications for the enlarged MCF approach:
- Small vestibular schwannomas reaching the fundus of the IAC with a CPA extension of less than 0.5 cm.
- Facial nerve tumors involving the nerve between the geniculate ganglion and IAC.
- Supralabyrinthine petrous bone cholesteatoma not eroding the labyrinth.

This approach is relatively contraindicated in patients over 60 years of age. In the elderly, the dura is less resistant and may be torn during elevation from the temporal bone.

6.1.2 Surgical Steps

See ▶ Fig. 6.7, ▶ Fig. 6.8, ▶ Fig. 6.9, ▶ Fig. 6.10, ▶ Fig. 6.11, ▶ Fig. 6.12, ▶ Fig. 6.13, ▶ Fig. 6.14, ▶ Fig. 6.15, ▶ Fig. 6.16, ▶ Fig. 6.17, ▶ Fig. 6.18, ▶ Fig. 6.19, ▶ Fig. 6.20, ▶ Fig. 6.21, ▶ Fig. 6.22, ▶ Fig. 6.23, ▶ Fig. 6.24, ▶ Fig. 6.25, ▶ Fig. 6.26, ▶ Fig. 6.27, ▶ Fig. 6.28, ▶ Fig. 6.29, ▶ Fig. 6.30, ▶ Fig. 6.31, ▶ Fig. 6.32, ▶ Fig. 6.33, ▶ Fig. 6.34, ▶ Fig. 6.35, ▶ Fig. 6.36, ▶ Fig. 6.37, ▶ Fig. 6.38, ▶ Fig. 6.39, ▶ Fig. 6.40, ▶ Fig. 6.41, ▶ Fig. 6.42, ▶ Fig. 6.43, ▶ Fig. 6.44, ▶ Fig. 6.45, ▶ Fig. 6.46, ▶ Fig. 6.47, ▶ Fig. 6.48, ▶ Fig. 6.49, ▶ Fig. 6.50, ▶ Fig. 6.51.

1. An ample quadrangular craniotomy measuring 4×5 cm is made. The craniotome is generally used for this step; however, if the instrument is not available, the craniotomy can be carried out using a drill. Craniotomy is started using a medium-sized cutting burr, and when the dura begins to show through the transparency of the bone, the burr is exchanged for a small diamond one. The lower edge of the craniotomy should be at the level of the base of the zygoma in order to be approximately at the level of the floor of the MCF. The craniotomy should lie two-thirds in front and one-third behind the external auditory canal.

2. The bone flap is then separated from the underlying dura using a septal raspatory. Care should be taken during this step so as not to injure the dura.

3. Elevation of the dura from the superior surface of the temporal bone is now started under microscopic magnification. Dural elevation should progress carefully from lateral to medial and from posterior to anterior. The importance of careful dural elevation cannot be overemphasized in live surgery, because of the risk of injury to the facial nerve (FN) caused by stretching the greater superficial petrosal nerve or injuring the geniculate ganglion (GG), which is dehiscent in 10 to 15% of cases.

4. While the procedure progresses, the following landmarks should be identified: the arcuate eminence, the middle meningeal artery, the greater superficial petrosal nerve, and the GG if dehiscent.

5. The medial limit of dural elevation should reach up to the border of the ridge of the petrous bone, which corresponds to the level of the superior petrosal sinus.

6. As dural elevation progresses, the middle fossa retractor is used to retract the dura, providing the necessary working space. The position of the retractor is changed to correspond to the point at which dural elevation is taking place. In its final position, the tip of the retractor should be lodged between the superior petrosal sinus and the border of the petrous bone. The middle meningeal artery forming the anterior limit of exposure should be kept intact.

7. At this point, the next step depends on the extent of the tumor. In tumors limited to the IAC, with or without limited extension to the CPA as in vestibular schwannomas, the bone drilling should uncover the IAC from the porus to the fundus. The position of the IAC is indicated by a line bisecting the angle formed by the arcuate eminence and the greater superficial petrosal nerve.

8. Four different methods are available for identifying the IAC. The House method (▶ Fig. 6.3b) puts the facial nerve at risk, and requires the utmost care and skill, while the major disadvantages of the Fisch method (▶ Fig. 6.3a) are the variable angle between the superior semicircular canal and the IAC and the need to blue-line the superior semicircular canal, with the risk of opening it. The method we use identifies the canal at the bisection of the greater superficial petrosal nerve and superior semicircular canal, as proposed by Garcia Ibanez (1980) (▶ Fig. 6.3c); however, we start drilling medially (▶ Fig. 6.3d) at the level of the porus.

9. Identification of the IAC is started medially at the expected level of the porus of the IAC near the superior petrosal sinus.

A large diamond drill is used, and drilling is carried out carefully at and around the predicted level of the porus.

10. Once the canal has been identified, bone removal should be continued until wide exposure of the dura has been achieved both anterior and posterior to the IAC, leaving only a thin shell of bone.

11. Drilling is now continued laterally to identify the full length of the IAC. In order to avoid injury to IAC, the drill should be moved in a direction parallel to the IAC and never crossing its longitudinal axis. Note that the exposure of the canal laterally is less than what can be achieved medially. This is due to the presence of the cochlea and vestibule, respectively, anterior and posterior to the lateral half of the IAC.

12. Once the whole length of the IAC has been identified, the last shell of bone covering the canal and the dura is removed. In live surgery, a small hole is created in the posterior fossa dura posterior to the IAC to allow for cerebrospinal fluid (CSF) escape, thus reducing the tension within the dura and improving exposure.

13. A small diamond burr is used to identify Bill's bar at the level of the fundus. The level of exposure achieved up to this point is sufficient to remove tumors situated within the IAC.

14. Using a pair of microscissors, the dura of the IAC is opened. In live surgery, the suction tube must be exchanged at this step for a Brackmann suction.

15. The tumor usually originates from the inferior vestibular nerve, pushing the facial nerve superiorly and putting it at greater risk. The superior vestibular nerve is first dislocated using a small hook, and the tumor is then dealt with carefully so as not to injure the facial nerve lying between the surgeon and the tumor.

6.1.3 Hints and Pitfalls

- The craniotomy should be placed at the level of the root of the zygoma. This will reduce the amount of temporal lobe retraction.
- If air cells were opened either anteriorly at the level of the root of the zygoma or posteriorly at the level of the supramastoid crest, bone wax should be used to close them carefully to avoid CSF leakage.
- The dural elevation should reach medially to the level of the superior petrosal sinus. Failure to do this can lead to more lateral drilling, jeopardizing vital structures.
- Identification of Bill's bar at the level of the fundus is important for positive identification of the facial nerve.
- The IAC dura is opened posteriorly in order to avoid injuring the anteriorly lying facial nerve.
- In a few cases, the loop of the anterior inferior cerebellar artery may be encountered within the canal. The utmost care must be taken to avoid injuring it.

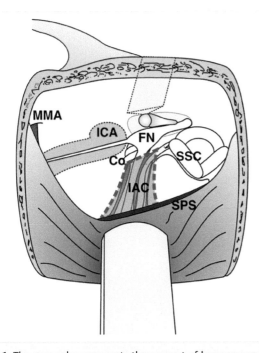

Fig. 6.1 The gray color represents the amount of bone removal using the classic middle cranial fossa approach. Note that the only bone overlying the internal auditory canal is removed. This technique is indicated in the case of facial nerve decompression or in vestibular neurectomy. Co cochlea; FN, facial nerve; ICA, internal carotid artery; MMA, middle meningeal artery; SPS, superior petrosal sinus; SSC, superior semicircular canal.

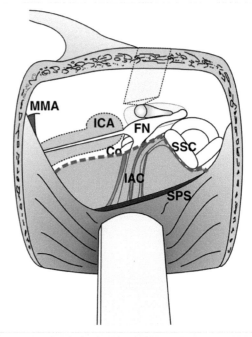

Fig. 6.2 The gray color represents the amount of bone removal using the enlarged middle cranial fossa approach. We would use this approach for the removal of small vestibular schwannomas reaching the fundus of the internal auditory canal with CPA extension of less than 0.5 cm, when hearing preservation is aimed for. For abbreviations see ► Fig. 6.1.

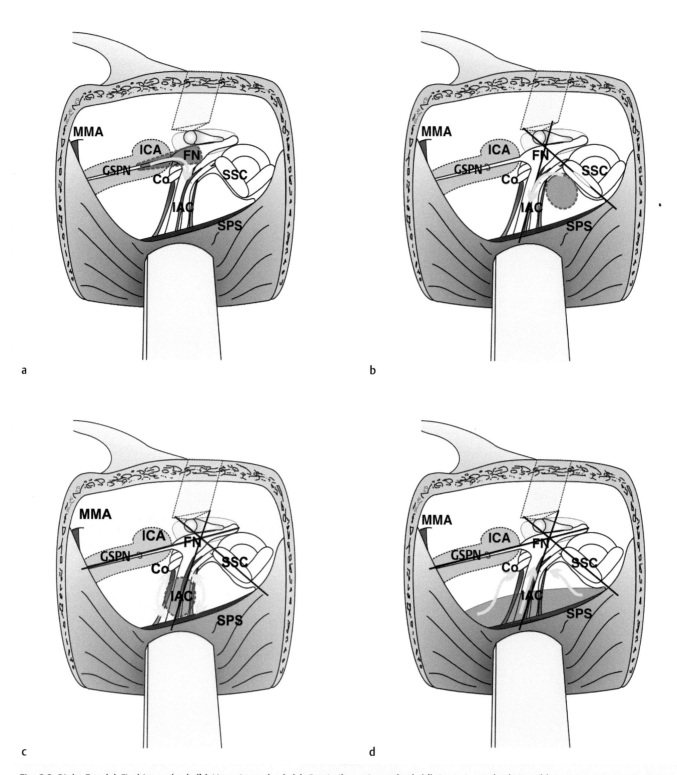

a

b

c

d

Fig. 6.3 Right Ear. **(a)** Fisch's method. **(b)** House's method. **(c)** Garcia Ibanez's method. **(d)** Sanna's method. For abbreviations see ▶ Fig. 6.1.

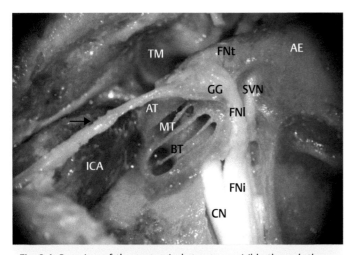

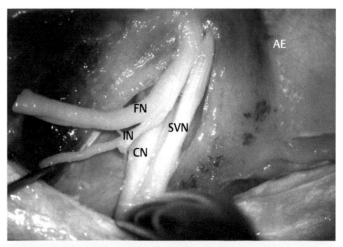

Fig. 6.4 Overview of the anatomical structures visible through the middle cranial fossa approach. Right ear. AE, arcuate eminence; arrow, greater superficial petrosal nerve; BT, basal turn of the cochlea; CN, cochlear neve; FN(i), internal auditory canal portion of the facial nerve; FN(l), labyrinthine segment of the facial nerve; FN(t) tympanic segment of the facial nerve; GG, geniculate ganglion; MT, middle turn of the cochlea; SVN, superior vestibular nerve (cut); TM, tympanic membrane.

Fig. 6.5 Anatomy of the internal auditory canal seen from a middle cranial fossa approach. AE arcuate eminence; CN, cochlear nerve; FN, facial nerve; IN, intermediate nerve; SVN, superior vestibular nerve.

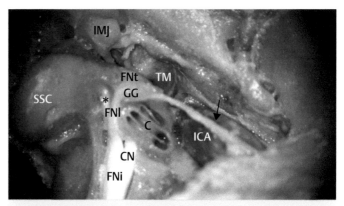

Fig. 6.6 Similar anatomical overview of ▶ Fig. 6.4. Left ear. *, superior vestibular nerve (cut), arrow; greater superficial petrosal nerve; C, cochlea; CN, cochlear neve; FN(i), internal auditory canal portion of the facial nerve; FN(l), labyrinthine segment of the facial nerve; FN(t), tympanic segment of the facial nerve; GG, geniculate ganglion; ICA, internal carotid artery; IMJ, incudomalleolar joint; SSC, superior semicircular canal; TM, tympanic membrane.

Fig. 6.7 (a) Skin incision; (b) craniotomy.

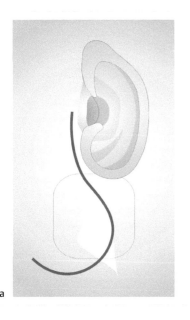

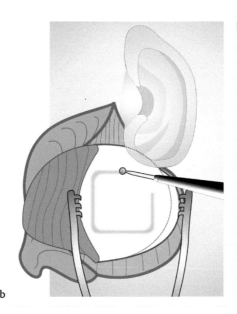

a

b

Left Ear

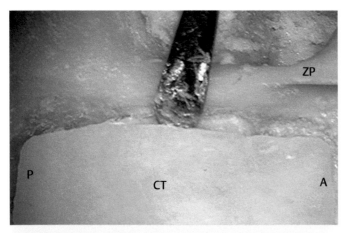

Fig. 6.8 After the craniotomy flap (CT) has been created in a left temporal bone, a septal raspatory is carefully used to separate the bony flap from the middle fossa dura. A, anterior; P, posterior; ZP, base of the zygomatic process.

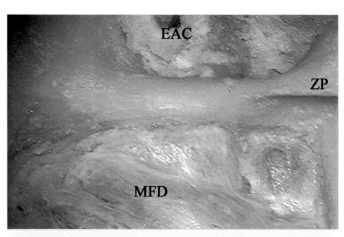

Fig. 6.9 The craniotomy is successfully elevated from the middle fossa dura (MFD). EAC, external auditory canal; ZP, base of the zygomatic process.

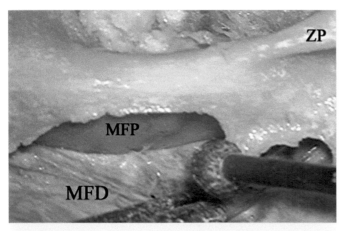

Fig. 6.10 The sharp bony edges are smoothed using a diamond burr while the middle fossa dura (MFD) is being retracted using the suction tube. MFP, middle fossa plate; ZP, base of the zygomatic process.

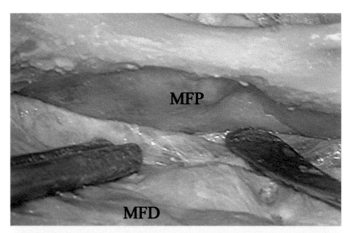

Fig. 6.11 Elevation of the middle fossa dura (MFD) from the middle fossa plate (MFP).

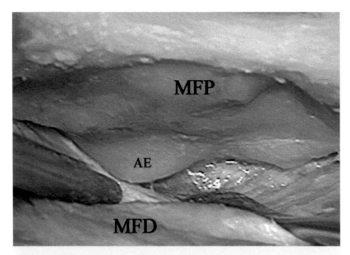

Fig. 6.12 The first landmark to be identified is the arcuate eminence (AE). MFD, middle fossa dura; MFP, middle fossa plate.

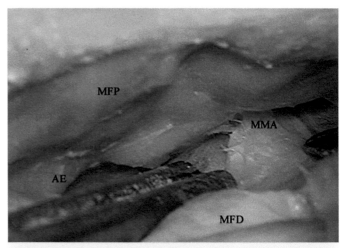

Fig. 6.13 As dural elevation advances anteriorly, the middle meningeal artery (MMA) is identified next. AE, arcuate eminence; MFD, middle fossa dura; MFP, middle fossa plate.

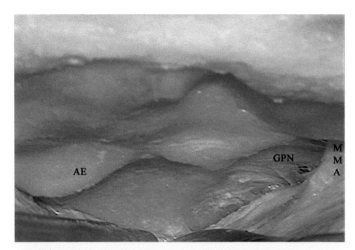

Fig. 6.14 The greater petrosal nerve (GPN) is identified next. AE, arcuate eminence; MMA, middle meningeal artery.

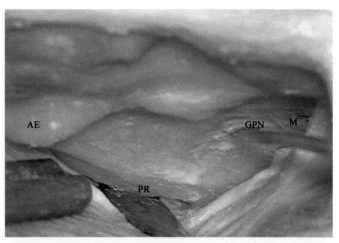

Fig. 6.15 The middle fossa retractor is fixed at the petrous ridge (PR). AE, arcuate eminence; GPN, greater petrosal nerve; M, middle meningeal artery.

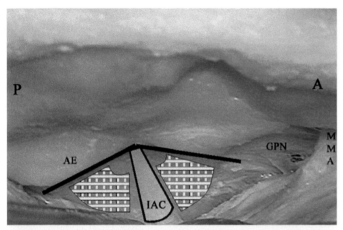

Fig. 6.16 The expected location of the internal auditory canal (IAC). The bar-shaded areas are the locations for drilling. A, anterior; AE, arcuate eminence; GPN, greater petrosal nerve; MMA, middle meningeal artery; P, posterior.

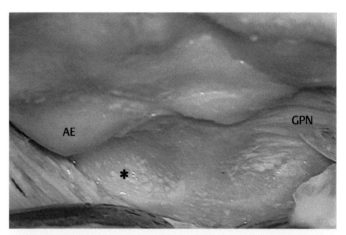

Fig. 6.17 Identification of the internal auditory canal is started by drilling between the arcuate eminence (AE) and the expected level of the internal auditory meatus (*) using a large burr. GPN, greater petrosal nerve.

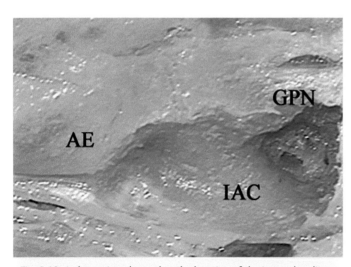

Fig. 6.18 A closer view shows that the location of the internal auditory canal (IAC) has been identified. AE, arcuate eminence; GPN, greater petrosal nerve.

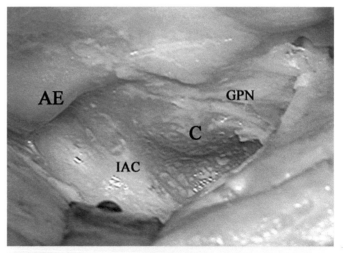

Fig. 6.19 The dura of the internal auditory canal (IAC) can be seen through the thin bone covering. The arcuate eminence (AE) and the cochlea (C) have been well skeletonized to gain the maximum space. GPN, greater petrosal nerve.

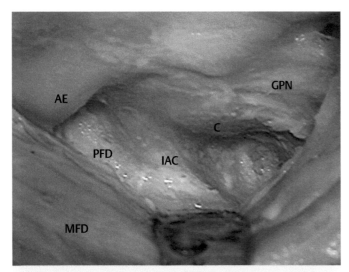

Fig. 6.20 Further drilling identifies the posterior fossa dura (PFD) under the thin bone covering. AE, arcuate eminence; C, cochlea, GPN, greater petrosal nerve; IAC, internal auditory canal; MFD, middle fossa dura.

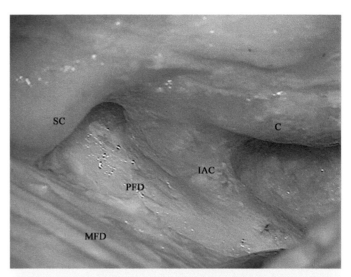

Fig. 6.21 The last shell of bone is to be dissected from the dura using a hook or a dissector. C, cochlea; IAC, internal auditory canal; MFD, middle fossa dura; PFD, posterior fossa dura; SC, superior semicircular canal.

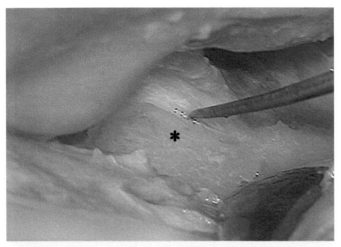

Fig. 6.22 The bony covering of the posterior fossa dura (*) is being removed.

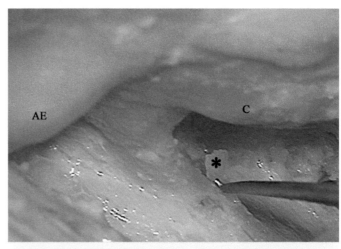

Fig. 6.23 The bony covering of the internal auditory canal and the posterior fossa dura anterior to the canal (*) is being removed. AE, arcuate eminence; C, cochlea.

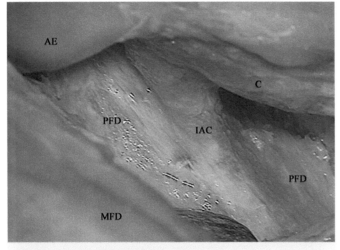

Fig. 6.24 The last bony shell has been removed. AE, arcuate eminence; C, cochlea; IAC, internal auditory canal; MFD, middle fossa dura; PFD, posterior fossa dura.

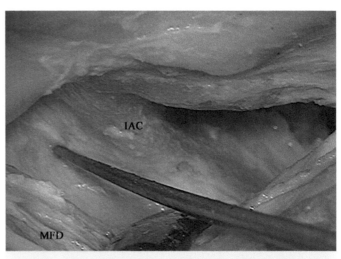

Fig. 6.25 A hook is used to create a hole in the posterior fossa dura. This step is useful in live surgery, to reduce intracranial pressure. IAC, internal auditory canal; MFD, middle fossa dura.

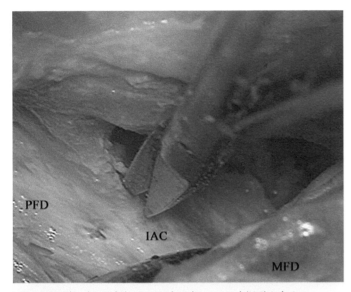

Fig. 6.26 The dura of the internal auditory canal (IAC) is being opened. MFD, middle fossa dura; PFD, posterior fossa dura.

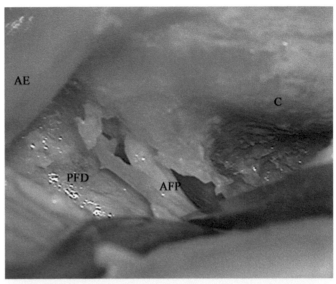

Fig. 6.27 The acousticofacial bundle (AFP) can be seen within the opened internal auditory canal. AE, arcuate eminence; C, cochlea; PFD, posterior fossa dura.

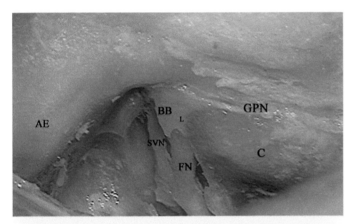

Fig. 6.28 The dura of the internal auditory canal has been further removed. Bill's bar (BB) can be seen at the level of the fundus. AE, arcuate eminence; C, cochlea; FN, facial nerve within the internal auditory canal; GPN, greater petrosal nerve; L, labyrinthine segment of the facial nerve; SVN, superior vestibular nerve.

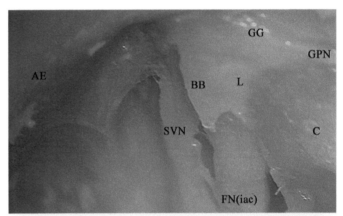

Fig. 6.29 The dura of the internal auditory canal has been further removed. Bill's bar (BB) can be seen at the level of the fundus. AE, arcuate eminence; C, cochlea; FN(iac), facial nerve within the internal auditory canal; GPN, greater petrosal nerve; L, labyrinthine segment of the facial nerve; SVN, superior vestibular nerve.

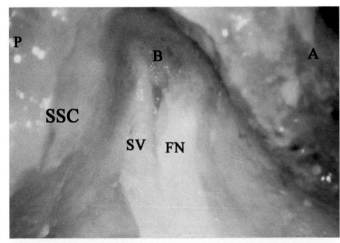

Fig. 6.30 A case of simple middle cranial fossa approach has been established, and the internal auditory canal dura has been opened. A, anterior; B, Bill's bar; FN, facial nerve; P, posterior; SSC, superior semicircular canal; SV, superior vestibular nerve.

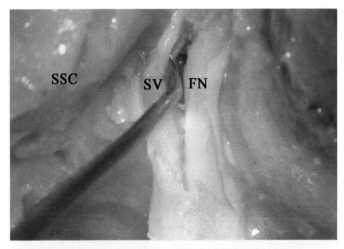

Fig. 6.31 A small hook is used carefully to dislodge the superior vestibular nerve (SV), which is usually free of tumor involvement. FN, facial nerve; SSC, superior semicircular canal.

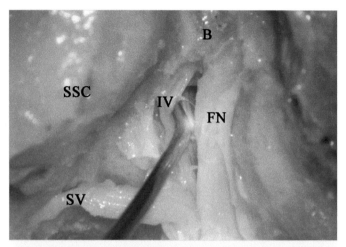

Fig. 6.32 The superior vestibular nerve (SV) has been dissected away, and the hook now is being used to dissect the inferior vestibular nerve (IV). B, Bill's bar; FN, facial nerve; SSC, superior semicircular canal.

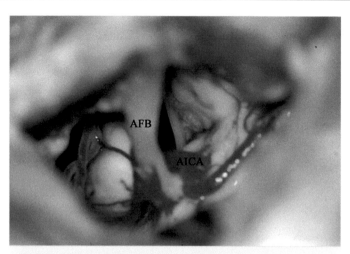

Fig. 6.33 This figure shows the intradural structures that can be seen using a simple middle cranial fossa approach. AFB, acousticofacial bundle; AICA, anterior inferior cerebellar artery.

Right Ear

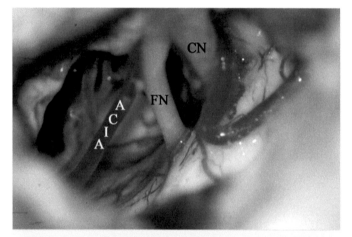

Fig. 6.34 The acousticofacial bundle components have been separated. Both the facial nerve (FN) and cochlear nerve (CN) can now be seen. AICA, anterior inferior cerebellar artery.

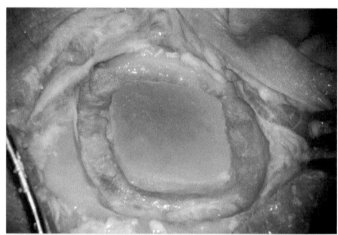

Fig. 6.35 The craniotomy flap has been created.

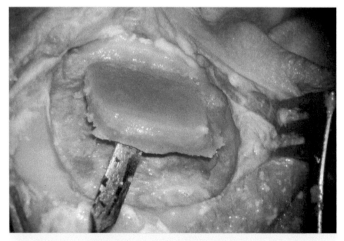

Fig. 6.36 The bony flap is separated from the dura using a raspatory.

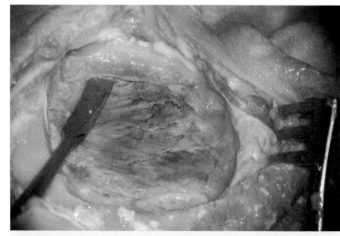

Fig. 6.37 The dura is gently detached from the base of the zygoma using a raspatory.

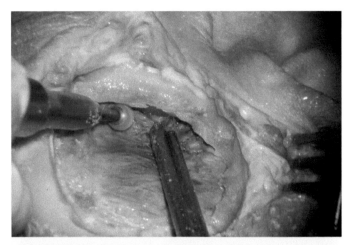

Fig. 6.38 The base of the zygoma is further drilled to keep the edge smoother. The dura is protected from the burr by gently depressing with the suction irrigator.

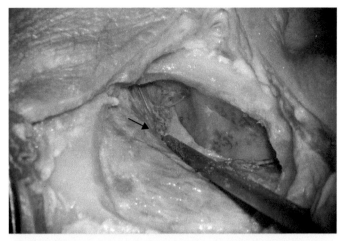

Fig. 6.39 Elevation of the dura from the superior surface of the temporal bone. Note the petrous venous plexus on the middle fossa dura (*arrow*).

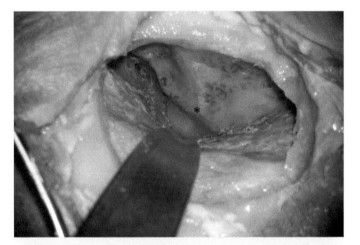

Fig. 6.40 The dura of the middle fossa has been elevated and kept in place with a retractor. The arcuate eminence is under view (*).

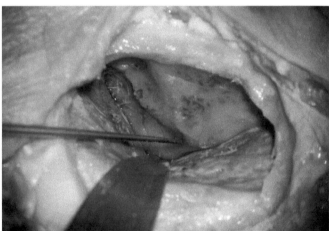

Fig. 6.41 Further retraction of the middle fossa dura to expose the assumed level of the internal auditory canal. The arcuate eminence is indicated with a hook.

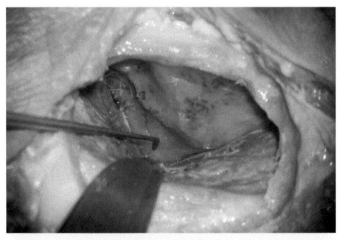

Fig. 6.42 The direction of the internal auditory canal is indicated with a hook.

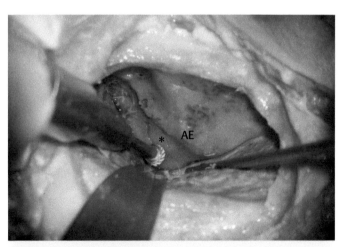

Fig. 6.43 Drill starts between the arcuate eminence (AE) and the expected level of the internal auditory meatus (*).

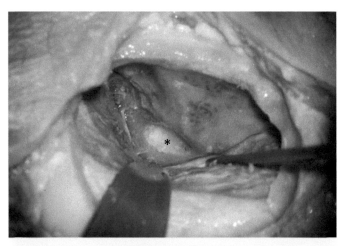

Fig. 6.44 The internal auditory canal (*) is starting to be seen.

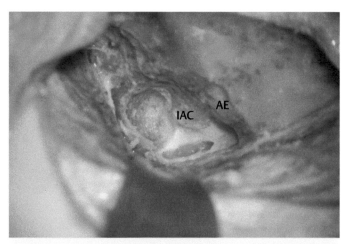

Fig. 6.45 Further drilling anterior and posterior to the internal auditory canal (IAC). AE, arcuate eminence.

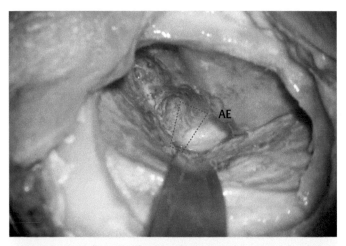

Fig. 6.46 At smaller magnification, the course of the internal auditory canal is under view (*red dashed line*). AE, arcuate eminence.

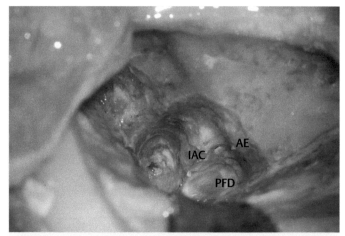

Fig. 6.47 Bigger magnification. The dura of the internal auditory canal (IAC) and posterior fossa (PFD) can be seen. AE, arcuate eminence.

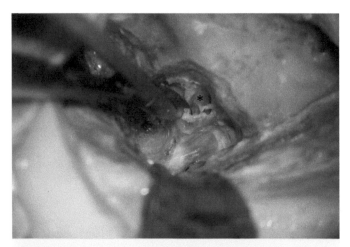

Fig. 6.48 The dura of the internal auditory canal is starting to be opened and the acousticofacial bundle (*) can be seen.

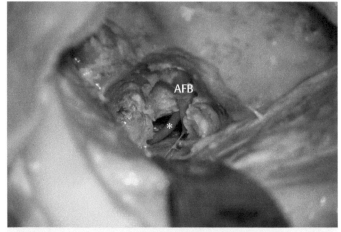

Fig. 6.49 The dura of the internal auditory canal has been completely opened. The acousticofacial bundle (AFB) can be seen with the anterior inferior cerebellar artery (AICA, *) behind.

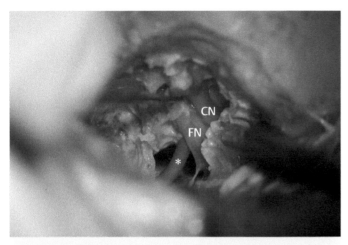

Fig. 6.50 At higher magnification, the facial nerve (FN) and cochlear nerve (CN) can be appreciated. The vestibular nerves have been resected. AICA, (*) forms a loop between the two nerves.

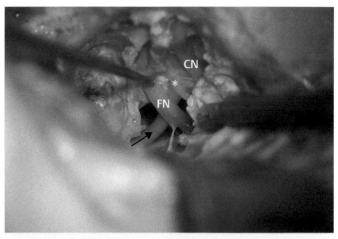

Fig. 6.51 The facial nerve is displaced anteriorly so the AICA loop (*arrow*) can be completely seen. *, intermediate nerve; CN, cochlear nerve; FN, facial nerve.

6.2 Middle Cranial Fossa Approach for Tumors of the Labyrinthine Segment of the Facial Nerve

6.2.1 Surgical Steps

See ▶ Fig. 6.52, ▶ Fig. 6.53, ▶ Fig. 6.54, ▶ Fig. 6.55 ▶ Fig. 6.55, ▶ Fig. 6.56, ▶ Fig. 6.57, ▶ Fig. 6.58, ▶ Fig. 6.59, ▶ Fig. 6.60, ▶ Fig. 6.61, ▶ Fig. 6.62, ▶ Fig. 6.63, ▶ Fig. 6.64, ▶ Fig. 6.65, ▶ Fig. 6.66, ▶ Fig. 6.67.

1. In contrast to vestibular schwannoma surgery, in which it is adequate for exposing the IAC, exposure for FN tumors should be extended distally to encompass the intralabyrinthine segment, GG, and the beginning of the tympanic segment of the FN. This level of exposure is essential for two reasons: firstly, to obtain adequate control of the extent of the tumor in order to achieve tumor-free margins, and secondly, to allow easy reconstruction of the FN after tumor excision.
2. The first structure to be identified is the GG, if not already dehiscent. To identify it, the greater superficial petrosal nerve is followed posteriorly to where it emerges from the bone. A large diamond drill is used to thin the bone in that area until the GG starts to show through the bone. Once the exact position of the GG has been identified, the drilling area is widened to encompass the whole of the GG, leaving a thin shell of bone overlying it.
3. The FN is now followed proximally toward the intralabyrinthine segment. The beginning of this segment is identified at the most medial part of the GG, where the anterior and posterior margins of the GG join to form an acute angle.

A diamond drill is used to remove the overlying bone. Extreme care should be taken while carrying out this step, since this segment is closely related to the cochlea, which lies anteriorly, and the superior semicircular canal, which lies posteriorly. When the fundus of the IAC is reached, Bill's bar can be identified separating the FN from the superior vestibular nerve.
4. In live surgery, further exposure of the proximal course of the FN, when indicated by the extent of the pathology, can be achieved using this approach by identifying and uncovering the IAC as described previously.
5. The next step is to identify the beginning of the tympanic segment of the FN. This step is started by drilling the roof of the middle ear, lying posterolateral to the GG. Drilling in this area should be carried out carefully in order not to touch the intact ossicular chain with the rotating burr.
6. Once the ossicular chain has been identified at the level of the incudomalleolar joint, drilling the roof of the middle ear can be safely continued posteriorly to identify the beginning of the horizontal segment of the FN.

6.2.2 Hints and Pitfalls

- This approach is used to resect a facial nerve tumor centered on the labyrinthine segment of the facial nerve. For reconstruction purposes, the facial nerve must be exposed both proximally and distally.
- Sometimes the facial nerve canal is found to be dehiscent due to tumor erosion. If additional drilling is needed, care should be taken not to injure the surrounding vital structures in altered anatomy of this type.
- Since hearing and the ossicular chain are both intact in these cases, extreme care should be taken to avoid touching the ossicular chain with the rotating burr while drilling the roof of the middle ear.

Left Ear

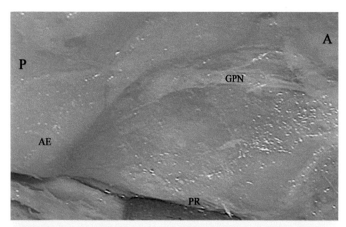

Fig. 6.52 The middle fossa dura of a left temporal bone has been elevated, the greater petrosal nerve (GPN) and the arcuate eminence (AE) identified, and the retractor fixed at the petrous ridge (PR). A, anterior; P, posterior.

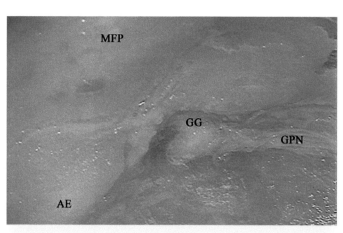

Fig. 6.53 Following the greater petrosal nerve (GPN) and drilling at its root identifies the geniculate ganglion (GG). AE, arcuate eminence; MFP, middle fossa plate.

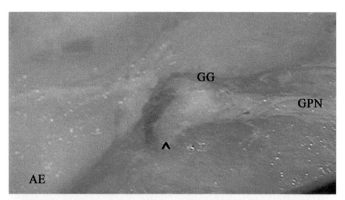

Fig. 6.54 The geniculate ganglion (GG) has been fully exposed, and the beginning of the labyrinthine segment of the facial nerve at the acute angle (^) can be seen. AE, arcuate eminence; GPN, greater petrosal nerve.

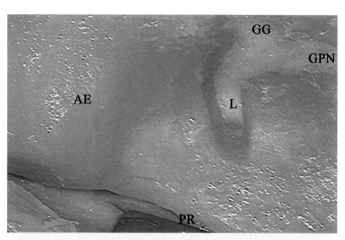

Fig. 6.55 The labyrinthine segment of the facial nerve (L) is followed to the internal auditory canal. AE, arcuate eminence; GG, geniculate ganglion; GPN, greater petrosal nerve; PR, petrous ridge.

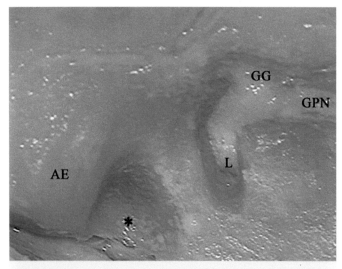

Fig. 6.56 The area (*) between the expected position of the internal auditory canal and the arcuate eminence (AE) is drilled using a large burr. GG, geniculate ganglion; GPN, greater petrosal nerve; L, labyrinthine segment of the facial nerve.

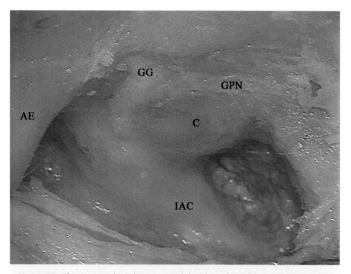

Fig. 6.57 The internal auditory canal (IAC) and cochlea (C) have been identified. AE, arcuate eminence; GG, geniculate ganglion; GPN, greater petrosal nerve.

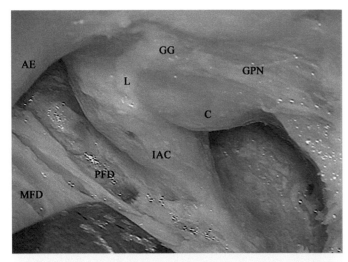

Fig. 6.58 The last shell of bone covering the posterior fossa dura (PFD) and the internal auditory canal (IAC). AE, arcuate eminence; C, cochlea; GG, geniculate ganglion; GPN, greater petrosal nerve; L, labyrinthine segment of the facial nerve; MFD, middle fossa dura.

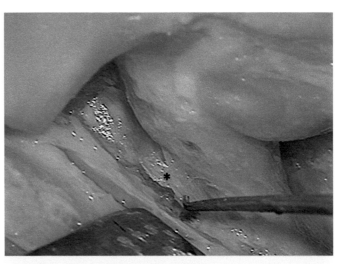

Fig. 6.59 Removal of the last bony shell (*).

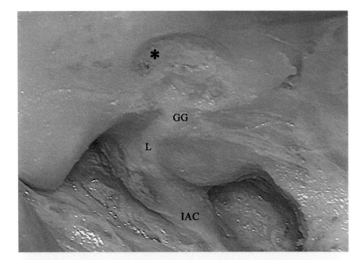

Fig. 6.60 Drilling is now shifted to the middle fossa plate (*), posterolateral to the geniculate ganglion (GG), to identify the head of the malleus and the tympanic segment of the facial nerve. IAC, internal auditory canal; L, labyrinthine segment of the facial nerve.

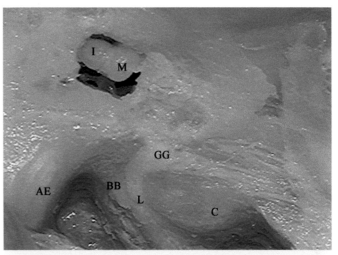

Fig. 6.61 The head of the malleus (M) and body of the incus (I) have been identified in the attic. AE, arcuate eminence; BB, Bill's bar; C, cochlea; GG, geniculate ganglion; L, labyrinthine segment of the facial nerve.

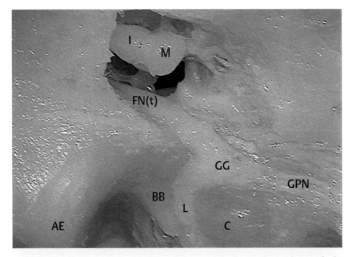

Fig. 6.62 After adequate drilling of the middle fossa plate (the roof of the middle ear), the tympanic segment of the facial nerve (FN[t]) has been identified. AE, arcuate eminence; BB, Bill's bar; C, cochlea; GG, geniculate ganglion; GPN, greater petrosal nerve; I, body of the incus; L, labyrinthine segment of the facial nerve; M, head of the malleus.

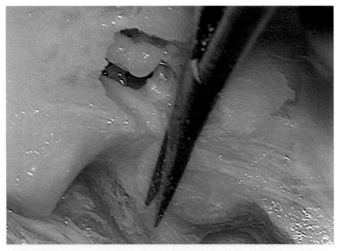

Fig. 6.63 The dura of the internal auditory canal is being opened.

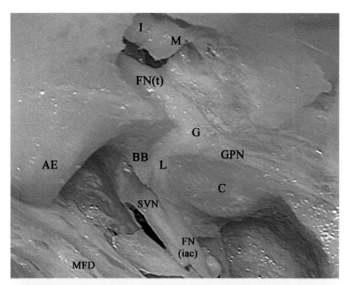

Fig. 6.64 The view after completion of the approach. AE, arcuate eminence; BB, Bill's bar; C, cochlea; FN(iac), internal auditory canal segment of the facial nerve; FN(t), tympanic segment of the facial nerve; G, geniculate ganglion; GPN, greater petrosal nerve; I, body of the incus; L, labyrinthine segment of the facial nerve; M, head of the malleus; MFD, middle fossa dura; SVN, superior vestibular nerve.

Right Ear

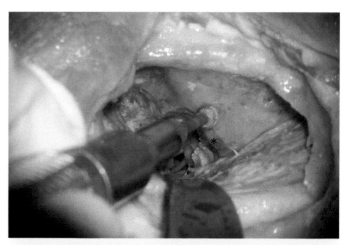

Fig. 6.65 Dissection continues from ▶ Fig. 6.51. In this case the greater superficial petrosal nerve is not under view. Drilling is shifted to the middle fossa plate, in an anterosuperior direction from the arcuate eminence (*).

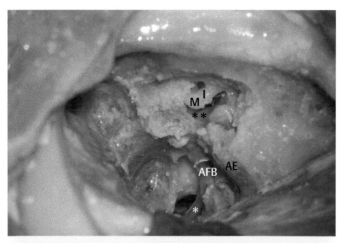

Fig. 6.66 The head of the malleus (M) and the body of the incus (I) have been identified in the attic. The second portion of the facial nerve is starting to be seen (**). The acousticofacial bundle (AFB) and the AICA (*) are exposed. AE, arcuate eminence.

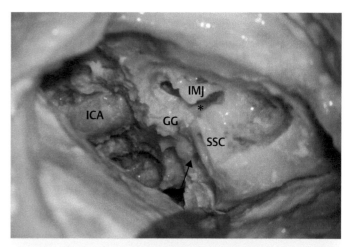

Fig. 6.67 The facial nerve has been further exposed from the internal auditory canal (*arrow*) to the geniculate ganglion (GG) and the tympanic portion (*). Superior semicircular canal (SSC) has been opened and the petrous apex drilled with exposure of the horizontal portion of the internal carotid artery (ICA). IMJ, incudomalleolar joint.

6.3 Combined Middle Cranial Fossa Transpetrous Approach

6.3.1 Indications

- Small petroclival tumors anterior to the IAC, when hearing preservation is planned.
- Small and moderate-sized tumors of the superior CPA, when hearing preservation is planned.

6.3.2 Surgical Steps

See ▶ Fig. 6.75, ▶ Fig. 6.76, ▶ Fig. 6.77, ▶ Fig. 6.78, ▶ Fig. 6.79, ▶ Fig. 6.80, ▶ Fig. 6.81, ▶ Fig. 6.82, ▶ Fig. 6.83, ▶ Fig. 6.84, ▶ Fig. 6.85, ▶ Fig. 6.86, ▶ Fig. 6.87, ▶ Fig. 6.88, ▶ Fig. 6.89, ▶ Fig. 6.90, ▶ Fig. 6.91, ▶ Fig. 6.92, ▶ Fig. 6.93, ▶ Fig. 6.94, ▶ Fig. 6.95, ▶ Fig. 6.96, ▶ Fig. 6.97, ▶ Fig. 6.98, ▶ Fig. 6.99, ▶ Fig. 6.100, ▶ Fig. 6.101, ▶ Fig. 6.102, ▶ Fig. 6.103, ▶ Fig. 6.104, ▶ Fig. 6.105, ▶ Fig. 6.106.

1. The craniotomy used for this approach is wider anteroposteriorly than that used for the simple MCF approach, to provide adequate control of the petrous apex.
2. Dural elevation proceeds in the same manner as in the simple MCF approach. The only difference is that the middle meningeal artery is coagulated and transected to provide adequate control over the petrous apex.
3. Identification of the internal auditory canal is achieved as previously described.

4. After the internal auditory canal has been completely skeletonized, the mandibular division of the trigeminal nerve is identified. To allow the drilling of the petrous apex to proceed anteriorly, the mandibular nerve should either be retracted anteriorly or transected, depending on the availability of space.
5. Drilling now proceeds carefully to identify and skeletonize the horizontal segment of the ICA. If the cavernous sinus is to be reached, then the mandibular nerve has to be sacrificed to obtain the required access.
6. Drilling should include the whole petrous apex, reaching to the clivus area.

6.3.3 Hints and Pitfalls

- Although this approach provides additional exposure of the petroclival area, the working area is narrow in comparison with the transcochlear approach, and the use of this approach should therefore be limited to selected cases.
- To achieve the additional anterior exposure, the middle meningeal artery and sometimes the mandibular division of the trigeminal nerve have to be sacrificed.
- Extreme care must be taken when drilling in the region of the internal carotid artery. Only diamond burrs moved parallel to the artery should be used.
- Bleeding encountered from the inferior petrosal sinus and from the clivus bone can be stopped using a diamond burr.
- The dura of the clivus is opened only after adequate drilling of the clivus bone. Care should be taken while opening the dura not to injure the abducent nerve as it passes through Dorello's canal.

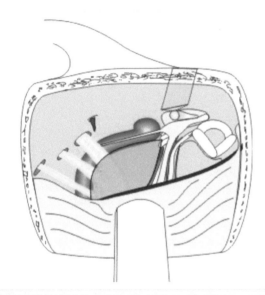

Fig. 6.68 An illustration of a right middle cranial fossa. The gray color represents the amount of petrous apex bone removal required to achieve a middle cranial fossa transpetrous approach.

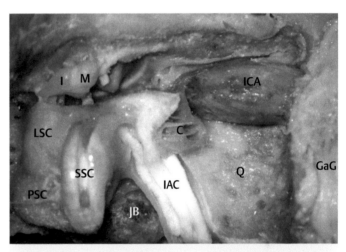

Fig. 6.69 Left ear. Middle cranial fossa transpetrous approach. The petrous apex is divided surgically into a posterior rhomboidal area and an anterior triangular area. The posterior rhomboid (Q) is bounded by the internal auditory canal (IAC) posteromedially, the cochlea (C) posterolaterally, the internal carotid artery (ICA) laterally, and the posterior border of the gasserian ganglion (GaG) anteriorly. The superior semicircular canal (SSC) and the cochlea have been opened. The greater superficial petrosal nerve and middle meningeal artery have been cut. I, incus; JB, jugular bulb; LSC, lateral semicircular canal; M, malleus; PSC, posterior semicircular canal.

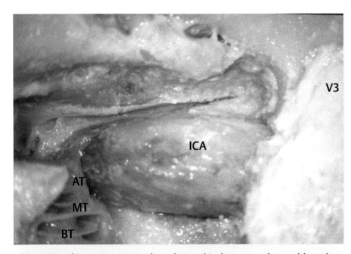

Fig. 6.70 Closer view. Note the relationship between the cochlea, the internal carotid artery (ICA), and the third division of the trigeminal nerve (V3). AT, apical turn of the cochlea; BT, basal turn of the cochlea; MT, middle turn of the cochlea.

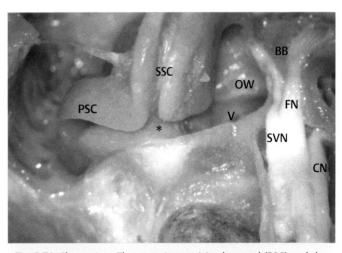

Fig. 6.71 Closer view. The posterior semicircular canal (PSC) and the vestibule (V) have been opened. *, common crus; BB, Bill's bar; CN, cochlear nerve; FN, facial nerve; JB, jugular bulb; OW, oval window (medial view); SVN, superior vestibular nerve.

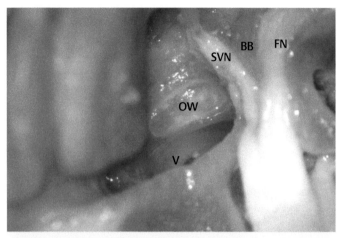

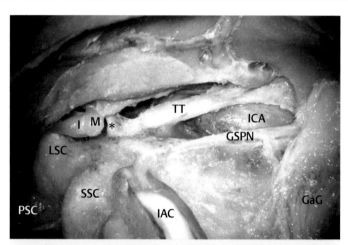

Fig. 6.72 Closer view inside the vestibule. BB, Bill's bar; FN, facial nerve; OW, oval window; V, vestibule.

Fig. 6.73 Another example of middle fossa transpetrous approach. Left ear. *, tensor tympani tendon; GaG, gasserian ganglion; GSPN, greater superficial petrosal nerve; I, incus; IAC, internal auditory canal; ICA, internal carotid artery; LSC, lateral semicircular canal; M, malleus; PSC, posterior semicircular canal; SSC, superior semicircular canal; TT, tensor tympani muscle.

Right Ear

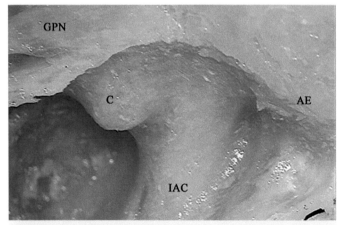

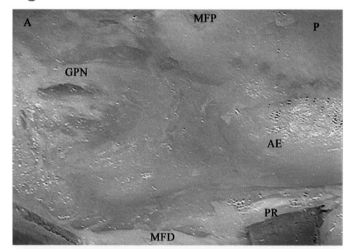

Fig. 6.74 Closer view. *, tensor tympani tendon; FN(l), labyrinthine portion of the facial nerve; FM(t), tympanic portion of the facial nerve; GG, geniculate ganglion; GSPN, greater superficial petrosal nerve; I, incus; LSC, lateral semicircular canal; M, malleus; PSC, posterior semicircular canal; SSC, superior semicircular canal; SVN, superior vestibular nerve; TT, tensor tympani muscle.

Fig. 6.75 The middle fossa dura (MFD) of a right temporal bone has been elevated from the middle fossa plate (MFP). Since wider exposure is needed in this case, the middle meningeal artery has been transected. A, anterior; AE, arcuate eminence; GPN, greater petrosal nerve; P, posterior; PR, petrous ridge.

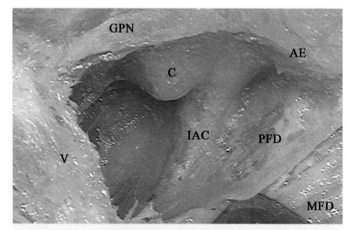

Fig. 6.76 The internal auditory canal (IAC) and cochlea (C) have been identified. Note that bone removal anterior to the canal is wider than in the simple middle fossa approach. AE, arcuate eminence; GPN, greater petrosal nerve.

Fig. 6.77 The last shell of bone covering the dura is to be dissected using a hook or a dissector. AE, arcuate eminence; C, cochlea; GPN, greater petrosal nerve; IAC, internal auditory canal; MFD, middle fossa dura; PFD, posterior fossa dura; V, trigeminal nerve.

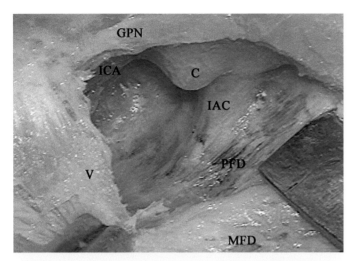

Fig. 6.78 The last bony shell has been removed. C, cochlea; GPN, greater petrosal nerve; IAC, internal auditory canal; ICA, internal carotid artery; MFD, middle fossa dura; PFD, posterior fossa dura; V, trigeminal nerve.

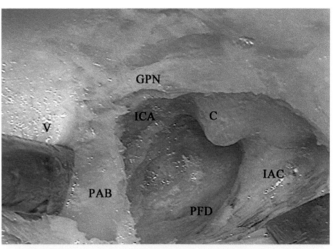

Fig. 6.79 The trigeminal nerve (V) is retracted in order to drill the petrous apex bone (PAB) lying underneath it. C, cochlea; GPN, greater petrosal nerve; IAC, internal auditory canal; ICA, internal carotid artery; PFD, posterior fossa dura.

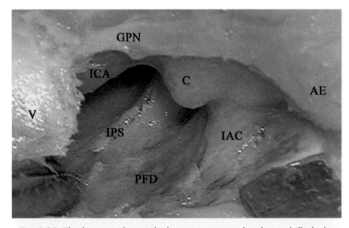

Fig. 6.80 The bone underneath the petrous apex has been drilled, the inferior petrosal sinus (IPS) has been identified, and the internal carotid artery (ICA) is better skeletonized. Note that the extent of bone removal at the petrous apex level is not yet sufficient to expose all the horizontal segment of the internal carotid artery. AE, arcuate eminence; C, cochlea; GPN, greater petrosal nerve; IAC, internal auditory canal; PFD, posterior fossa dura; V, trigeminal nerve.

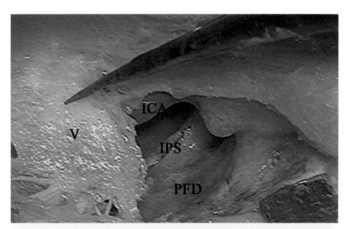

Fig. 6.81 To obtain access to the horizontal segment of the internal carotid artery (ICA), the mandibular branch of the trigeminal nerve (V) is being cut. IPS, inferior petrosal sinus; PFD, posterior fossa dura.

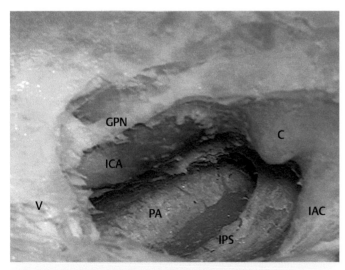

Fig. 6.82 The horizontal segment of the internal carotid artery (ICA) is better skeletonized, and the drilling is extended to the petrous apex (PA). C, cochlea; GPN, greater petrosal nerve; IAC, internal auditory canal; IPS, inferior petrosal sinus; V, trigeminal nerve.

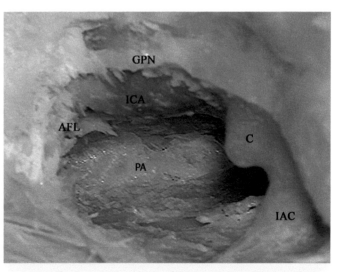

Fig. 6.83 The horizontal segment of the internal carotid artery (ICA) has been skeletonized up to the anterior foramen lacerum (AFL) and the petrous apex (PA) has been fully drilled. C, cochlea; GPN, greater petrosal nerve; IAC, internal auditory canal.

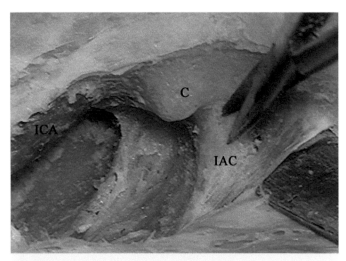

Fig. 6.84 The dura of the internal auditory canal (IAC) is being opened. C, cochlea; ICA, internal carotid artery.

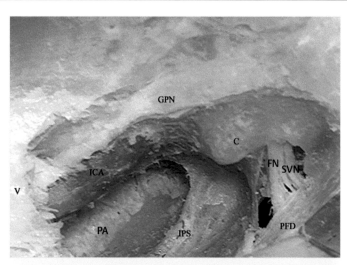

Fig. 6.85 The view after the completion of the approach. C, cochlea; FN, facial nerve; GPN, greater petrosal nerve; ICA, internal carotid artery; IPS, inferior petrosal sinus; PA, petrous apex; PFD, posterior fossa dura; SVN, superior vestibular nerve; V, trigeminal nerve.

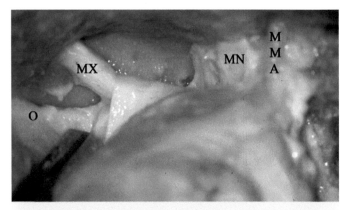

Fig. 6.86 To provide a clearer picture of the approach, the last part of the approach is shown here in a right-sided cadaveric dissection. Seen here are the middle meningeal artery (MMA) and the mandibular (MN), maxillary (MX), and ophthalmic (O) divisions of the trigeminal nerve as these enter their foramina.

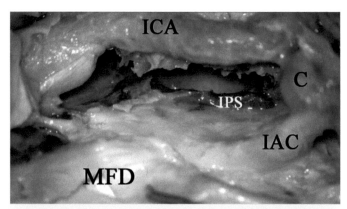

Fig. 6.87 The required bone drilling as described above has been carried out. C, cochlea; IAC, internal auditory canal; ICA, internal carotid artery; IPS, inferior petrosal sinus; MFD, middle fossa dura.

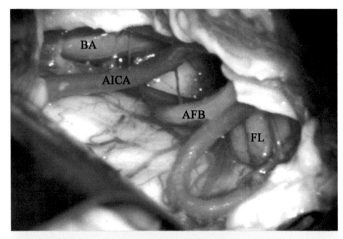

Fig. 6.88 The dura has been opened, and the cerebellopontine angle can be seen. AFB, acousticofacial bundle; AICA, anterior inferior cerebellar artery; BA, basilar artery; FL, flocculus.

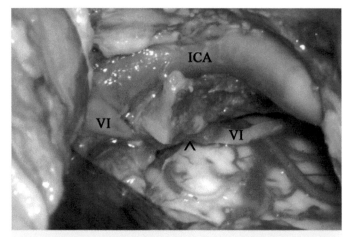

Fig. 6.89 Examining the anterior part of the approach, the abducens nerve (VI) can be seen entering Dorello's canal (^), and the internal carotid artery (ICA) can be seen entering the anterior foramen lacerum, passing to the cavernous sinus.

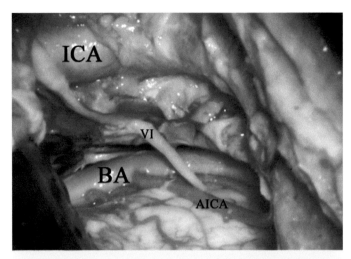

Fig. 6.90 The last piece of bone has been drilled away, and the approach is completed. Seen here is the prepontine cistern, which is the main target for which this approach is performed. AICA, anterior inferior cerebellar artery; BA, basilar artery; ICA, internal carotid artery; VI, abducens nerve.

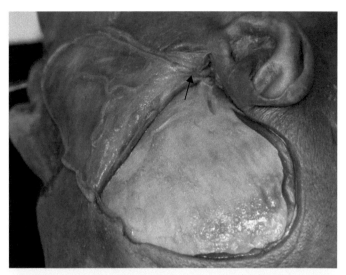

Fig. 6.91 Right ear. Another example of middle cranial fossa transpetrous approach with orbitozygomatic extension. Incision is similar to ▶ Fig. 6.7 with further anterior extension. The superficial temporal artery and vein are under view (*arrow*).

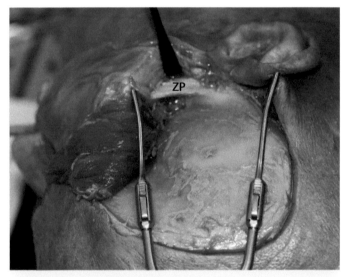

Fig. 6.92 The musculoperiosteal flap has been created and displaced anteriorly. ZP, zygomatic process.

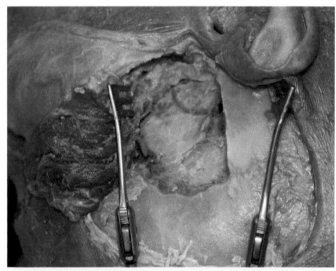

Fig. 6.93 The craniotomy flap with the zygomatic process has been removed. The dura of the temporal lobe is exposed.

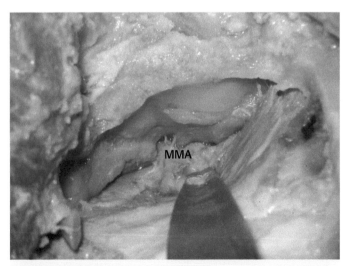

Fig. 6.94 The middle fossa dura is elevated with exposure of the middle meningeal artery (MMA) which goes through the foramen spinosum.

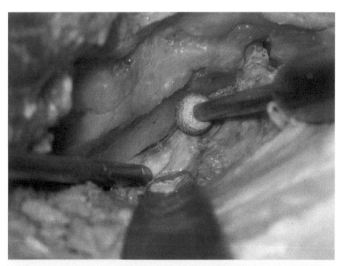

Fig. 6.95 The bone is drilled corresponding to the area of the foramen ovalis to show the third division of the trigeminal nerve (mandibular nerve, V3).

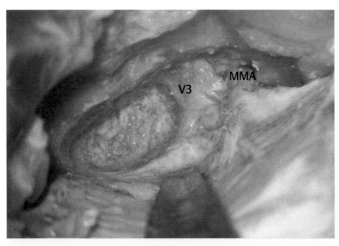

Fig. 6.96 The third division of the trigeminal nerve (V3) in under view. MMA, middle meningeal artery.

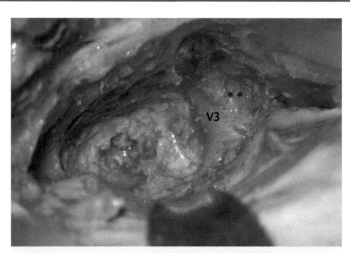

Fig. 6.97 Closer view. The third division of the trigeminal nerve (V3) and the accessory meningeal artery (**) are exposed. The bone anterior to V3 is further drilled to show the second division of the trigeminal nerve (maxillary nerve, V2).

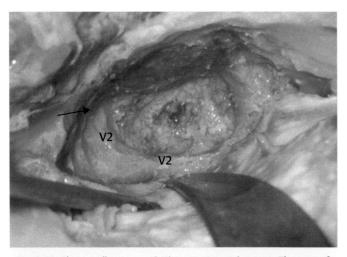

Fig. 6.98 The maxillary nerve (V2) is starting to be seen. The area of the foramen rotundum is marked with an arrow.

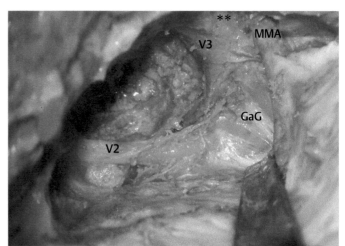

Fig. 6.99 Closer view. V3, V2, accessory meningeal artery (**), the gasserian ganglion (GaG), and the middle meningeal artery (MMA) are shown.

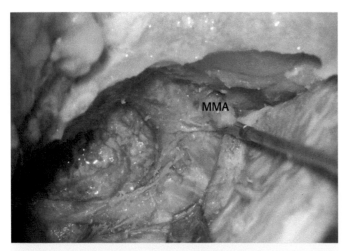

Fig. 6.100 The middle meningeal artery (MMA) is cut.

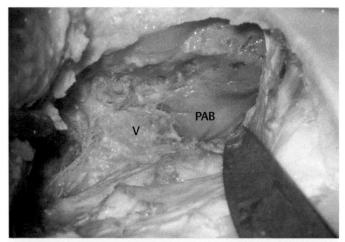

Fig. 6.101 The middle meningeal artery has been cut and the trigeminal nerve (V) displaced anteriorly, exposing the petrous apex bone (PAB).

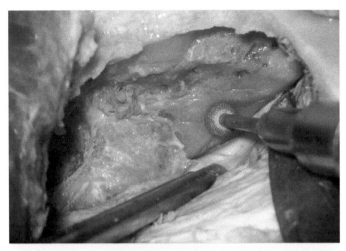

Fig. 6.102 The petrous apex bone is drilled to expose the horizontal portion of the internal carotid artery. In about 15% of cases this portion of the artery is uncovered from bone.

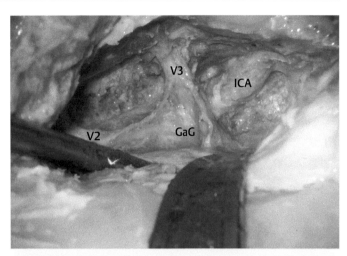

Fig. 6.103 After removal of the petrous apex bone, the horizontal portion of the internal carotid artery (ICA) can be seen under the mandibular branch of the trigeminal nerve (V3). GaG, gasserian ganglion; V2, maxillary nerve.

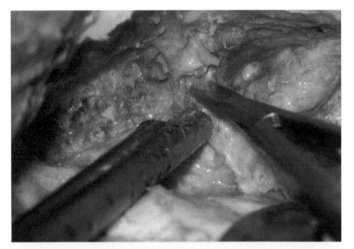

Fig. 6.104 V3 and gasserian ganglion are cut to expose the anterior foramen lacerum and precavernous portion of the internal carotid artery.

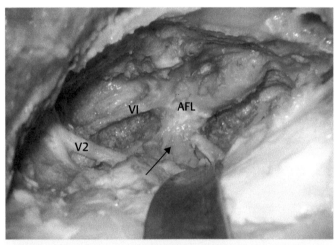

Fig. 6.105 The anterior foramen lacerum (AFL) and the precavernous portion of the internal carotid artery (*arrow*) are shown. The abducens nerve (sixth cranial nerve, VI) crosses the carotid laterally on its precavernous portion. Through the Dorello's canal the nerve merges with the cavernous sinus. It then enters the orbit through the superior orbital fissure with the first division of the trigeminal nerve (ophthalmic nerve, V1). V2, maxillary nerve.

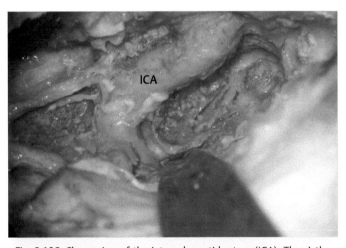

Fig. 6.106 Closer view of the internal carotid artery (ICA). The sixth cranial nerve has been cut.

6.4 Combined Transmastoid Middle Cranial Fossa Approach

6.4.1 Indications

The aim of this approach is to achieve adequate exposure of the full length of the intratemporal facial nerve without compromising preoperatively preserved hearing.

- Facial nerve tumors centered on the geniculate ganglion and extending both proximally and distally.
- Exploration of the facial nerve after a temporal bone fracture.

6.4.2 Surgical Steps

See ► Fig. 6.107, ► Fig. 6.108, ► Fig. 6.109, ► Fig. 6.110, ► Fig. 6.111, ► Fig. 6.112, ► Fig. 6.113, ► Fig. 6.114, ► Fig. 6.115, ► Fig. 6.116, ► Fig. 6.117, ► Fig. 6.118, ► Fig. 6.119, ► Fig. 6.120.

1. The mastoid cavity is prepared in the same manner as in the closed tympanoplasty approach. The only difference here is that extra care is taken to maintain the integrity of the middle fossa dural plate. For this reason, the plate is not thinned too much here.

2. The same craniotomy as that used in the MCF is carried out here. In this approach, evaluating the lower limit is easier than in the regular MCF approach, as the level of the MCF plate can be actively visualized after the mastoidectomy. It is important to ensure that the lateral edge of the middle fossa plate contains no ridges or bony overhangs from either side, to allow simultaneous visualization of structures on both sides of the plate.

3. Once the dura has been elevated and the middle fossa retractor applied, a connection between the two approaches is established by drilling a small hole at the middle fossa plate at the level of the head of the malleus. This connection, in addition to facilitating surgical manipulation of the perigeniculate portion of the facial nerve, also provides a valuable guide to the position of the geniculate ganglion, since it can be seen in the attic.

4. The subsequent steps are the same as those described in the MCF approach for facial nerve tumors.

6.4.3 Hints and Pitfalls

- The middle fossa plate will form the barrier between the intracranial cavity and the mastoid cavity created in this approach. The utmost care should be taken to preserve its integrity, to avoid CSF leakage and meningoencephalic herniation.
- If difficulties are encountered in identifying the geniculate ganglion, the level of the head of the malleus as seen from the atticotomy can be a useful guide for the location of the ganglion.
- At the end of the procedure, cartilage and fibrin glue are used to reconstruct the defect created in the middle fossa plate.

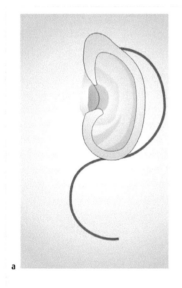
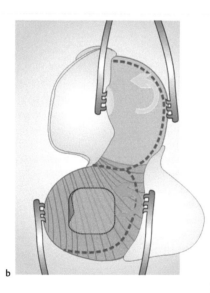

Fig. 6.107 **(a)** S-shape skin incision. **(b)** Elevation of the skin and muscular flaps. **(c)** A schematic view of the combined transmastoid–middle cranial fossa approach.

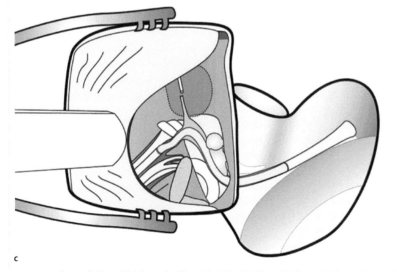

c

Left Ear

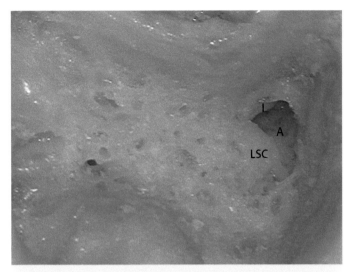

Fig. 6.108 The lateral semicircular canal (LSC) and the short process of the incus (I) have been identified within the mastoid antrum (A) of a left temporal bone.

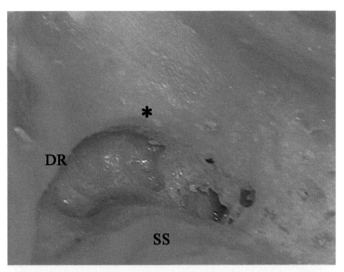

Fig. 6.109 The digastric ridge (DR) can be seen, pointing toward the facial nerve at the level of the stylomastoid foramen (*). SS, sigmoid sinus.

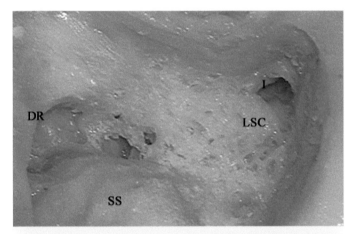

Fig. 6.110 The mastoid segment of the facial nerve, extending from between the lateral semicircular canal (LSC) and short process of the incus (I) to the anterior edge of the digastric ridge (DR), is to be skeletonized. SS, sigmoid sinus.

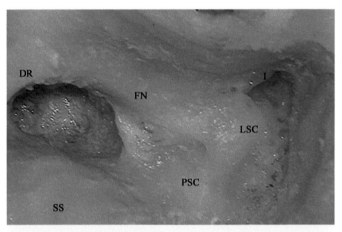

Fig. 6.111 The mastoid segment of the facial nerve (FN) has been identified. DR, digastric ridge; I, short process of the incus; LSC, lateral semicircular canal; PSC, posterior semicircular canal; SS, sigmoid sinus.

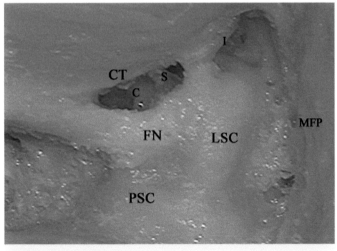

Fig. 6.112 A posterior tympanotomy has been carried out. C, cochlea; CT, chorda tympani; FN, facial nerve; I, short process of the incus; LSC, lateral semicircular canal; MFP, middle fossa plate; PSC, posterior semicircular canal; S, stapes.

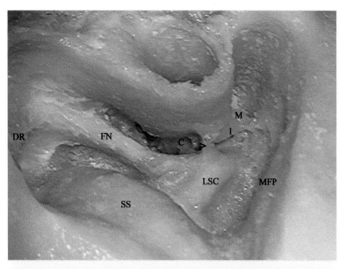

Fig. 6.113 The posterior tympanotomy has been extended toward the hypotympanum and an atticotomy has been carried out. The last strut of bone (>) left to protect the incus from the drill should be removed using a curette. C, cochlea; DR, digastric ridge; FN, facial nerve; I, incus; LSC, lateral semicircular canal; M, malleus; MFP, middle fossa plate; SS, sigmoid sinus.

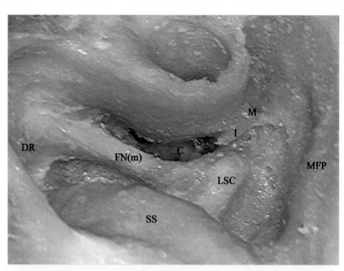

Fig. 6.114 After the removal of the last strut of bone, the tympanic segment of the facial nerve (*) can be seen. C, cochlea; DR, digastric ridge; FN(m), mastoid segment of the facial nerve; I, incus; LSC, lateral semicircular canal; M, malleus; MFP, middle fossa plate; S, stapes; SS, sigmoid sinus.

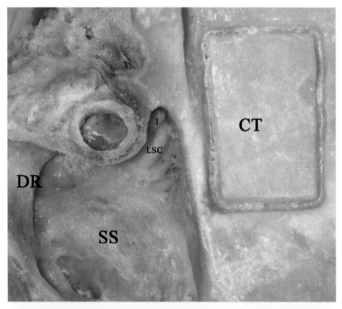

Fig. 6.115 Attention is now shifted to the middle cranial fossa component of the approach. The craniotomy (CT) is created. Note that the middle fossa plate is less beveled than in a regular closed tympanoplasty. DR, digastric ridge; I, incus; LSC, lateral semicircular canal; SS, sigmoid sinus.

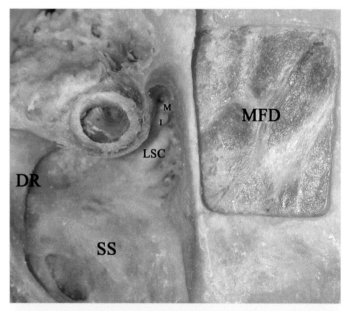

Fig. 6.116 The craniotomy bone has been separated from the middle fossa dura (MFD). DR, digastric ridge; I, incus; LSC, lateral semicircular canal; M, malleus; SS, sigmoid sinus.

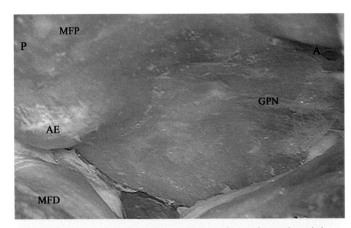

Fig. 6.117 The middle fossa dura (MFD) has been elevated, and the greater petrosal nerve (GPN) and the arcuate eminence (AE) have been identified. A, anterior; MFP, middle fossa plate; P, posterior.

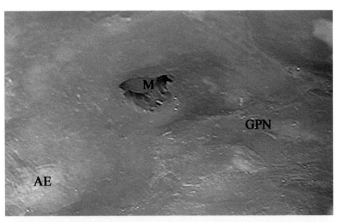

Fig. 6.118 The middle fossa plate has been drilled over the location of the malleus head (M), as judged from the middle ear. AE, arcuate eminence; GPN, greater petrosal nerve.

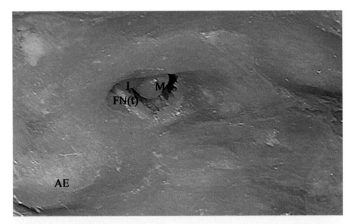

Fig. 6.119 Further removal of the middle fossa plate exposes the tympanic segment of the facial nerve (FN[t]). AE, arcuate eminence; I, incus; M, malleus.

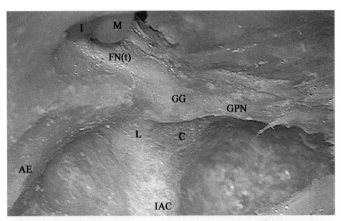

Fig. 6.120 The full course of the facial nerve has now been identified. Further steps depend on the extent of the pathology being treated. AE, arcuate eminence; C, cochlea; FN(t), tympanic segment of the facial nerve; GG, geniculate ganglion; GPN, greater petrosal nerve; I, incus; IAC, internal auditory canal; L, labyrinthine segment of the facial nerve; M, malleus.

7 Retrosigmoid–Retrolabyrinthine Approach

Abstract

The retrosigmoid approach is a technical modification of the suboccipital approach to the cerebellopontine angle. This approach carries the craniotomy more anterolaterally, to lie just posterior to the sigmoid sinus. This approach provides access to the cerebellopontine angle without sacrificing the labyrinth.

Keywords: retrosigmoid–retrolabyrinthine approach, hearing preservation

7.1 Indications

- Hearing preservation surgery for small vestibular schwannomas (< 2 cm) with absence of involvement of the fundus of the internal auditory canal.
- Hearing preservation surgery for other cerebellopontine angle tumors in which the major part of the tumor is located posterior to the internal auditory canal.

7.2 Surgical Steps

See ▶ Fig. 7.1, ▶ Fig. 7.2, ▶ Fig. 7.3, ▶ Fig. 7.4, ▶ Fig. 7.5, ▶ Fig. 7.6, ▶ Fig. 7.7, ▶ Fig. 7.8, ▶ Fig. 7.9, ▶ Fig. 7.10, ▶ Fig. 7.11, ▶ Fig. 7.12, ▶ Fig. 7.13, ▶ Fig. 7.14, ▶ Fig. 7.15, ▶ Fig. 7.16, ▶ Fig. 7.17, ▶ Fig. 7.18, ▶ Fig. 7.19, ▶ Fig. 7.20, ▶ Fig. 7.21, ▶ Fig. 7.22, ▶ Fig. 7.23, ▶ Fig. 7.24, ▶ Fig. 7.25, ▶ Fig. 7.26, ▶ Fig. 7.27, ▶ Fig. 7.28, ▶ Fig. 7.29.

1. The supine position is used. A retroauricular skin incision is performed as shown.

2. A U-shaped, inferiorly based musculoperiosteal flap is elevated.

3. An extended mastoidectomy is carried out. The bone covering the middle fossa dura is removed for a distance of 1 to 2 cm. In contrast to the translabyrinthine approach, the bony covering of the posterior fossa dura is removed here up to the posterior edge of the sigmoid sinus only; removal is not extended posteriorly beyond this level. The mastoid emissary vein is skeletonized and closed.

4. All the air cells in the mastoid cavity should be removed and the semicircular canals identified. In cases of extensive pneumatization, as many perilabyrinthine air cells as possible should be drilled out. Any remaining air cells in the region should be occluded using bone wax. This step is extremely important for avoiding postoperative cerebrospinal fluid (CSF) leakage in live surgery.

5. Since the aim of this operation is to preserve hearing, the utmost care must be taken when carrying out the retrolabyrinthine part of the approach. Drilling must always be parallel to the semicircular canal being identified, and the overlying bone should not be overthinned in order not to risk opening the labyrinth.

6. A 5 × 5 cm craniotomy is carried out using a diamond burr. The sigmoid sinus is followed to the transverse sinus, and the craniotomy should be located posterior to the sigmoid sinus and inferior to the transverse sinus.

7. The bone flap is separated from the underlying dura using a septal dissector. The lower edge of the craniotomy is trimmed using a rongeur. The sigmoid sinus is also uncovered. The bone flap is then removed and placed in a saline solution.

8. The dura is held using a toothed forceps, and a small incision is made. In live surgery, Merocel is inserted between the dura and the cerebellum in the lines of the incision, to provide protection for the cerebellum.

9. Once the dura has been opened, the dural flaps are retracted using stay sutures.

10. In live surgery, the cerebellum lies just underneath the dura, narrowing the approach. Gentle retraction of the cerebellum allows space for identifying the cistern. Opening of the arachnoid of the cistern should be carried out carefully, parallel to the direction of the lower cranial nerves and above the level of the glossopharyngeal nerve. This step results in the escape of the CSF and therefore shrinkage of the cerebellum, providing the necessary space for tumor removal.

11. An inverted U-shaped dural flap is outlined on the posterior surface of the petrous bone. The long limbs lie a few millimeters inferior and superior to the internal auditory canal porus. The dura is incised using a sharp dissector or a Beaver knife. The dural flap is elevated from the underlying bone to the level of the porus. The flap can then be excised.

12. In live surgery, Gelfoam is inserted far anteriorly into the cerebellopontine angle and around the porus of the internal auditory canal, to prevent bone dust from falling into the cisterns.

13. Using a diamond burr, drilling of the posterior wall of the internal auditory canal now begins, starting from the porus and moving laterally.

14. Drilling continues until the common crus is blue-lined. The superior and posterior semicircular canals are also blue-lined just before they join into the common crus. This is the most lateral limit of drilling. If there is any doubt, examining the retrolabyrinthine part of the approach provides an adequate idea of the position of the canals.

15. The posterior wall of the internal auditory canal (as far as the blue-lined common crus) is now completely drilled. The internal auditory canal dura is opened next.

16. In live surgery, the tumor inside the internal auditory canal is removed from medial to lateral. If there is still residual tumor in the fundus area, angled instruments are used to remove it. At the end, an endoscope is used to ascertain that no residual tumor has been left behind.

17. If the tumor extends more laterally into the internal auditory canal, beyond the limit of visual control, then tumor removal can be carried out using one of the following methods:

    - Exposing the fundus at the superior aspect of the internal auditory canal. To achieve this additional exposure, the dura overlying the petrous ridge and the superior surface of the petrous bone should be carefully elevated. Drilling is then shifted to the anterosuperior aspect of the internal auditory canal. The superior semicircular canal is then skeletonized. Following the anterior surface of the superior semicircular canal will lead to the fundus. The problem with this extension is the fact that the additional exposure of the fundus is very narrow and the procedure itself caries a risk of opening the labyrinth, resulting in hearing loss.

- Labyrinth drill-out. This is only applicable in cases of doubt. However, it is the surest way of eliminating the risk of residual tumor.
18. After tumor removal from the internal auditory canal, fibrin glue and a free muscle graft are used to close the internal auditory canal, while bone wax is used to close all the open air cells to avoid postoperative CSF leakage.
19. Watertight closure of the dura should be attempted, to reduce the risk of postoperative CSF leakage. If a small dural defect is noticed, a piece of muscle can be used to seal the defect, and can be fixed with a transfixion suture.
20. The bone flap (craniotomy) is turned back. This prevents contact between the muscles of the neck and the posterior fossa dura, reducing the incidence of postoperative headache.
21. Abdominal fat is used to obliterate the mastoid cavity.

7.3 Hints and Pitfalls

- Most surgeons use a vertical or slightly curved skin incision. The exposure required is achieved using retractors, which have the disadvantage of making the surgical field deeper and the working angle more acute. We prefer a wide C-shaped incision and suturing the edges of the incision. Although this is more time-consuming, it removes the need for retractors.
- Complete exposure of the sigmoid sinus allows it to be displaced forward with the dural flap, thus providing wider exposure. Exposure of the transverse sinus allows the surgeon to be aware of the exact upper limit of the approach.
- Combining a retrolabyrinthine mastoidectomy with dural exposure to the retrosigmoid has several advantages:
  ○ The most important is the reduction of the incidence of CSF leakage. The removal of the air cells in this area interrupts potential pathways between the intradural cavity and the middle ear, and filling the cavity with fat at the end of the approach adds to the seal.
  ○ Another advantage of this combination is the fact that the sigmoid sinus and the attached dura can be retracted anteriorly, adding to the available space.
  ○ The semicircular canal can be located more easily through the retrolabyrinthine part of the approach.

- If deep perilabyrinthine air cells are present, bone wax is used to seal them.
- Before drilling is started in the posterior wall of the internal auditory canal, the Merocel strips are removed to prevent them from becoming entangled in the burr. Gelfoam is placed in the angle and around the internal auditory canal mainly inferior to it, to avoid dispersion of bone dust in the cistern. The cerebellum is gently retracted, a large diamond burr is used, and drilling is carried out under continuous suction irrigation. Drilling should be carried out parallel to the direction of the internal auditory canal and from medial to lateral.
- Various landmarks have been proposed to help avoid injury to the labyrinth during drilling of the posterior wall of the internal auditory canal. These include the singular canal, the transverse crest, and the vestibular aqueduct. We find that the vestibular aqueduct is a constant landmark, since it lies immediately medial and inferior to the common crus. However, during surgery, identification of the vestibular aqueduct may be difficult. In such cases, we prefer blue-lining of the common crus. This method involves a risk of opening the labyrinth while blue-lining it. Another method is to follow the dura of the canal and drill laterally (about 6–7 mm) until the dura becomes narrower. This method lacks any specific landmark for the point at which drilling should stop. It does not provide the maximum possible exposure of the internal auditory canal, but involves less risk to the labyrinth. Residual tumor at the level of the fundus can be checked by endoscopy.
- While the internal auditory canal is being drilled, a wide area of bone should be removed—i.e., superior and inferior to the canal, rather than just exposing only the posterior wall. This allows more space for safer tumor removal, and reduces the risk to the facial nerve.
- A high jugular bulb reaching up to the level of the inferior border of the internal auditory canal is present in about 10% of cases. In these cases, the bulb may be injured while the posterior wall of the internal auditory canal is being drilled, with subsequent profuse bleeding that may even make it necessary to terminate the procedure.

Retrosigmoid-retrolabyrinthine approach

Fig. 7.1 The structures controlled by the combined retrosigmoid–retrolabyrinthine approach. See ▶ Fig. 4.1 for key to abbreviations.

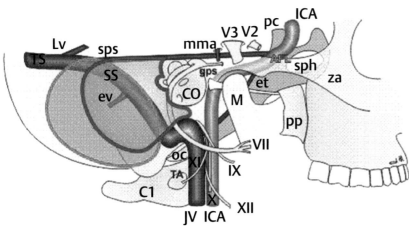

Retrosigmoid   Retrolabyrinthine

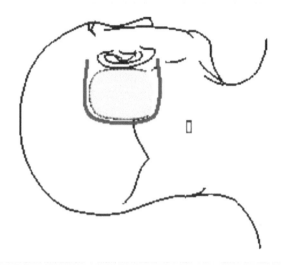

Fig. 7.2 The skin incision is made as shown.

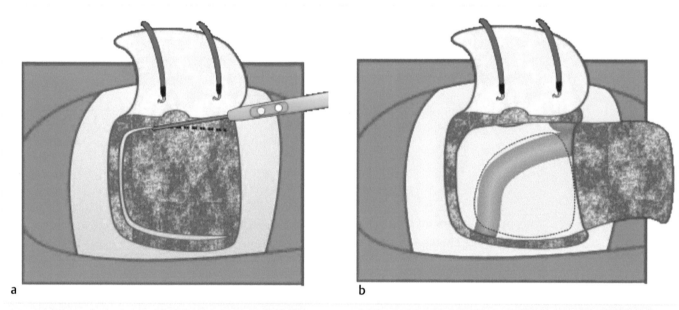

a

b

Fig. 7.3 (a) Inverted U inferiorly based musculoperiosteal flap. (b) Elevation of the musculoperiosteal flap and area of the craniotomy (*dashed lines*).

Left Ear

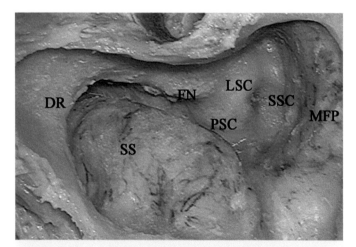

Fig. 7.4 An extended mastoidectomy has been achieved in a left temporal bone. DR, digastric ridge; FN, facial nerve; LSC, lateral semicircular canal; MFP, middle fossa plate; PSC, posterior semicircular canal; SS, sigmoid sinus; SSC, superior semicircular canal.

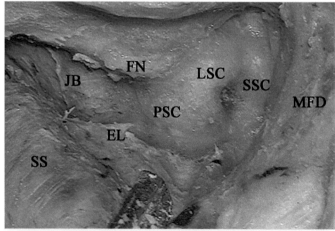

Fig. 7.5 The dura has been uncovered from the overlying bone. Note the high jugular bulb (JB), touching the posterior semicircular canal (PSC). EL, endolymphatic duct; FN, facial nerve; LSC, lateral semicircular canal; MFD, middle fossa dura; SS, sigmoid sinus; SSC, superior semicircular canal.

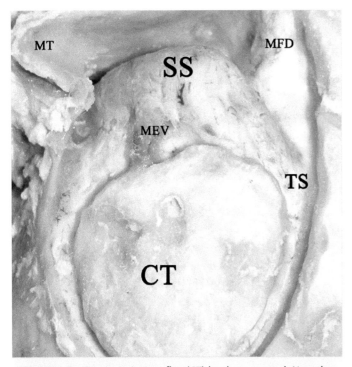

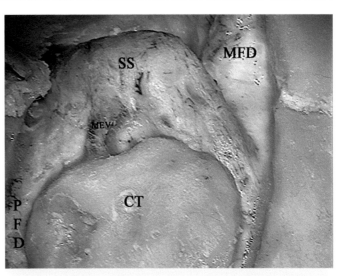

Fig. 7.7 At higher magnification. CT, craniotomy; MEV, mastoid emissary vein; MFD, middle fossa dura; PFD, posterior fossa dura; SS, sigmoid sinus.

Fig. 7.6 A 5-×5-cm craniotomy flap (CT) has been created. Note that the craniotomy should be located posterior to the sigmoid sinus (SS) and inferior to the transverse sinus (TS). MEV, mastoid emissary vein; MFD, middle fossa dura; MT, mastoid tip.

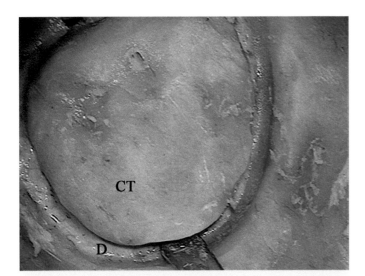

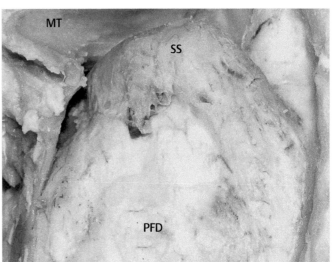

Fig. 7.8 A septal raspatory is used to detach the craniotomy flap (CT) from the underlying posterior fossa dura (D).

Fig. 7.9 The craniotomy flap is separated from the dura. Then, an anteriorly based flap is created in the posterior fossa dura (PFD). MT, mastoid tip; SS, sigmoid sinus.

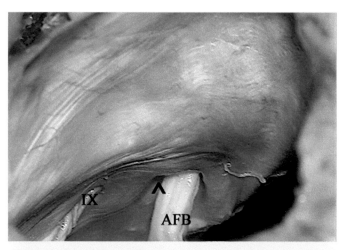

Fig. 7.10 Through the craniotomy, the acousticofacial bundle (AFB) can be seen entering the internal auditory canal (^). IX, glossopharyngeal nerve.

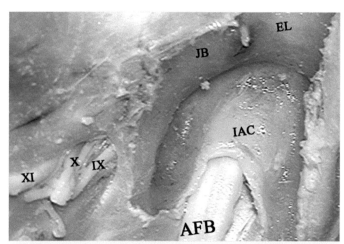

Fig. 7.11 Identification of the internal auditory canal (IAC) has been achieved by following the porus medially until the endolymphatic duct (EL) started to show through the bone laterally. Note the high jugular bulb (JB). AFB, acousticofacial bundle; IX, glossopharyngeal nerve; X, vagus nerve; XI, accessory nerve.

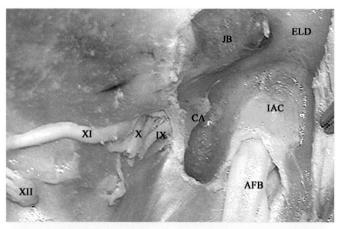

Fig. 7.12 Drilling has been carried out more inferiorly to identify the cochlear aqueduct (CA). Note the proximity of the aqueduct to the glossopharyngeal nerve (IX). AFB, acousticofacial bundle; ELD, endolymphatic duct; IAC, internal auditory canal; JB, jugular bulb; X, vagus nerve; XI, accessory nerve; XII, hypoglossal nerve.

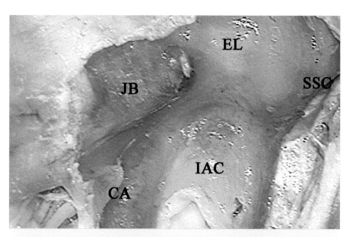

Fig. 7.13 The dura overlying the superior aspect of the internal auditory canal (IAC) has been elevated, and identification of the superior semicircular canal (SSC) has been started in order to reach to the fundus. CA, cochlear aqueduct; EL, endolymphatic duct; JB, jugular bulb.

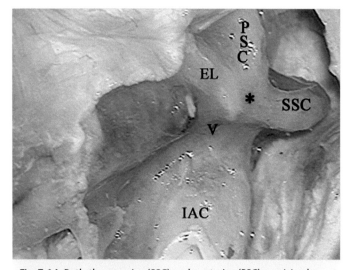

Fig. 7.14 Both the superior (SSC) and posterior (PSC) semicircular canals have been skeletonized. The endolymphatic duct (EL) can be seen lying posterior to the junction of the common crus (*), with the vestibule (V). IAC, internal auditory canal.

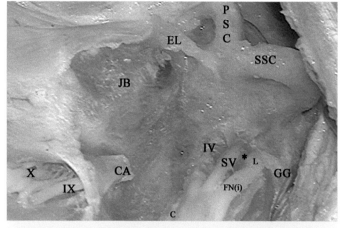

Fig. 7.15 At the fundus, Bill's bar (*) can be seen separating the labyrinthine segment of the facial nerve (L) from the superior vestibular nerve (SV). C, cochlear nerve; CA, cochlear aqueduct; EL, endolymphatic duct; FN(i), internal auditory canal segment of the facial nerve; GG, geniculate ganglion; IV, inferior vestibular nerve; IX, glossopharyngeal nerve; JB, jugular bulb; PSC, posterior semicircular canal; SSC, superior semicircular canal; X, vagus nerve.

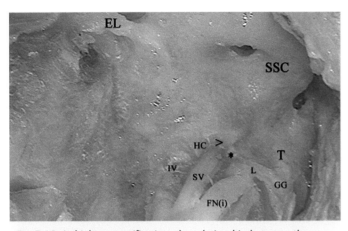

Fig. 7.16 At higher magnification, the relationship between the nerves in the fundus area can be better appreciated. *, Bill's bar; >, superior ampullary canal; EL, endolymphatic duct; FN(i), internal auditory canal segment of the facial nerve; GG, geniculate ganglion; HC, horizontal crest; IV, inferior vestibular nerve; L, labyrinthine segment of the facial nerve; SSC, superior semicircular canal; SV, superior vestibular nerve entering the superior ampullary canal; T, tympanic segment of the facial nerve.

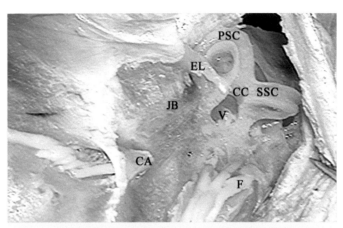

Fig. 7.17 The superior semicircular canal (SSC) and posterior semicircular canal (PSC) have been opened and can be seen as these join to form the common crus (CC) and enter the vestibule. CA, cochlear aqueduct; EL, endolymphatic duct; F, facial nerve; JB, jugular bulb; V, vestibule.

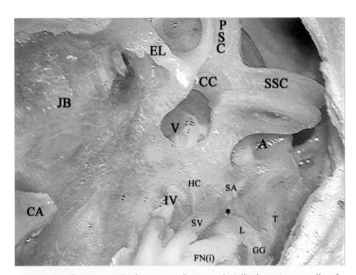

Fig. 7.18 The view at higher magnification. *, Bill's bar; A, ampulla of the superior canal; CA, cochlear aqueduct; CC, common crus; EL, endolymphatic duct; FN(i), internal auditory canal segment of the facial nerve; GG, geniculate ganglion; HC, horizontal crest; IV, inferior vestibular nerve; JB, jugular bulb; L, labyrinthine segment of the facial nerve; PSC, posterior semicircular canal; SA, superior ampullary nerve; SSC, superior semicircular canal; SV, superior vestibular nerve; T, tympanic segment of the facial nerve; V, vestibule.

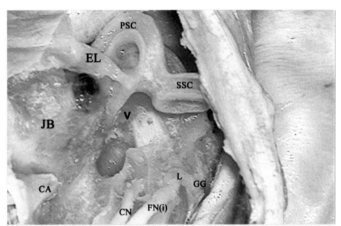

Fig. 7.19 The vestibular nerves have been removed, the vestibule (V) has been completely opened, and the cochlear nerve entering the modiolus (C) is visible inside. CA, cochlear aqueduct; CN, cochlear nerve within the internal auditory canal; EL, endolymphatic duct; FN(i), internal auditory canal segment of the facial nerve; GG, geniculate ganglion; JB, jugular bulb; L, labyrinthine segment of the facial nerve; PSC, posterior semicircular canal; SSC, superior semicircular canal.

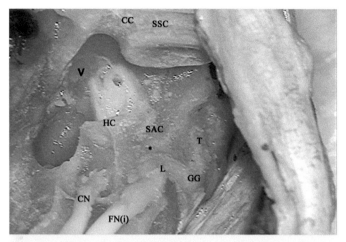

Fig. 7.20 The view at higher magnification. *, Bill's bar; C, cochlear nerve entering the modiolus; CC, common crus; CN, cochlear nerve within the internal auditory canal; FN(i), internal auditory canal segment of the facial nerve; GG, geniculate ganglion; HC, horizontal crest; L, labyrinthine segment of the facial nerve; SAC, saccule; SSC, superior semicircular canal; T, tympanic segment of the facial nerve; V, vestibule.

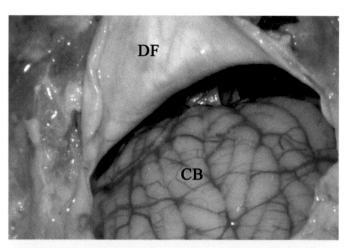

Fig. 7.21 A cadaveric dissection to show the intradural structures exposed by this approach. The dural flap (DF) has been created and reflected anteriorly, and the cerebellum (CB) can be seen.

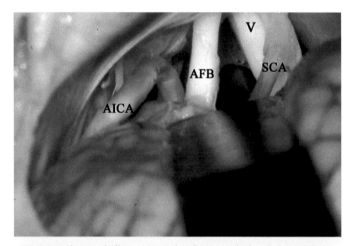

Fig. 7.22 The cerebellar retractor has been applied and the cerebellopontine angle opened. AFB, acousticofacial bundle; AICA, anterior inferior cerebellar artery; SCA, superior cerebellar artery; V, trigeminal nerve.

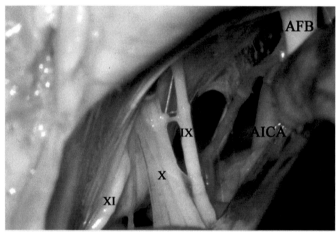

Fig. 7.23 The lower cranial nerves are visible in the lower part of the approach. AFB, acousticofacial bundle; AICA, anterior inferior cerebellar artery; IX, glossopharyngeal nerve; X, vagus nerve; XI, accessory nerve.

Right Ear

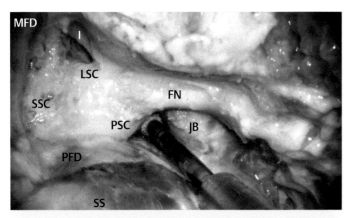

Fig. 7.24 A simple retrolabyrinthine approach has been performed in a right temporal bone. The cells between the jugular bulb (JB) and the posterior semicircular canal (PSC) are starting to be drilled. FN, facial nerve; I, incus; LSC, lateral semicircular canal; MFD, middle fossa dura; PFD, posterior fossa dura; SS, sigmoid sinus; SSC, superior semicircular canal.

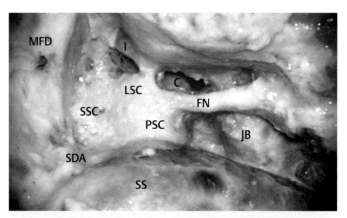

Fig. 7.25 Note the space between the jugular bulb (JB) and the posterior semicircular canal (PSC). Extended posterior tympanotomy and subfacial tympanotomy have been performed just for dissection purposes. C, cochlea (promontory); FN, facial nerve; I, incus; LSC, lateral semicircular canal; MFD, middle fossa dura; SDA, sinodural angle; SS, sigmoid sinus; SSC, superior semicircular canal.

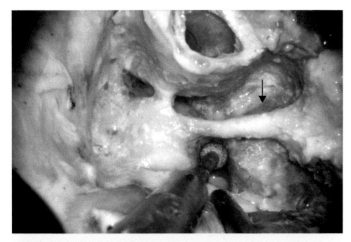

Fig. 7.26 The jugular bulb is further skeletonized. The posterior tympanotomy has been extended to the hypotympanum (note the portion of the sigmoid sinus anterior to the facial nerve, *black arrow*). The suction irrigator is pushing against the posterior fossa dura to avoid damage during drilling (*red arrow*).

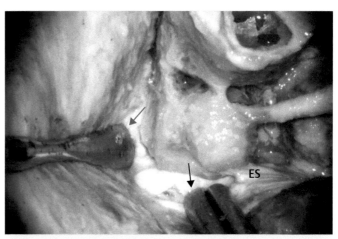

Fig. 7.27 The middle fossa dura (*red arrow*) and the posterior fossa dura (*black arrow*) are retracted. The labyrinthine block is completely skeletonized. ES, endolymphatic sac.

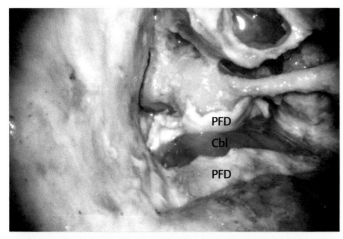

Fig. 7.28 The posterior fossa dura (PFD) has been opened. The cerebellum (Cbl) is under view.

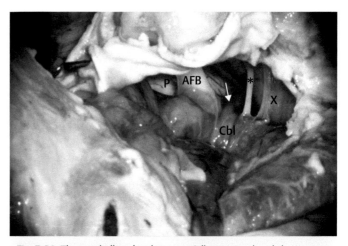

Fig. 7.29 The cerebellum has been partially retracted and the content of the cerebellopontine angle is under view. Arrow, posterior inferior cerebellar artery; asterisk, glossopharyngeal nerve; AFB, acousticofacial bundle; Cbl, cerebellum; P, pons; X, vagus nerve.

8 Transotic Approach

Abstract

The transotic approach represents an anterior extension of the translabyrinthine approach at the expense of the cochlea without mobilization of the facial nerve. The external auditory canal (EAC) and the middle ear are removed.

Keywords: transotic approach, internal carotid artery

8.1 Indications

- Some cases of cerebellopontine angle tumor with anterior extension and normal facial nerve function preoperatively (e. g., epidermoids).
- Some cases of petrous bone cholesteatoma.
- Some cases of petrous bone tumor with normal facial nerve function preoperatively.
- Some cases of vestibular schwannoma with invasion of the turns of the cochlea.

8.2 Surgical Steps

See ► Fig. 8.1, ► Fig. 8.2, ► Fig. 8.3, ► Fig. 8.4, ► Fig. 8.5, ► Fig. 8.6, ► Fig. 8.7, ► Fig. 8.8, ► Fig. 8.9, ► Fig. 8.10, ► Fig. 8.11, ► Fig. 8.12, ► Fig. 8.13, ► Fig. 8.14, ► Fig. 8.15, ► Fig. 8.16, ► Fig. 8.17, ► Fig. 8.18, ► Fig. 8.19, ► Fig. 8.20, ► Fig. 8.21, ► Fig. 8.22, ► Fig. 8.23, ► Fig. 8.24, ► Fig. 8.25, ► Fig. 8.26, ► Fig. 8.27, ► Fig. 8.28, ► Fig. 8.29, ► Fig. 8.30, ► Fig. 8.31, ► Fig. 8.32, ► Fig. 8.33, ► Fig. 8.34, ► Fig. 8.35, ► Fig. 8.36, ► Fig. 8.37, ► Fig. 8.38, ► Fig. 8.39, ► Fig. 8.40, ► Fig. 8.41, ► Fig. 8.42, ► Fig. 8.43, ► Fig. 8.44, ► Fig. 8.45, ► Fig. 8.46, ► Fig. 8.47, ► Fig. 8.48, ► Fig. 8.49, ► Fig. 8.50, ► Fig. 8.51, ► Fig. 8.52, ► Fig. 8.53.

1. Skin incision is the same as for the translabyrinthine approach (see ► Fig. 4.2), but the external auditory canal is transected and blind-sac is closed. After the blind-sac closure of the external auditory canal (EAC), the remaining skin covering the bony portion of the canal is removed together with the tympanic membrane and ossicular chain. This step is carried out under the microscope in order to avoid leaving any skin remnants.

2. A canal wall–down mastoidectomy is carried out, with additional skeletonization of the middle fossa dura, the sigmoid sinus, and the posterior fossa dura. These structures are only skeletonized; the decision on whether or not to remove the overlying bone depends on the level of exposure required and is judged in accordance with the pathology being treated.

3. The facial nerve (FN) is skeletonized from the stylomastoid foramen to the geniculate ganglion (GG) without removing the overlying bone, which serves to protect the nerve later on.

4. Labyrinthectomy and skeletonization of the internal auditory canal (IAC) are carried out in the same manner as in the translabyrinthine and transcochlear approaches.

5. After the complete skeletonization of the IAC, the infralabyrinthine air cells are drilled out using a diamond burr of the appropriate size. Care should be taken when performing this step to avoid injuring the jugular bulb, lying inferiorly, and the posterior fossa dura, lying medially. It should also be noted that the medial aspect of the fallopian canal should not be overthinned, as it acts as the main support for the nerve after the approach has been completed.

6. Drilling of the inferior tympanic bone and the anterior wall is carried out.

7. Drilling now is started in the area anterior to the mastoid segment of the FN. Extreme care should be taken when carrying out the subsequent steps to avoid injuring this segment of the nerve. In general, injury to the mastoid segment rarely results directly from the rotating burr, as surgeons pay good attention to this. However, the rotating shaft of the burr is often forgotten. When there is prolonged contact between it and the nerve, it can result in heat injury to the nerve. Sometimes an instrument introduced wrongly into the middle ear space medial or lateral to the skeletonized nerve can fracture the bony covering and lead to FN paralysis. For this reason, adequate attention to these steps cannot be overemphasized.

8. Identification of the ICA can be started from the eustachian tube, which lies superior lateral to the artery or just at the anterior border of the cochlea, the middle turn of which lies behind the genu of the artery. Care should be taken when drilling in the area of the eustachian tube, as the bony septum between the two is sometimes dehiscent and injury to the artery can be sustained. For this reason, a large diamond burr should be used whenever drilling in the region of the ICA.

9. After identification of the ICA, the cochlea is drilled. The reason for this sequence is that being aware of the location of the artery helps to avoid injury to it. Drilling of the cochlea is started using a medium-sized cutting burr. When the middle turn is reached, the burr is exchanged for a diamond one to ensure the safety of the ICA. The remaining part of the cochlea and the bone overlying the posterior fossa dura and lying anterior to the IAC is removed, thus completing the skeletonization of the canal.

10. Further skeletonization of the ICA is continued if required.

11. At the end of the approach, the facial nerve is seen lying as a bridge in the middle of the approach.

8.3 Hints and Pitfalls

- When drilling anterior to the facial nerve, care should be taken to avoid injuring the nerve with the rotating shaft of the burr.
- In some cases, bone removal superior to the IAC is needed to obtain proper control of the superior pole of the tumor. Because of the proximity of the middle fossa dura, this may prove difficult. The middle fossa dura is therefore completely uncovered and gently retracted with suction aspiration.
- The transotic approach avoids facial nerve mobilization and therefore makes it possible to preserve perfect function.
- The facial nerve is left like a bridge in the middle of the approach. This limits the control of the ICA and petrous apex. In addition, the nerve itself may be endangered if rough manipulations break the fallopian canal.

Transotic approach

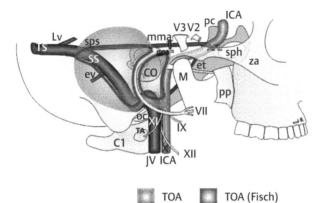

TOA   TOA (Fisch)

Fig. 8.1 The structures exposed by the transotic approach (TOA). Note that the amount of bone removed in the extended transotic approach (*green shaded area*) provides wider exposure in comparison with the classic transotic approach developed by Fisch. VII, facial nerve; IX, glossopharyngeal nerve; X, vagus nerve; XI, accessory nerve; XII, hypoglossal nerve; AFL, anterior foramen lacerum; C1, atlas; CO, cochlea; et, eustachian tube; ev, emissary vein; gps, greater superficial petrosal nerve; ICA, internal carotid artery; JV, jugular vein; Lv, Labbé's vein; M, mandible; mma, middle meningeal artery; oc, occipital condyle; pc, posterior clinoid; pp, pterygoid process; sph, sphenoid sinus; sps, superior petrosal sinus; SS, sigmoid sinus; TA, lateral process of the atlas; TS, transverse sinus; V2, second division of the trigeminal nerve; V3, third division of the trigeminal nerve; za, zygomatic arch.

Left Ear

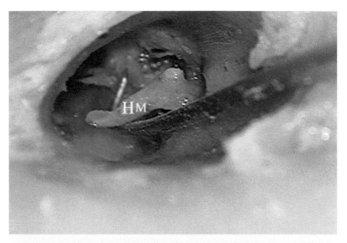

Fig. 8.2 The skin of the external auditory canal of a left temporal bone has been removed, and the handle of the malleus (HM) is being pulled using a hook.

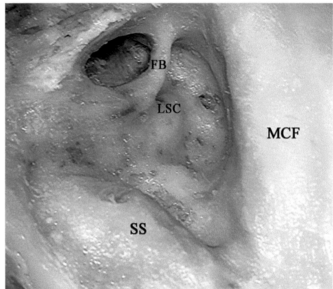

Fig. 8.4 The mastoid cavity has been drilled out, and the posterior and superior canal walls have been lowered. FB, facial bridge; LSC, lateral semicircular canal; MCF, middle cranial fossa; SS, sigmoid sinus.

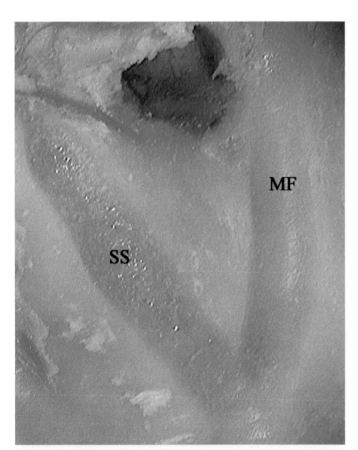

Fig. 8.3 The expected levels of the middle cranial fossa (MF) and sigmoid sinus (SS) have been identified.

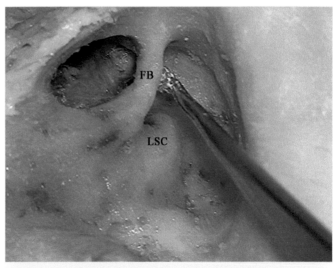

Fig. 8.5 The mastoid cavity has been drilled out, and the posterior and superior canal walls have been lowered. FB, facial bridge; LSC, lateral semicircular canal; MCF, middle cranial fossa; SS, sigmoid sinus.

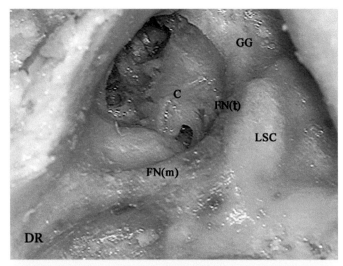

Fig. 8.6 The facial nerve has been skeletonized from the digastric ridge (DR) to the geniculate ganglion (GG). C, basal turn of the cochlea (promontory); FN(m), mastoid segment of the facial nerve; FN(t), tympanic segment of the facial nerve; LSC, lateral semicircular canal.

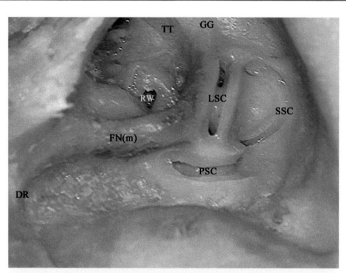

Fig. 8.7 The lateral semicircular canal (LSC), posterior semicircular canal (PSC), and superior semicircular canal (SSC) have been opened. DR, digastric ridge; FN(m), mastoid segment of the facial nerve; GG, geniculate ganglion; RW, round window; TT, tensor tympani.

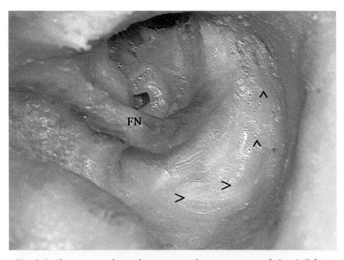

Fig. 8.8 The arrows show the semicircular movement of the drill for skeletonization of the internal auditory canal. FN, facial nerve.

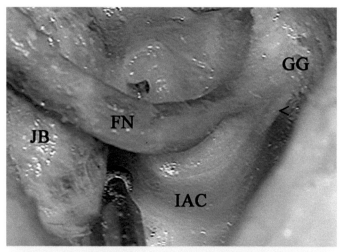

Fig. 8.9 The internal auditory canal (IAC) has been identified. Note the high jugular bulb (JB), almost touching the canal. Drilling of the intervening bone should proceed with extreme caution, using a small diamond drill. <, labyrinthine segment of the facial nerve; FN, facial nerve; GG, geniculate ganglion.

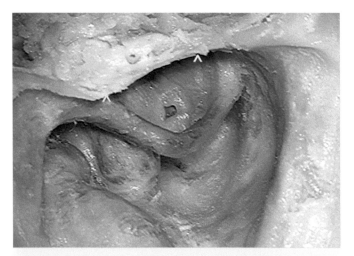

Fig. 8.10 Note that the inferior and anterior canal wall (^ ^) are overhanging here, obscuring the required view.

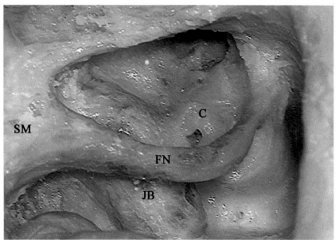

Fig. 8.11 The overhanging part of the canal wall has been drilled. The jugular bulb (JB) anterior to the facial nerve (FN) and the location of the internal carotid (*) artery are now visible. C, basal turn of the cochlea (promontory); SM, stylomastoid foramen.

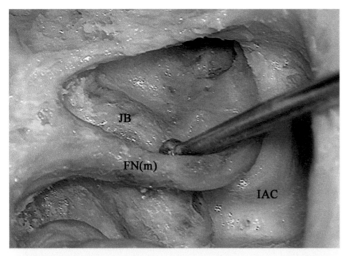

Fig. 8.12 Note that the contact seen here between the burr shaft and the facial nerve (FN[m]) is extremely dangerous and should be avoided. IAC, internal auditory canal; JB, jugular bulb.

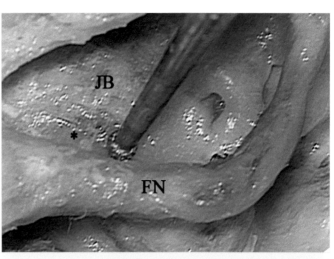

Fig. 8.13 The bone (*) between the jugular bulb (JB) and facial nerve (FN) is carefully removed using an appropriately sized diamond burr.

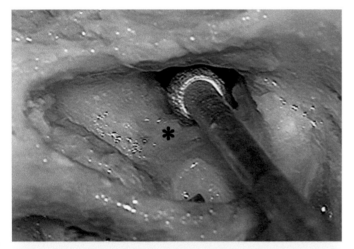

Fig. 8.14 Identification of the internal carotid artery is either started from the eustachian tube, where the burr is located, or at the anteroinferior limit of the promontory (*). A diamond burr should be used in both cases.

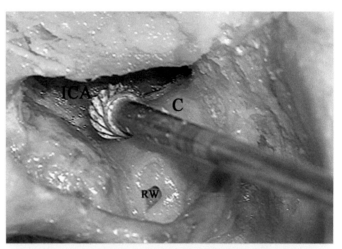

Fig. 8.15 After identification of the internal carotid artery (ICA), a cutting burr is used initially to open the cochlea (C). RW, round window.

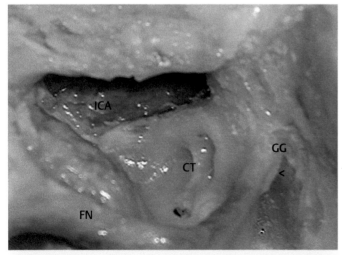

Fig. 8.16 Because of its proximity to the internal carotid artery (ICA), the last part of the cochlea (CT) should be drilled away using a small diamond burr. <, labyrinthine segment of the facial nerve; FN, facial nerve.

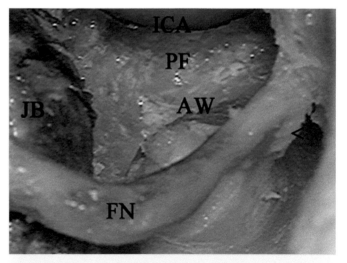

Fig. 8.17 The cochlea has been drilled out, the anterior wall of the internal auditory canal (AW) has been skeletonized, and the posterior fossa dura (PF) has been identified. <, labyrinthine segment of the facial nerve; FN, facial nerve; ICA, internal carotid artery; JB, jugular bulb.

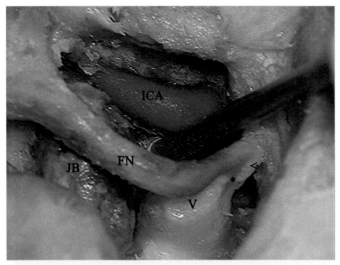

Fig. 8.18 If necessary, further drilling of the bone medial to the internal carotid artery (ICA) can be carried out. *, Bill's bar; <, labyrinthine segment of the facial nerve; FN, facial nerve; JB, jugular bulb; V, vestibule.

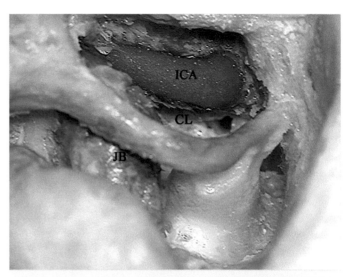

Fig. 8.19 The clivus bone (CL) can be seen medial to the internal carotid artery (ICA). JB, jugular bulb.

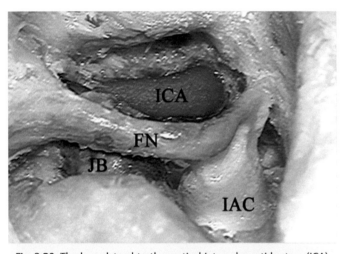

Fig. 8.20 The bone lateral to the vertical internal carotid artery (ICA) has also been drilled. FN, facial nerve; IAC, internal auditory canal; JB, jugular bulb.

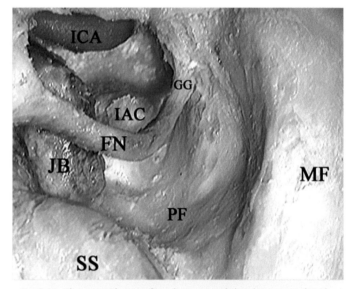

Fig. 8.21 The vertical view after the approach has been completed. Note that the facial nerve (FN) lies like a bridge in the middle of the field, limiting the surgical access. GG, geniculate ganglion; IAC, internal auditory canal; ICA, internal carotid artery; JB, jugular bulb; MF, middle fossa level; PF, posterior fossa; SS, sigmoid sinus.

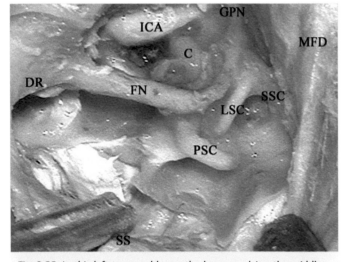

Fig. 8.22 In this left temporal bone, the bone overlying the middle fossa dura (MFD), sigmoid sinus (SS), and posterior fossa dura has already been uncovered and removed, and the facial nerve (FN), internal carotid artery (ICA), and lateral (LSC), posterior (PSC), and superior (SSC) semicircular canals have been skeletonized. C, cochlea; DR, digastric ridge; GPN, greater petrosal nerve.

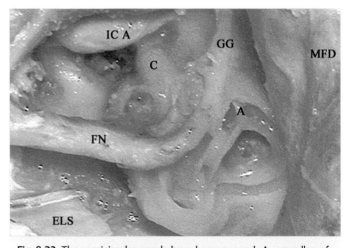

Fig. 8.23 The semicircular canals have been opened. A, ampullae of the lateral and superior semicircular canals; C, cochlea; ELS, cut endolymphatic sac; FN, facial nerve; GG, geniculate ganglion; ICA, internal carotid artery; MFD, middle fossa dura.

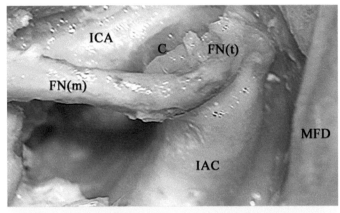

Fig. 8.24 Labyrinthectomy has been completed and the internal auditory canal (IAC) has been skeletonized. C, cochlea; FN(m), mastoid segment of the facial nerve; FN(t), tympanic segment of the facial nerve; ICA, internal carotid artery; MFD, middle fossa dura.

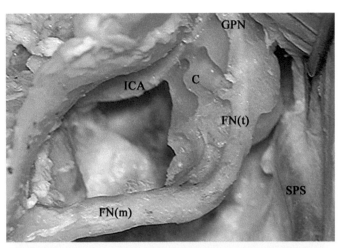

Fig. 8.25 The cochlea (C) has been opened. FN(m), mastoid segment of the facial nerve; FN(t), tympanic segment of the facial nerve; GPN, greater petrosal nerve; ICA, internal carotid artery; SPS, superior petrosal sinus.

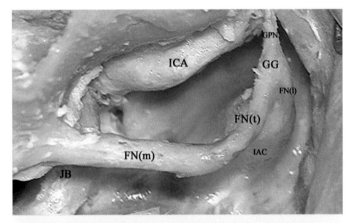

Fig. 8.26 The cochlea has been completely drilled away, and the vertical portion of the internal carotid artery (ICA) has been skeletonized. FN(l), labyrinthine segment of the facial nerve; FN(m), mastoid segment of the facial nerve; FN(t), tympanic segment of the facial nerve; GG, geniculate ganglion; GPN, greater petrosal nerve; IAC, internal auditory canal; JB, jugular bulb.

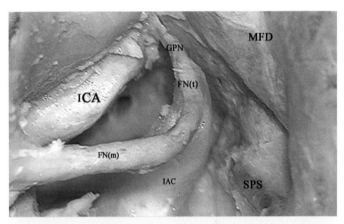

Fig. 8.27 The view after the approach has been completed. FN(m), mastoid segment of the facial nerve; FN(t), tympanic segment of the facial nerve; GPN, greater petrosal nerve; IAC, internal auditory canal; ICA, internal carotid artery; MFD, middle fossa dura; SPS, superior petrosal sinus.

Right Ear

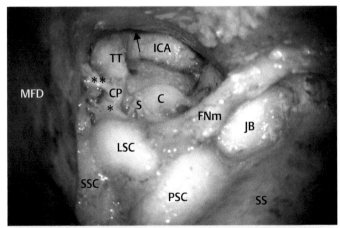

Fig. 8.28 Right ear. Subtotal petrosectomy has been completed. *, tympanic portion of the facial nerve; **, cog; arrow, eustachian tube; C, cochlea (promontory); CP, cochleariform process; FN(m), mastoid portion of the facial nerve; ICA, internal carotid artery; JB, jugular bulb; LSC, lateral semicircular canal; MFD, middle fossa dura; PSC, posterior semicircular canal; S, stapes; SS, sigmoid sinus; SSC, superior semicircular canal; TT, tensor tympani.

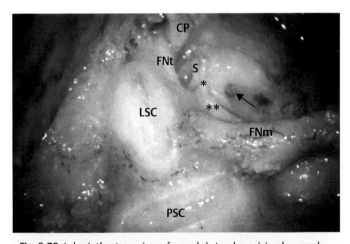

Fig. 8.29 Labyrinthectomy is performed. Lateral semicircular canal (LSC) and posterior semicircular canal (PSC) are blue-lined. Arrow, round window; *, pyramidal eminence with the stapedius muscle tendon; **, stapedius muscle; CP, cochleariform process; FN(m), mastoid portion of the facial nerve; FN(t), tympanic portion of the facial nerve.

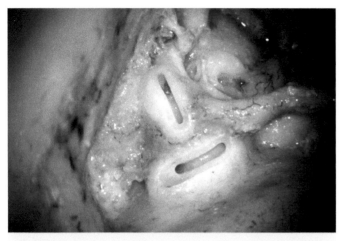

Fig. 8.30 Lateral semicircular canal and posterior semicircular canal are opened.

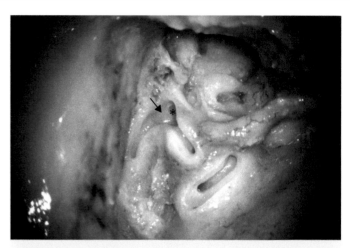

Fig. 8.31 The superior semicircular canal is opened from the ampullary end (*arrow*), following the ampulla of the lateral semicircular canal. *, joint of lateral and superior ampullae.

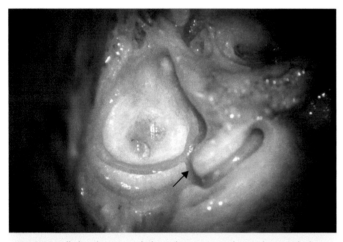

Fig. 8.32 All the three canals have been opened into the vestibule. Arrow, area of the common crus.

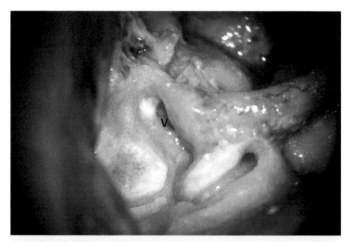

Fig. 8.33 Drilling of the canals proceeds to open the vestibule (V).

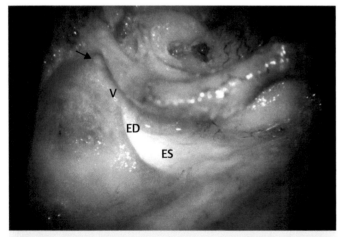

Fig. 8.34 The canals have been drilled and the vestibule (V) opened. The vestibule represents the roof of the internal auditory canal. The ampulla of the superior canal (*arrow*) has been left as a landmark to the superior edge of the internal auditory canal. Removal of the posterior semicircular canal allows visualization of the course of the endolymphatic duct (ED), from the vestibule to the endolymphatic sac (ES).

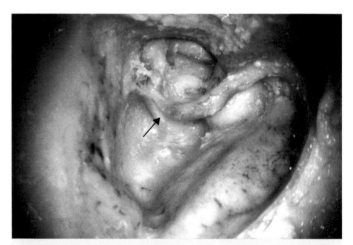

Fig. 8.35 Identification of the internal auditory canal (*arrow*) has been completed.

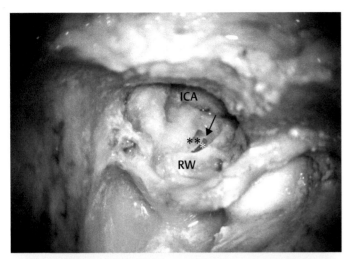

Fig. 8.36 Drilling of the cochlea has been started from the basal turn (*arrow*). *, scala tympani; **, scala vestibuli; ICA, internal carotid artery; RW, round window.

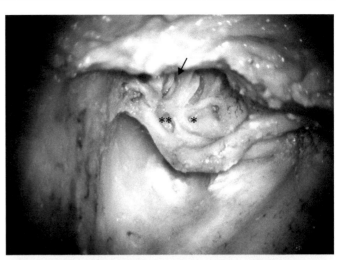

Fig. 8.37 The middle turn of the cochlea has been opened (*arrow*) and the stapes removed. Complete removal of the cochlea is going to be accomplished to identify the anterior wall of the internal auditory canal and the clivus. **, oval window; *, round window.

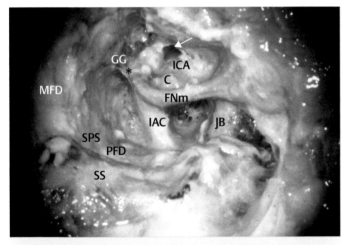

Fig. 8.38 Another example of a transotic approach in a right temporal bone. Identification of the internal auditory canal (IAC) has been completed and drilling of the cochlea is going to be performed. *, tympanic portion of the facial nerve; arrow, eustachian tube; C, cochlea (promontory); FN(m), mastoid portion of the facial nerve; GG, geniculate ganglion; ICA, internal carotid artery; JB, jugular bulb; MFD, middle fossa dura; PFD, posterior fossa dura; SPS, superior petrosal sinus; SS, sigmoid sinus.

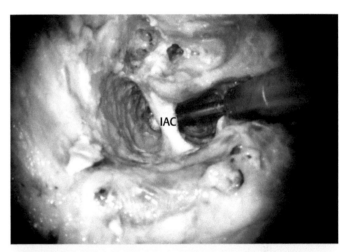

Fig. 8.39 The internal auditory canal (**IAC**) is drilled for 360 degrees of its circumference.

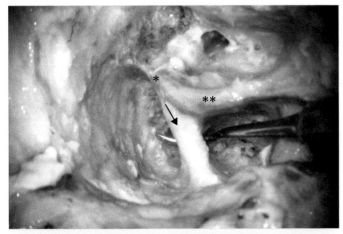

Fig. 8.40 Closer view. The internal auditory canal is free from bone. Note the course of the facial nerve. Arrow, direction of the first portion of the facial nerve; *, second portion of the facial nerve (tympanic portion); **, third portion of the facial nerve (mastoid).

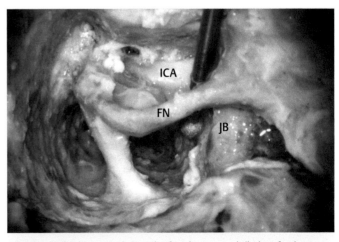

Fig. 8.41 The bone medial to the facial nerve is drilled to further skeletonize the internal carotid artery (ICA) and jugular bulb (JB). FN, facial nerve.

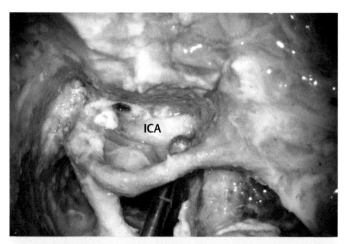

Fig. 8.42 The vertical portion of the petrous internal carotid artery (ICA) is decompressed.

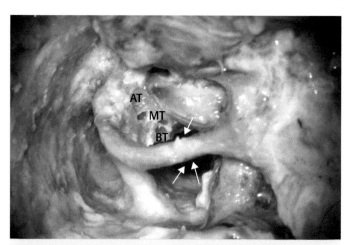

Fig. 8.43 The cochlea has been opened in the basal (BT) and middle (MT) turns. The apical turn (AT) is still intact. The petrous apex is exposed medial to the facial nerve, in the area between the cochlea, the internal carotid artery, and the jugular bulb (*arrows*).

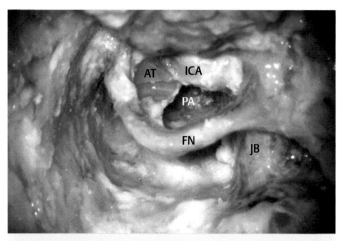

Fig. 8.44 Further drilling of the cochlea exposes the petrous apex (PA). The apical turn of the cochlea (AT) is still intact. FN, facial nerve; ICA, internal carotid artery; JB, jugular bulb.

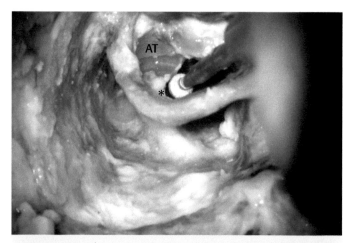

Fig. 8.45 The remaining part of the cochlea is removed, exposing the anterior wall of the internal auditory canal (*). AT, apical turn of the cochlea.

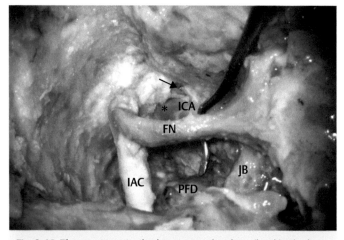

Fig. 8.46 The specimen is tilted to expose the clivus (hook). The bone of the petrous apex has been removed with exposure of the posterior fossa dura (PFD). The internal carotid artery (ICA) has been decompressed. The genu of the ICA (*) is under view. Arrow, eustachian tube; FN, facial nerve; IAC, internal auditory canal; JB, jugular bulb.

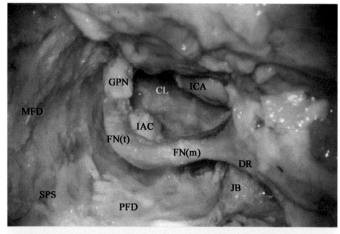

Fig. 8.47 At the end of the approach, the facial nerve is seen lying as a bridge in the middle of the approach. CL, clivus; DR, digastric ridge; FN(m), mastoid segment of the facial nerve; FN(t), tympanic segment of the facial nerve; GPN, greater petrosal nerve; IAC, internal auditory canal; ICA, internal carotid artery; JB, jugular bulb; MFD, middle fossa dura; PFD, posterior fossa dura; SPS, superior petrosal sinus.

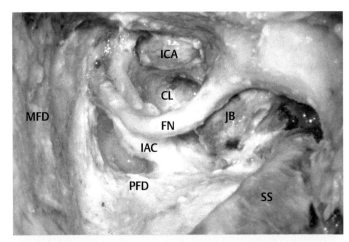

Fig. 8.48 Similar case of ▶ Fig. 8.47. The clivus (CL) is exposed. Note that the jugular bulb (JB) is high, almost reaching the inferior border of the internal auditory canal (IAC). FN, facial nerve; ICA, internal carotid artery; MFD, middle fossa dura; PFD, posterior fossa dura; SS, sigmoid sinus.

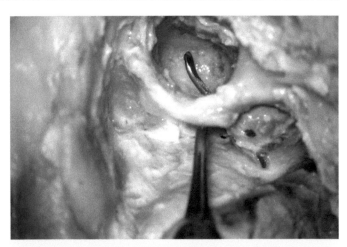

Fig. 8.49 Closer view. The clivus is indicated with a hook.

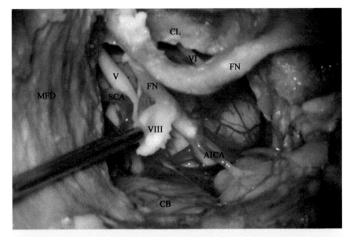

Fig. 8.50 The intracranial structures that can be seen using the transotic approach. Note that the facial nerve lies like a bridge in the middle of the approach, obstructing access to the cerebellopontine angle. AICA, anterior inferior cerebellar artery; CB, cerebellum; CL, clivus bone; FN, facial nerve; MFD, middle fossa dura; SCA, superior cerebellar artery; V, trigeminal nerve; VI, abducens nerve; VIII, cochlear nerve.

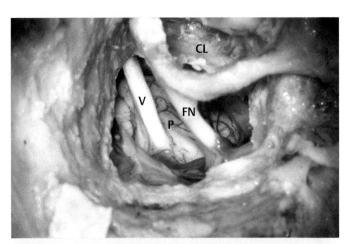

Fig. 8.51 Closer view. Note the relationship between the facial nerve (FN) and the trigeminal nerve (V). CL, clivus; P, pons.

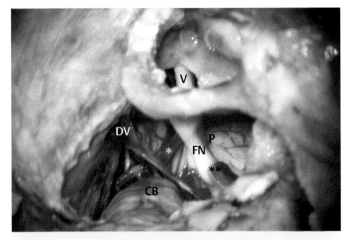

Fig. 8.52 The specimen is tilted to show the Dandy's vein (DV). *, superior cerebellar artery (SCA); **, anterior inferior cerebellar artery (AICA); CB, cerebellum; FN, facial nerve; P, pons; V, trigeminal nerve.

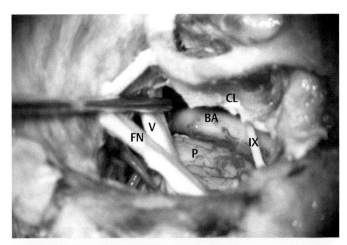

Fig. 8.53 The facial nerve (FN) and trigeminal nerve (V) are retracted, exposing the basilar artery (BA). CL, clivus; P, pons; IX, glossopharyngeal nerve.

9 Modified Transcochlear Approach (Type A)

Abstract

The modified transcochlear approach combines the removal of the external auditory canal (EAC) and middle ear with posterior rerouting of the facial nerve (FN), thus removing the major impediment to anterior extension of the approach. This allows better control of the vertical and horizontal intrapetrous internal carotid artery and facilitates total removal of the petrous apex. The extensive anterior bone removal provides excellent control of the ventral surface of the brainstem without cerebellar and brainstem retraction.

Keywords: transcochlear approach, posterior facial nerve rerouting

9.1 Indications

- *Extradural lesions:* extensive petrous apex lesions with preoperative FN and inner ear loss of function:
  - Petrous bone cholesteatoma of the massive, infralabyrinthine apical and (less commonly) supralabyrinthine types.
  - Recurrent acoustic neurinoma with petrous bone invasion and FN paralysis.
  - Extensive FN tumors.
- *Intradural lesions:*
  - Large clival and petroclival lesions lying ventral to the brainstem, for example, petroclival meningiomas.
  - Residual or recurrent nonacoustic lesions of the posterior fossa with anterior extension into the prepontine cistern, particularly those with encasement of the vertebrobasilar artery or perforating arteries, or both; for example, huge posterior fossa epidermoids.
  - Recurrent acoustic neurinomas with FN paralysis.
- *Transdural lesions:* invading the petrous apex as en plaque meningiomas, or primary clival or temporal bone lesions with secondary posterior fossa extension such as chordomas, chondrosarcomas, and extensive glomus jugulare tumors.

9.2 Surgical Steps

See ▶ Fig. 9.1, ▶ Fig. 9.2, ▶ Fig. 9.3, ▶ Fig. 9.4, ▶ Fig. 9.5, ▶ Fig. 9.6, ▶ Fig. 9.7, ▶ Fig. 9.8, ▶ Fig. 9.9, ▶ Fig. 9.10, ▶ Fig. 9.11, ▶ Fig. 9.12, ▶ Fig. 9.13, ▶ Fig. 9.14, ▶ Fig. 9.15, ▶ Fig. 9.16, ▶ Fig. 9.17, ▶ Fig. 9.18, ▶ Fig. 9.19, ▶ Fig. 9.20, ▶ Fig. 9.21, ▶ Fig. 9.22, ▶ Fig. 9.23, ▶ Fig. 9.24, ▶ Fig. 9.25, ▶ Fig. 9.26, ▶ Fig. 9.27, ▶ Fig. 9.28, ▶ Fig. 9.29, ▶ Fig. 9.30, ▶ Fig. 9.31, ▶ Fig. 9.32, ▶ Fig. 9.33, ▶ Fig. 9.34, ▶ Fig. 9.35, ▶ Fig. 9.36, ▶ Fig. 9.37, ▶ Fig. 9.38, ▶ Fig. 9.39, ▶ Fig. 9.40, ▶ Fig. 9.41, ▶ Fig. 9.42, ▶ Fig. 9.43, ▶ Fig. 9.44, ▶ Fig. 9.45, ▶ Fig. 9.46, ▶ Fig. 9.47, ▶ Fig. 9.48, ▶ Fig. 9.49, ▶ Fig. 9.50, ▶ Fig. 9.51, ▶ Fig. 9.52, ▶ Fig. 9.53, ▶ Fig. 9.54, ▶ Fig. 9.55, ▶ Fig. 9.56, ▶ Fig. 9.57, ▶ Fig. 9.58, ▶ Fig. 9.59, ▶ Fig. 9.60.

1. Skin incision is the same as for the translabyrinthine approach (see ▶ Fig. 4.2), but the EAC is transected and blind-sac is closed. After blind-sac closure of the external auditory canal, the skin covering the bony part of the EAC should be removed under the microscope. Mastoidectomy is started by creating the triangle of attack; the middle fossa dura and the sigmoid sinus are identified, and the posterior canal wall is thinned and lowered to the level of the annulus.

2. The remnants of the tympanic membrane and the ossicles are removed.

3. The digastric ridge is identified and the FN is skeletonized.

4. The nerve can now be seen extending from the stylomastoid foramen at the anterior edge of the digastric ridge to the second genu, housed within the curvature of the lateral semicircular canal (LSC). From here, the tympanic segment of the FN runs anteriorly under the LSC to reach the geniculate ganglion (GG) superior to the cochleariform process.

5. Depending on the pathology being treated and thus the level of exposure required, a decision is taken on whether to uncover the middle fossa dura and sigmoid sinus. Whether these structures are to be uncovered or not, the edges of the cavity should be rounded and smoothed, and the bone overlying the dura and sinus should be thinned to a very fine shell.

6. If these structures are to be uncovered, a Freer periosteal elevator is used to separate the dura from the remaining bony shell, in the same way as in the translabyrinthine approach.

7. Labyrinthectomy is started by drilling the LSC. Care must be taken at this point not to injure the second genu of the FN, which lies within the curvature of the canal. Leaving the inferior wall of the canal intact will provide the necessary protection.

8. Following the cavity of the LSC superiorly will lead to the joint ampulla of the lateral and superior canals. From here, the cavity of the superior semicircular canal (SSC) can be followed posteriorly to reach common crus, which is formed by the union of the nonampullated ends of the superior and posterior canals.

9. Leaving the anterior wall of the ampulla of the superior semicircular canal (SSC) intact serves to protect the tympanic and labyrinthine segments of the nerve from drilling injury, as well as providing a sign for the upper border of the internal auditory canal (IAC).

10. Following the posterior canal at this point will lead to its ampullated end, which lies a few millimeters medial to the mastoid segment of the FN. Again, care must be taken here to avoid injuring the nerve.

11. The endolymphatic sac is encountered between the sigmoid sinus (SS) and the posterior semicircular canal (PSC). Passing from behind and medial to the canal to enter between the layers of the dura, this structure exerts tension, hampering the dural retraction. In order to release the dura at this position, a Beaver knife with the sharp border directed against the bone is used to cut the endolymphatic duct.

12. The vestibule is now opened carefully. Since the genu of the FN lies at its lateral wall and the fundus of the IAC lies at its medial wall, the direction of drilling in this area should be parallel to these walls in a superior to inferior direction, or vice versa, and never from medial to lateral. The posterior edge of the lateral wall of the vestibule should be cautiously reduced. Although a very small amount of bone needs to be removed at this location, its removal is crucial for adequate visualization of the IAC.

13. The ampulla of the SSC serves as the landmark for the level of the superior border of the IAC. The bone between the middle fossa dura and the IAC is now drilled using an appropriately sized diamond drill. Drilling in this area should proceed from medial to lateral. Care must be taken not to injure the dura or open the wall of the IAC, jeopardizing the FN lying within. In order to avoid such mishaps, a septal dissector is used to separate the dura from the bone to be drilled. During drilling, the dura should be retracted superiorly using suction irrigation. In live surgery, the middle fossa dura can be shrunk using bipolar coagulation under irrigation, adding to the dural retraction.

14. The inferior border of the IAC is then identified by drilling the retrofacial air cells lying between that border and the jugular bulb (JB) inferiorly. During drilling in this area, the cochlear aqueduct is identified. The importance of this structure lies in the fact that it serves as a landmark for the glossopharyngeal nerve, which lies just inferior to its level. Thus, identifying the cochlear aqueduct during drilling means that the lower limit of drilling has been reached. Opening the cochlear aqueduct in live surgery also helps to allow cerebrospinal fluid (CSF) to escape, relaxing the intradural tension and improving exposure.

15. Once the IAC has been identified, drilling is continued using an appropriately sized diamond burr, moving in a semicircular fashion from superior to posterior to inferior until only a transparent shell of bone is left covering the IAC.

16. Skeletonization of the mastoid and tympanic segments of the FN is started using an appropriately sized diamond burr, moving in a direction parallel to the nerve under ample suction irrigation. Drilling should be continued until only a thin, transparent bony covering is left overlying the nerve. The bone overlying the area of the stylomastoid foramen should be completely removed, especially at the posterior aspect, in order to prevent the sharp bony remnants from injuring the FN while it is being rerouted.

17. On the posterior surface of the IAC fundus, the transverse crest is identified. This crest is the bar of bone separating the superior vestibular nerve and FN, lying superior to it, from the inferior vestibular nerve and cochlear nerve, lying inferior to it. Following the superior vestibular nerve from the superior level of the transverse crest laterally to the superior ampulla will lead to the canal of the superior ampullary nerve, which forms a very important landmark for safe identification of the FN at the fundus. At this level, Bill's bar lies anterior to the superior ampullary nerve, protecting the FN from injury while the former is dislodged from its canal. A small cutting burr is used carefully to open the canal of the superior vestibular nerve. Drilling in the expected position of the canal is carried out until the whitish color of the canal starts to appear.

18. Bill's bar is identified using a small diamond drill. The suction irrigation tube at this step helps to irrigate the field and to retract the dura away from the drill to prevent injury to it. While the dura is retracted, drilling is advanced to identify the labyrinthine segment of the FN. Again, adequate suction irrigation is vital to avoid injury. The drill should be moved parallel to the course of this segment, and the direction of rotation of the burr should be away from the nerve.

19. The bone overlying the GG is drilled using the same diamond drill. Adequate removal of the bone lying anterior to the GG and the sharp angle of bone lying between the labyrinthine segment and the GG is important to avoid injury to the nerve while it is being rerouted posteriorly.

20. The greater superficial petrosal nerve is followed from the anterior border of the GG, and the bone overlying it is drilled to uncover the nerve. In live surgery, the nerve is sharply cut after bipolar coagulation to prevent bleeding, since the major blood supply to the FN is carried via the petrosal branch of the middle meningeal artery, following the nerve.

21. The last shell of bone overlying the full course of the FN is now removed using a double-curved hook.

22. The decision to open the dura of the IAC depends on the extent of the pathology. In the cases where the intracanalicular portion of the FN is not involved, maintaining the integrity of the dura will help to maintain the blood supply to the remaining portion of the nerve and to prevent postoperative CSF leakage.

23. At the level of the fundus of the IAC, the inferior vestibular nerve is dislodged using a double-curved hook.

24. This is followed by dislodging the superior ampullary nerve from its canal using a small hook. The superior ampullary nerve is then dissected medially until the superior vestibular nerve is reached and the FN can be identified anterior to it.

25. Rerouting of the FN is started at the level of the GG. Using an angled pick and a Brackmann suction tube, the GG is dislodged and followed carefully to the labyrinthine segment of the nerve. This step is the most delicate step in the rerouting, and the facial nerve is most liable to injury at this level. This is because the labyrinthine segment is the thinnest part of the FN, due to the absence of an epineural covering, and due to the sharp bony angle between the GG and labyrinthine segment, which can injure this segment if extreme care is not taken.

26. The tympanic segment is next dissected free from the canal.

27. The fibrous and vascular attachments of the mastoid segment of the facial nerve to the medial aspect of the fallopian canal should be sharply dissected. The mastoid segment of the nerve should be freed down to the stylomastoid foramen.

28. The labyrinthine segment of the FN is followed as far as the IAC. If a decision not to open the dura has been made, the cochlear nerve is freed from its attachment at the fundus, and the dura covering the anterior wall of the IAC is elevated. The whole contents of the IAC, together with the rest of the FN, are now rerouted posteriorly and laid on the posterior fossa dura just anterior to the sigmoid sinus. A piece of aluminum obtained from the covering of the surgical threads is used to protect the rerouted nerve from injury during further manipulations and drilling.

29. The remaining part of the fallopian canal is removed either using a rongeur or using a large cutting burr, and the inferior part of the tympanic ring is widely drilled.

30. Drilling the cochlea is started using a large cutting burr. When the middle turn of the cochlea is reached, the burr is exchanged for a diamond burr, since at this level the amount of bone separating the drill from the internal carotid artery is very thin. Using the diamond burr and sufficient suction irrigation, drilling is continued to remove the remaining part of the cochlea and identify the vertical segment of the ICA.

31. The petrous apex is drilled as far as the level of the midclivus, exposing the dura of the posterior surface of the temporal bone. For extradural pathologies, removal of the disease is started after this step. On the other hand, if the pathology shows intradural extension, the dura is opened after bipolar coagulation.

9.3 Hints and Pitfalls

- Special care should be taken in the region of the GG. All bone should be removed here to avoid injury to the nerve during transposition.
- The vertical segment of the FN has tough fibrous attachments to the fallopian canal, and sharp dissection is therefore needed to avoid stretching the nerve at this level. By contrast, the tympanic and labyrinthine segments are delicate and require fine manipulation.

- Failure to free the FN up to the level of the stylomastoid foramen would leave the most distal part of its mastoid segment in situ. This part would obstruct complete control of the jugular bulb and preclude visualization of the lower pole of the tumor.
- While rerouting the FN, cottonoids are used to protect it against direct suction. Brackmann suction tips can be used instead.
- This approach provides excellent control of the intrapetrous ICA, and the extent to which it should be exposed depends on the extent needed for tumor removal. The artery may be merely skeletonized, or can be exposed for 360 and 270 degrees in its vertical and horizontal segments, respectively.
- The approach allows wide exposure of the cerebellopontine angle and prepontine cistern without cerebellar and brainstem retraction. It also makes it possible to remove the infiltrated dura and bone.
- Facial nerve rerouting leads to postoperative paralysis, which usually recovers to grade III.

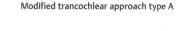
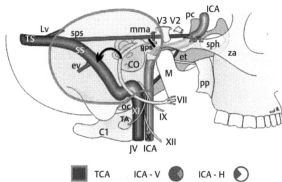

Fig. 9.1 The extent of bone removal and the structures controlled with the transcochlear approach. See VII, facial nerve; IX, glossopharyngeal nerve; X, vagus nerve; XI, accessory nerve; XII, hypoglossal nerve; AFL, anterior foramen lacerum; C1, atlas; CO, cochlea; et, eustachian tube; ev, emissary vein; gps, greater superficial petrosal nerve; ICA, internal carotid artery; JV, jugular vein; Lv, Labbé's vein; M, mandible; mma, middle meningeal artery; oc, occipital condyle; pc, posterior clinoid; pp, pterygoid process; sph, sphenoid sinus; sps, superior petrosal sinus; SS, sigmoid sinus; TA, lateral process of the atlas; TS, transverse sinus; V2, second division of the trigeminal nerve; V3, third division of the trigeminal nerve; za, zygomatic arch.

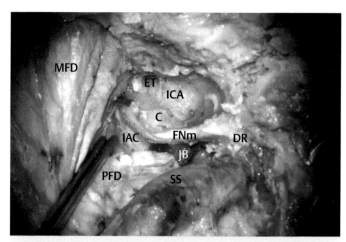

Fig. 9.2 The main difference between the modified transcochlear approach and the transotic approach is the posterior rerouting of the facial nerve. In the following figures, the steps of this procedure will be shown in a right temporal bone. Cochlea (C) is still intact. DR, digastric ridge; ET, eustachian tube; FN(m), mastoid portion of the facial nerve; IAC, internal auditory canal; ICA, internal carotid artery; JB, jugular bulb; MFD, middle fossa dura; PFD, posterior fossa dura; SS, sigmoid sinus.

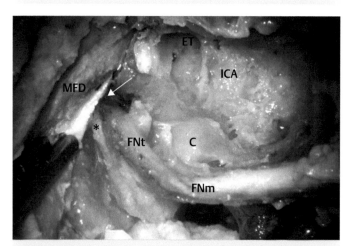

Fig. 9.3 The middle fossa dura (MFD) is elevated to expose the geniculate ganglion area (arrow). The facial nerve has been decompressed and the mastoid (FN[m]), tympanic (FN[t]), and labyrinthine (*) portions are visible. C, cochlea; ET, eustachian tube; ICA, internal carotid artery.

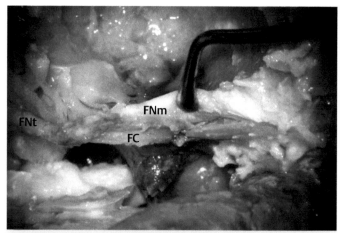

Fig. 9.4 The mastoid portion of the facial nerve (FN[m]) is progressively detached from the fallopian canal (FC). FN(t), tympanic portion of the facial nerve.

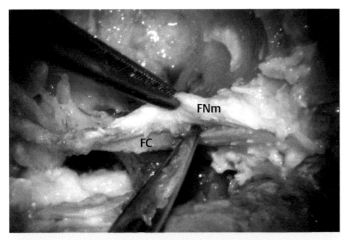

Fig. 9.5 The fibrovascular adhesions between the mastoid segment of the facial nerve (FN[m]) and the fallopian canal (FC) are cut.

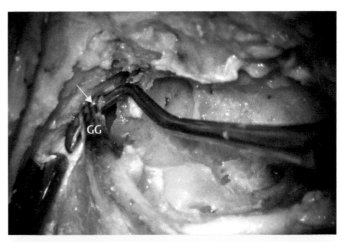

Fig. 9.6 The greater superficial petrosal nerve (*arrow*) is dissected and cut. GG, geniculate ganglion.

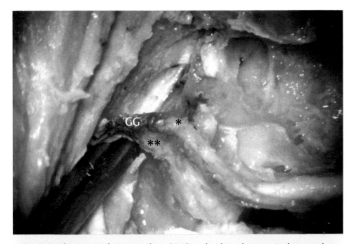

Fig. 9.7 The geniculate ganglion (GG) is displaced posteriorly together with the tympanic portion of the facial nerve (*) and the labyrinthine segment (**).

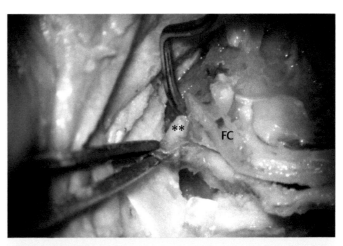

Fig. 9.8 The labyrinthine segment of the facial nerve (**) is dissected. FC, fallopian canal.

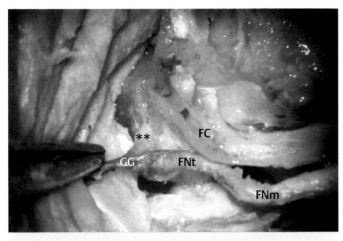

Fig. 9.9 The labyrinthine segment of the facial nerve (**) has been completely dissected. FC, fallopian canal; FN(m), mastoid portion of the facial nerve; FN(t), tympanic portion of the facial nerve; GG, geniculate ganglion.

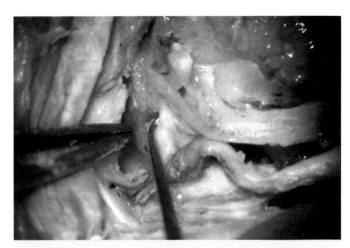

Fig. 9.10 Dissection proceeds to the internal auditory canal.

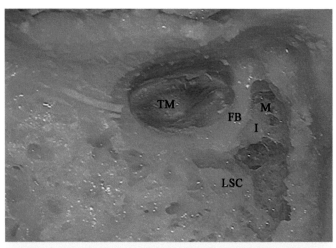

Fig. 9.11 The facial nerve has been posteriorly rerouted from the mastoid (*yellow arrow*) to the internal auditory canal (*red arrow*) segments.

Left Ear

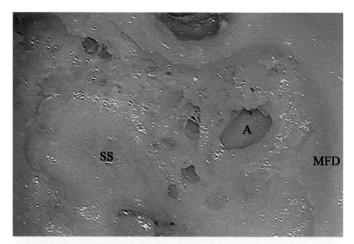

Fig. 9.12 In a left temporal bone, the mastoidectomy has been started and the mastoid antrum (A) has been identified. MFD, level of the middle fossa dura; SS, sigmoid sinus.

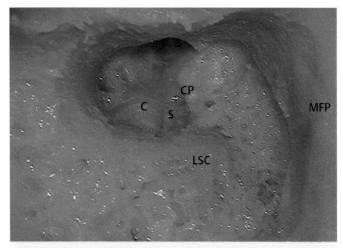

Fig. 9.13 The posterior and superior canal walls have been lowered down to the level of the annulus. FB, facial bridge; I, incus; LSC, lateral semicircular canal; M, malleus; TM, tympanic membrane.

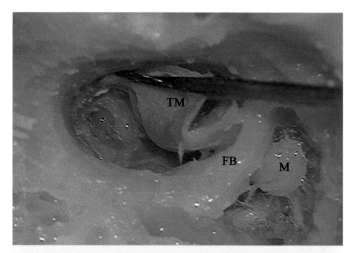

Fig. 9.14 Removal of the incus has been carried out. The tympanic membrane (TM) and malleus (M) are being removed. FB, facial bridge.

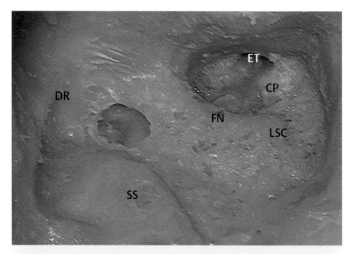

Fig. 9.15 The cavity after removal of the facial bridge. C, basal turn of the cochlea (promontory), CP, cochleariform process; LSC, lateral semicircular canal; MFP, middle fossa plate; S, stapes.

Fig. 9.16 The mastoid segment of the facial nerve (FN) has been identified. CP, cochleariform process; DR, digastric ridge; ET, eustachian tube; LSC, lateral semicircular canal; SS, sigmoid sinus.

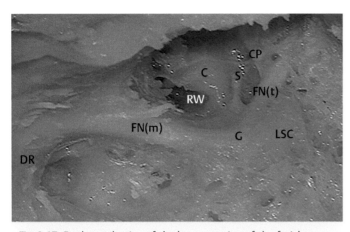

Fig. 9.17 Further reduction of the bony covering of the facial nerve has been carried out. C, basal turn of the cochlea (promontory); CP, cochleariform process; DR, digastric ridge; FN(m), mastoid segment of the facial nerve; FN(t), tympanic segment of the facial nerve; G, genu; LSC, lateral semicircular canal; RW, round window; S, stapes.

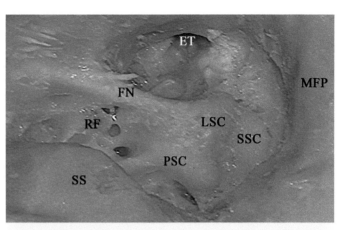

Fig. 9.18 The lateral semicircular canal (LSC), posterior semicircular canal (PSC), and superior semicircular canal (SSC) have been better identified. The retrofacial air cells (RF) are to be drilled away using a diamond burr to complete the skeletonization of the facial nerve (FN). ET, eustachian tube; MFP, middle fossa plate; SS, sigmoid sinus.

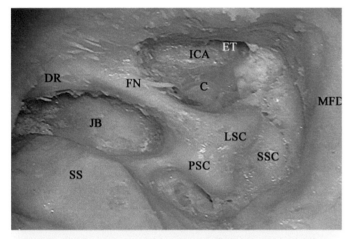

Fig. 9.19 The facial nerve (FN) has been well skeletonized, and the jugular bulb has been identified. The tympanic bone has been partially drilled away and the internal carotid artery (ICA) has been identified. C, basal turn of the cochlea (promontory); DR, digastric ridge; ET, eustachian tube; JB, jugular bulb; LSC, lateral semicircular canal; MFD, middle fossa dura; PSC, posterior semicircular canal; SS, sigmoid sinus; SSC, superior semicircular canal.

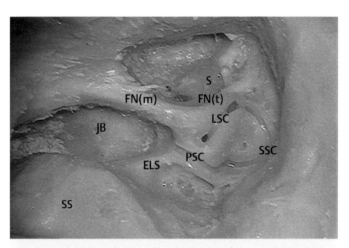

Fig. 9.20 The labyrinthectomy has been started. ELS, endolymphatic sac; FN(m), mastoid segment of the facial nerve; FN(t), tympanic segment of the facial nerve; JB, jugular bulb; LSC, lateral semicircular canal; PSC, posterior semicircular canal; S, stapes; SS, sigmoid sinus; SSC, superior semicircular canal.

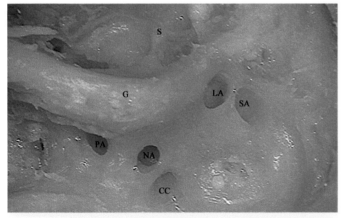

Fig. 9.21 Note the five openings into the vestibule. CC, common crus; G, genu of the facial nerve; LA, ampulla of the lateral canal; NA, nonampullated end of the lateral canal; PA, ampulla of the posterior canal; S, stapes; SA, ampulla of the superior canal.

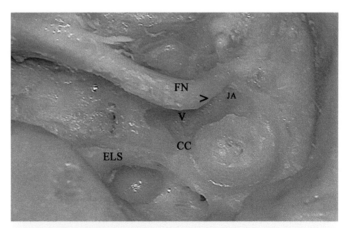

Fig. 9.22 The vestibule (V) has been opened. Note the thin amount of bone (>) separating the genu of the facial nerve (FN) from the vestibule. CC, common crus; ELS, endolymphatic sac; JA, joint lateral and superior ampullae.

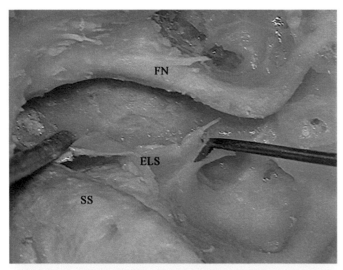

Fig. 9.23 The endolymphatic sac has been cut open and is being dissected away. ELS, endolymphatic sac; FN, facial nerve; SS, sigmoid sinus.

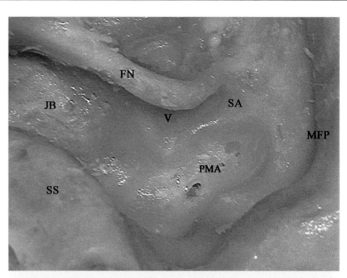

Fig. 9.24 Labyrinthectomy has been completed, and the internal auditory canal is to be identified next. FN, facial nerve; JB, jugular bulb; MFP, middle fossa plate; PMA, perimeatal air cells; SA, ampulla of the superior canal; SS, sigmoid sinus; V, vestibule.

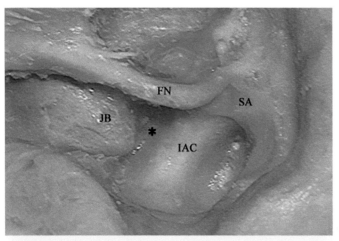

Fig. 9.25 The superior and posterior edges of the internal auditory canal (IAC) have been identified. The bone (*) between the canal and the jugular bulb (JB) is to be removed next. FN, facial nerve; SA, ampulla of the superior canal.

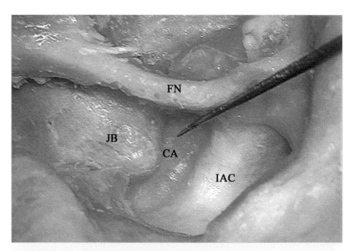

Fig. 9.26 The cochlear aqueduct (CA) has been identified. FN, facial nerve; IAC, internal auditory canal; JB, jugular bulb.

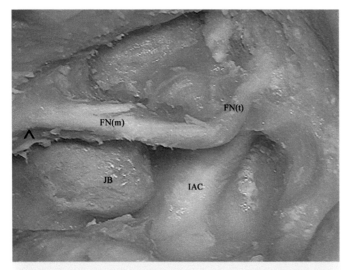

Fig. 9.27 Only a thin shell of bone is left covering the mastoid (FN[m]) and tympanic (FN[t]) segments of the facial nerve. The bone posterior to the facial nerve at the level of the digastric ridge (^) is to be further reduced. IAC, internal auditory canal; JB, jugular bulb.

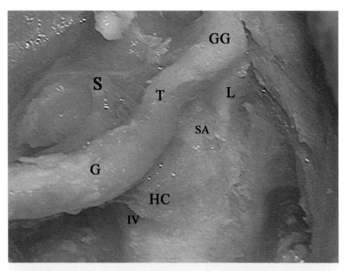

Fig. 9.28 The geniculate ganglion (GG) and labyrinthine segment (L) of the facial nerve have been identified. G, genu; HC, horizontal crest; IV, inferior vestibular nerve; S, stapes; SA, superior ampullary nerve; T, tympanic segment of the facial nerve.

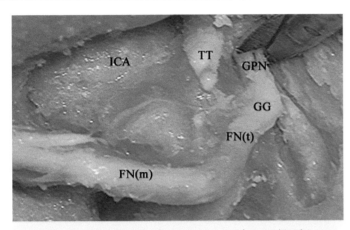

Fig. 9.29 After identification, the greater petrosal nerve (GPN) is now being cut. In live surgery, coagulation of this nerve should take place before it is cut. FN(m), mastoid segment of the facial nerve; FN(t), tympanic segment of the facial nerve; GG, geniculate ganglion; ICA, internal carotid artery; TT, tensor tympani muscle.

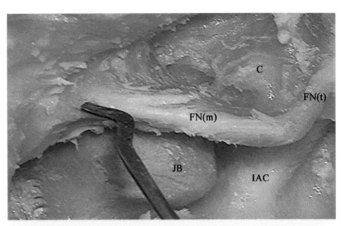

Fig. 9.30 The last shell of bone overlying the mastoid (FN[m]) and tympanic (FN[t]) segments of the facial nerve has been removed. The bone posterior to the facial nerve at the level of the digastric ridge is being removed to prevent injury to the nerve while it is being transposed. C, basal turn of the cochlea (promontory); IAC, internal auditory canal; JB, jugular bulb.

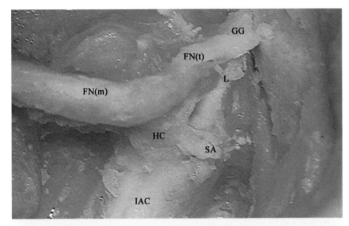

Fig. 9.31 The superior ampullary nerve (SA) has been dislocated from its canal. FN(m), mastoid segment of the facial nerve; FN(t), tympanic segment of the facial nerve; GG, geniculate ganglion; HC, horizontal crest; IAC, internal auditory canal; L, labyrinthine segment of the facial nerve.

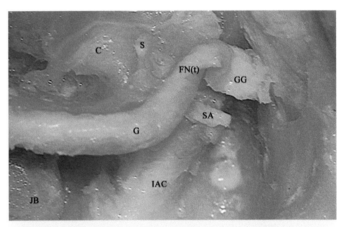

Fig. 9.32 Posterior rerouting of the facial nerve starts by the geniculate ganglion (GG). C, basal turn of the cochlea (promontory); FN(t), tympanic segment of the facial nerve; IAC, internal auditory canal; JB, jugular bulb; S, stapes; SA, superior ampullary nerve.

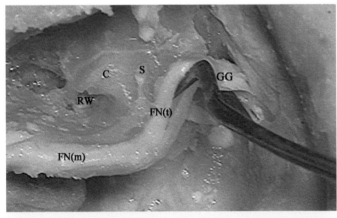

Fig. 9.33 The tympanic segment of the facial nerve (FN[t]) is being dissected from the canal. C, basal turn of the cochlea (promontory); FN(m), mastoid segment of the facial nerve; GG, geniculate ganglion; RW, round window; S, stapes.

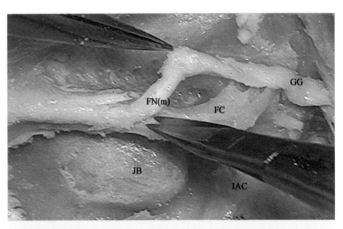

Fig. 9.34 Sharp cutting of the fibrovascular adhesions between the mastoid segment of the facial nerve (FN[m]) and the fallopian canal (FC). GG, geniculate ganglion; IAC, internal auditory canal; JB, jugular bulb.

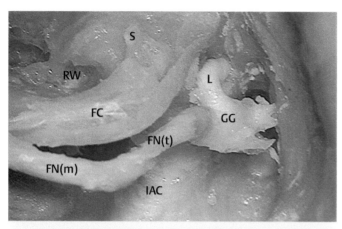

Fig. 9.35 The labyrinthine segment of the facial nerve (L) is being dissected from its canal. FC, fallopian canal; FN(m), mastoid segment of the facial nerve; FN(t), tympanic segment of the facial nerve; GG, geniculate ganglion; IAC, internal auditory canal; RW, round window; S, stapes.

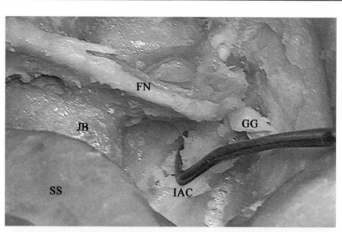

Fig. 9.36 Dislocating the inferior vestibular and cochlear nerves from the fundus. FN, facial nerve; GG, geniculate ganglion; IAC, internal auditory canal; JB, jugular bulb; SS, sigmoid sinus.

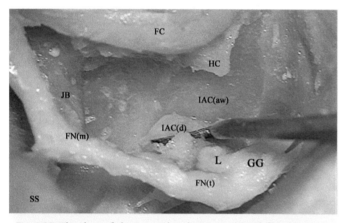

Fig. 9.37 The dura of the internal auditory canal (IAC[d]) is being dissected from the anterior wall of the canal (IAC[aw]). FC, fallopian canal; FN(m), mastoid segment of the facial nerve; FN(t), tympanic segment of the facial nerve; GG, geniculate ganglion; HC, horizontal crest; JB, jugular bulb; L, labyrinthine segment of the facial nerve; SS, sigmoid sinus.

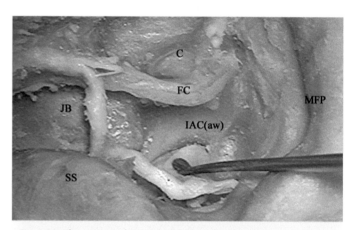

Fig. 9.38 The posteriorly rerouted facial nerve is placed between the jugular bulb (JB) and sigmoid sinus (SS). C, basal turn of the cochlea (promontory); FC, fallopian canal; IAC(aw), anterior wall of the internal auditory canal; MFP, middle fossa plate.

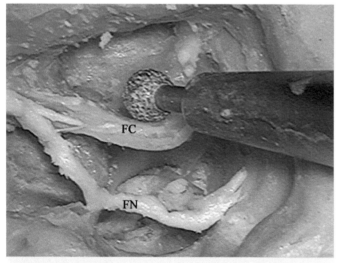

Fig. 9.39 A large diamond drill is used to remove the fallopian canal (FC). FN, facial nerve.

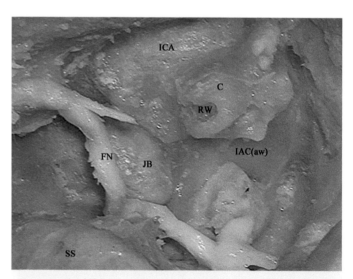

Fig. 9.40 The fallopian canal has been drilled away, and the cochlea (C) is to be removed next. FN, facial nerve; IAC(aw), anterior wall of the internal auditory canal; ICA, internal carotid artery; JB, jugular bulb; RW, round window; SS, sigmoid sinus.

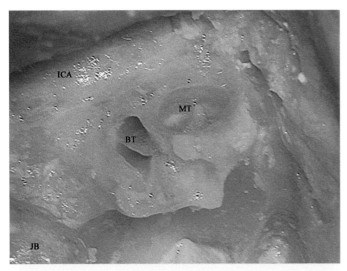

Fig. 9.41 The cochlea has been drilled open, and the basal turn (BT) and middle turn (MT) can be seen. ICA, internal carotid artery; JB, jugular bulb.

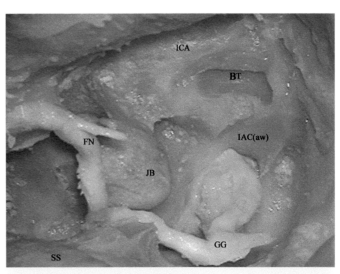

Fig. 9.42 Note the close relationship between the basal turn (BT) and the internal carotid artery (ICA). This part should be carefully removed using a small diamond burr. FN, facial nerve; GG, geniculate ganglion; IAC(aw), anterior wall of the internal auditory canal; JB, jugular bulb; SS, sigmoid sinus.

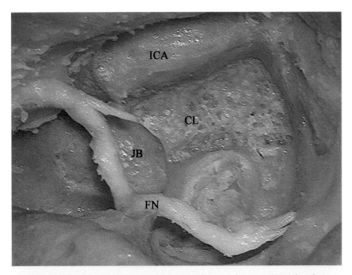

Fig. 9.43 The bone medial to the internal carotid artery (ICA) has been drilled and the clivus bone (CL) has been reached. FN, facial nerve; JB, jugular bulb.

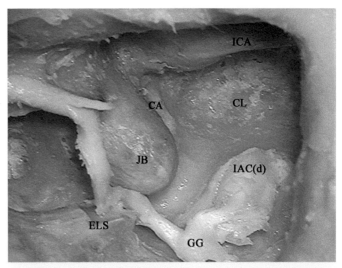

Fig. 9.44 The cochlear aqueduct (CA) can be seen in close relationship to the jugular bulb. CL, clivus; ELS, endolymphatic sac; GG, geniculate ganglion; IAC(d), dura of the internal auditory canal; ICA, internal carotid artery; JB, jugular bulb.

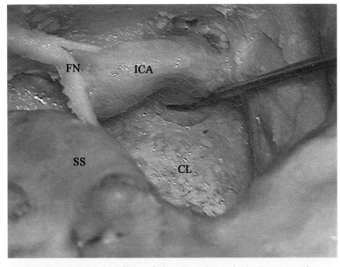

Fig. 9.45 For further drilling of the clivus bone (CL), the internal carotid artery (ICA) can be displaced laterally. FN, facial nerve; SS, sigmoid sinus.

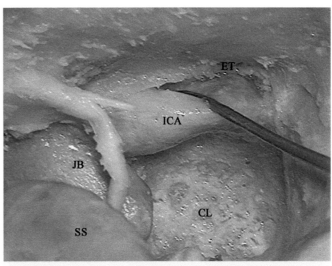

Fig. 9.46 If the bone lateral to the internal carotid artery (ICA) is to be removed, the artery can be displaced medially. CL, clivus; ET, eustachian tube; JB, jugular bulb; SS, sigmoid sinus.

Right Ear

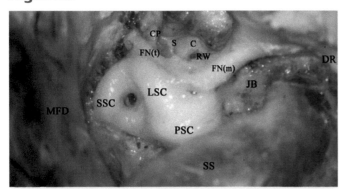

Fig. 9.47 The facial nerve of a right temporal bone has been identified from the stylomastoid foramen at the anterior border of the digastric ridge (DR) as far as the geniculate ganglion at the end of the tympanic segment of the nerve (FN[t]). C, cochlea; CP, cochleariform process; FN(m), mastoid segment of the facial nerve; JB, jugular bulb; LSC, lateral semicircular canal; MFD, middle fossa dura; PSC, posterior semicircular canal; RW, round window; S, stapes; SS, sigmoid sinus; SSC, superior semicircular canal.

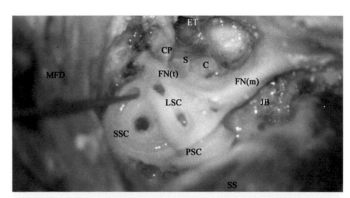

Fig. 9.48 The lateral (LSC), superior (SSC), and posterior (PSC) semicircular canals have been opened. The pointer has been introduced into the ampullae of the superior and lateral canals to show the relationship between these structures and the tympanic segment of the facial nerve (FN[t]). C, cochlea; CP, cochleariform process; ET, eustachian tube; FN(m), mastoid segment of the facial nerve; JB, jugular bulb; MFD, middle fossa dura; S, stapes; SS, sigmoid sinus.

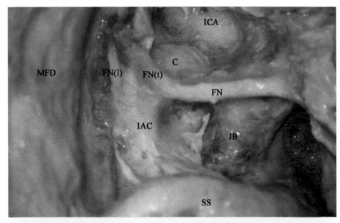

Fig. 9.49 Skeletonization of the whole intratemporal course of the facial nerve has been accomplished. C, cochlea; FN, mastoid segment of the facial nerve; FN(l), labyrinthine segment of the facial nerve; FN(t), tympanic segment of the facial nerve; IAC, internal auditory canal; ICA, internal carotid artery; JB, jugular bulb; MFD, middle fossa dura; SS, sigmoid sinus.

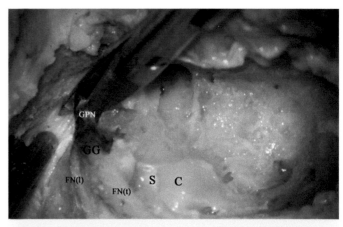

Fig. 9.50 The greater petrosal nerve (GPN) is being sharply cut following coagulation. C, cochlea; FN(l), labyrinthine segment of the facial nerve; FN(t), tympanic segment of the facial nerve; GG, geniculate ganglion; S, stapes.

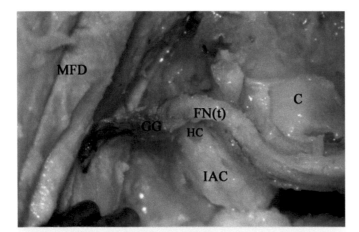

Fig. 9.51 Posterior rerouting is started by the rerouting of the geniculate ganglion (GG). C, cochlea; FN(t), tympanic segment of the facial nerve; HC, horizontal crest; IAC, internal auditory canal; MFD, middle fossa dura.

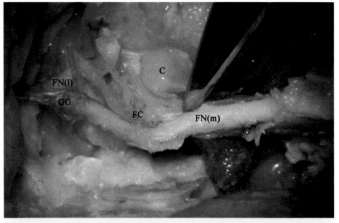

Fig. 9.52 The fibrovascular adhesions between the mastoid segment of the facial nerve (FN[m]) and the fallopian canal (FC) should be sharply cut. C, cochlea; FN(l), labyrinthine segment of the facial nerve; GG, geniculate ganglion.

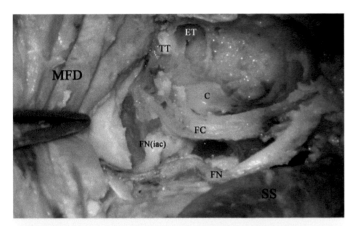

Fig. 9.53 Posterior rerouting of the facial nerve (FN) has been completed. C, cochlea; ET, eustachian tube; FC, fallopian canal; FN(iac), internal auditory canal segment of the facial nerve; MFD, middle fossa dura; SS, sigmoid sinus; TT, tensor tympani.

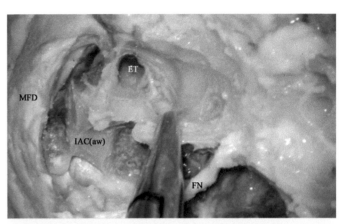

Fig. 9.54 A rongeur is used to remove the fallopian canal. ET, eustachian tube; FN, facial nerve; IAC(aw), anterior wall of the internal auditory canal; MFD, middle fossa dura.

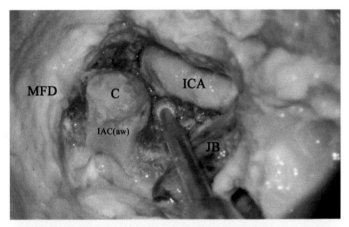

Fig. 9.55 A diamond drill of the appropriate size should be used for the drilling in the angle between the cochlea (C) and the internal carotid artery (ICA). IAC(aw), anterior wall of the internal auditory canal; JB, jugular bulb; MFD, middle fossa dura.

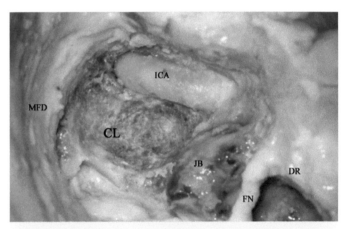

Fig. 9.56 The cochlea has been drilled out. CL, clivus; DR, digastric ridge; FN, facial nerve; ICA, internal carotid artery; JB, jugular bulb; MFD, middle fossa dura.

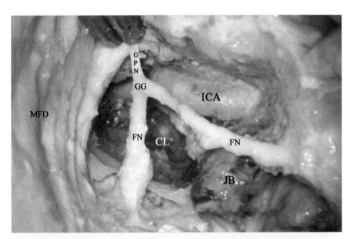

Fig. 9.57 The facial nerve (FN) has been returned into its original position, to compare the space provided by the approach before and after facial nerve rerouting. CL, clivus; GG, geniculate ganglion; GPN, greater petrosal nerve; ICA, internal carotid artery; JB, jugular bulb; MFD, middle fossa dura.

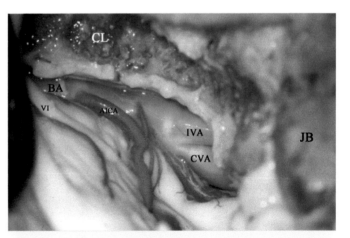

Fig. 9.58 The dura has been opened. Note the optimal control of the prepontine cistern provided by this approach. AICA, anterior inferior cerebellar artery; BA, basilar artery; CL, clivus; CVA, contralateral vertebral artery; IVA, ipsilateral vertebral artery; JB, jugular bulb; VI, Abducens nerve.

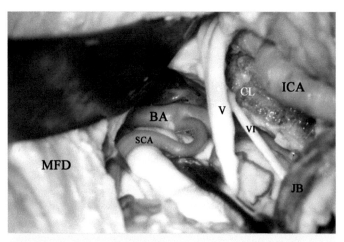

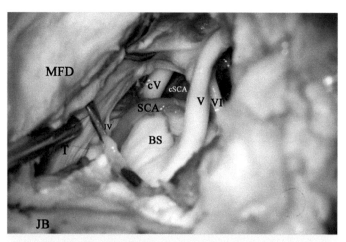

Fig. 9.59 In the upper part of the approach, the superior cerebellar artery (SCA) can be seen as it branches from the basilar artery (BA). CL, clivus; ICA, internal carotid artery; JB, jugular bulb; MFD, middle fossa dura; V, trigeminal nerve; VI, abducens nerve.

Fig. 9.60 The contralateral trigeminal nerve (cV) and contralateral superior cerebellar artery (cSCA), to indicate the excellent control of the prepontine cistern. BS, brainstem; IV, trochlear nerve; JB, jugular bulb; MFD, middle fossa dura; SCA. ipsilateral superior cerebellar artery; T, tentorium; V, ipsilateral trigeminal nerve; VI, abducens nerve.

10 Infratemporal Fossa Approaches

Abstract

The infratemporal fossa approach type A is designed to allow access to the jugular foramen area, the infralabyrinthine and apical compartments of the petrous bone, the vertical segment of the internal carotid artery (ICA), and the upper jugulocarotid space. The infratemporal fossa approach type B is an extralabyrinthine approach which is designed mainly for extradural lesions involving the petrous apex and midclivus.

Keywords: infratemporal fossa approach type A, anterior facial nerve rerouting, transcondylar–transtubercular extension, infratemporal fossa approach type B

10.1 Infratemporal Fossa Approach Type A

This approach is designed to allow access to the jugular foramen area (JF), the infralabyrinthine and apical compartments of the petrous bone, the vertical segment of the ICA, and the upper jugulocarotid space (▶ Fig. 10.1a). The approach is designed primarily for extensive extradural lesions involving these areas. The key point in this approach is the anterior transposition of the facial nerve, which provides optimal control of the infralabyrinthine and JF regions, as well as the vertical portion of the ICA (▶ Fig. 10.1b). The other structures that prevent lateral access to these areas are shown in ▶ Fig. 10.1c. Besides the facial nerve, these include the tympanic bone, the digastric muscle, and the styloid process. These structures are removed to allow unhindered lateral access.

10.1.1 Indications

- Lesions of the jugular foramen:
  - Types C and D paragangliomas (tympanojugular paragangliomas [TJPs]).
  - Lower cranial nerve schwannomas and meningiomas of the JF. However, in majority of these cases, we resort to the petro-occipital transsigmoid approach, with preservation of the middle ear function and without transposing the facial nerve.
- Lesions of the infralabyrinthine and apical compartments of the temporal bone:
  - Infralabyrinthine and some cases of apical cholesteatoma.
  - Lower clivus chordomas.

10.1.2 Surgical Anatomy

- The mastoid segment of the facial nerve is centered on the jugular bulb. In 60% of cases, half or more of the bulb lies anterior to the vertical plane of the nerve (▶ Fig. 10.2).
- When they exit from the skull base, the glossopharyngeal nerve is the most lateral, while the hypoglossal nerve is the most medial. The hypoglossal nerve turns inferiorly to run together with the vagus nerve for a short distance in the upper neck (▶ Fig. 10.3).
- The glossopharyngeal nerve is seen crossing the ICA anteriorly (▶ Fig. 10.3).
- More inferiorly, the hypoglossal nerve crosses the artery to go toward the tongue. The vagus nerve is seen coursing between the internal jugular vein and the ICA (▶ Fig. 10.4). The accessory nerve crosses the lateral surface of the internal jugular vein and travels posteriorly.
- In half of cases, the spinal accessory nerve crosses medial to the internal jugular vein. In all cases, it passes anterolateral to the transverse process of the atlas (▶ Fig. 10.5).
- Note the close relation between the vertebral artery and the internal jugular vein. TJPs with considerable extension into the neck may well involve the artery (▶ Fig. 10.5).
- The styloid process and its muscles separate the external carotid artery laterally from the ICA medially.
- The condylar emissary vein drains into the jugular bulb in 70% of cases, and the vein often has an intimate relation to the lower cranial nerves (X–XI) at their exit from the JF (▶ Fig. 10.6).
- After its origin from the external carotid artery, the occipital artery runs backward, lateral to the internal jugular vein and the accessory nerve in the neck. The ICA angles medially at its ingress into its bony canal at the skull base. The jugular bulb curves laterally before its exit into the neck to form the internal jugular vein (▶ Fig. 10.7).
- ▶ Fig. 10.1c shows the structures passing lateral to the great vessels at the base of the skull: the facial nerve, the styloid process and its attached ligaments and muscles, as well as the posterior belly of the digastric muscle and sternocleidomastoid muscle. For extensive JF tumors extending down to the neck, as in class C TJP, adequate control of this region from the lateral to medial aspect requires these structures to be either sacrificed or transposed.

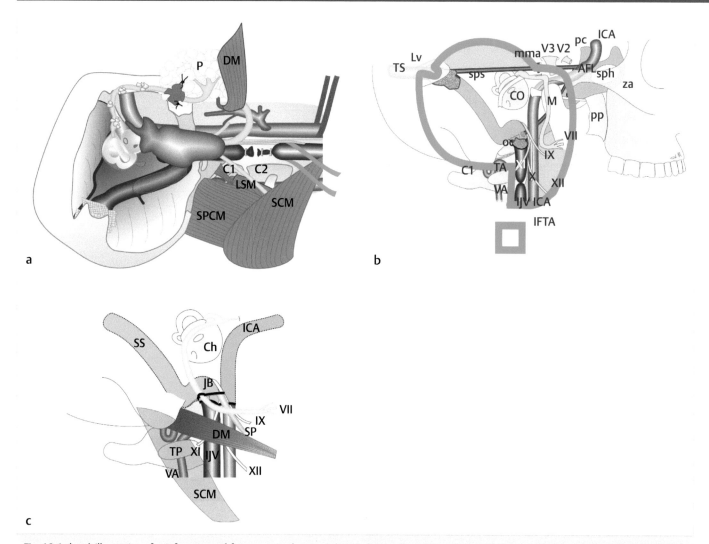

a

b

c

Fig. 10.1 (a–c) Illustrations for infratemporal fossa approach type A (ITFA). (a) An illustration of obstacles to approaching the jugular bulb. (b) An illustration of the surgical limit in ITFA. (c) An illustration of the surgical view in ITFA. AFL, anterior foramen lacerum; C1, atlas; C2, axis; Ch, cochlea; DM, posterior belly of the digastric muscle; ICA, internal carotid artery; IJV, internal jugular vein; JB, jugular bulb; LSM, levator scapulae muscle; Lv, vein of Labbé; mma, middle meningeal artery; M, mandible; OC, occipital condyle; P, parotid gland; pc, clinoid process; pp, pterygoid plate; SCM, sternocleidomastoid muscle; SP, styloid process; SPCM, splenius capitis muscle; sph, sphenoid sinus; sps, superior petrosal sinus; TP, transverse process of the atlas; TS, transverse sinus; V2, maxillary branch of the trigeminal nerve; V3, mandibular branch of the trigeminal nerve; za, zygomatic arch; VA, vertebral artery; VII, facial nerve; IX, glossopharyngeal nerve; XI, spinal accessory nerve; XII, hypoglossal nerve.

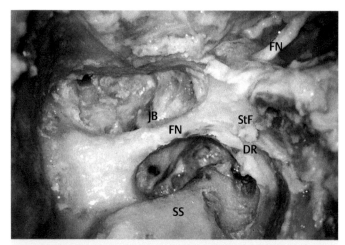

Fig. 10.2 DR, digastric ridge; FN, facial nerve; JB, jugular bulb; SS, sigmoid sinus; StF, stylomastoid foramen.

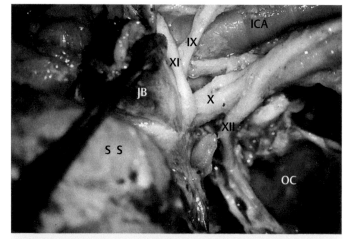

Fig. 10.3 ICA, internal carotid artery; IX, glossopharyngeal nerve; JB, jugular bulb; OC, occipital condyle; SS, sigmoid sinus; X, vagus nerve; XI, spinal accessory nerve; XII, hypoglossal nerve.

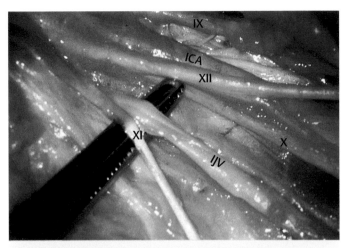

Fig. 10.4 ICA, internal carotid artery; IJV, internal jugular vein; IX, glossopharyngeal nerve; X, vagus nerve; XI, spinal accessory nerve; XII, hypoglossal nerve.

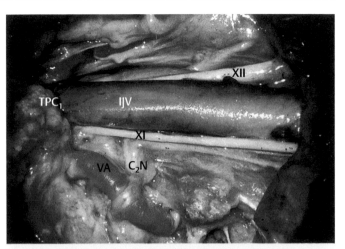

Fig. 10.5 C2N, C2 nerve; IJV, internal jugular vein; TPC1, transverse process of the atlas; VA, vertebral artery; XI, spinal accessory nerve; XII, hypoglossal nerve.

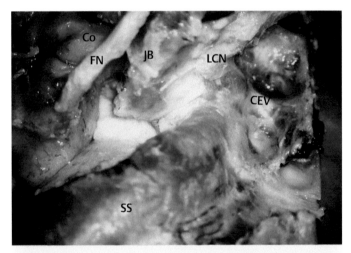

Fig. 10.6 CEV, condylar emissary vein; Co, cochlea; FN, facial nerve; JB, jugular bulb; LCN, lower cranial nerves; SS, sigmoid sinus.

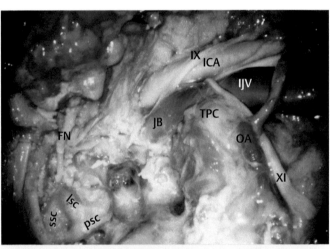

Fig. 10.7 FN, facial nerve; ICA, internal carotid artery; IJV, internal jugular vein; IX, glossopharyngeal nerve; JB, jugular bulb; Isc, lateral semicircular canal; OA, occipital artery; psc, posterior semicircular canal; ssc, superior semicircular canal; TPC, transverse process of the atlas (C1); XI, spinal accessory nerve.

10.1.3 Surgical Steps

Refer to ▶ Fig. 10.8, ▶ Fig. 10.9, ▶ Fig. 10.10, ▶ Fig. 10.11, ▶ Fig. 10.12, ▶ Fig. 10.13, ▶ Fig. 10.14, ▶ Fig. 10.15, ▶ Fig. 10.16, ▶ Fig. 10.17, ▶ Fig. 10.18, ▶ Fig. 10.19, ▶ Fig. 10.20, ▶ Fig. 10.21, ▶ Fig. 10.22, ▶ Fig. 10.23, ▶ Fig. 10.24, ▶ Fig. 10.25, ▶ Fig. 10.26, ▶ Fig. 10.27, ▶ Fig. 10.28, ▶ Fig. 10.29, ▶ Fig. 10.30, ▶ Fig. 10.31, ▶ Fig. 10.32.

1. A postauricular skin incision is made.
2. A small, anteriorly based musculoperiosteal flap is elevated to help in closure afterward. The external auditory canal is transected as before.
3. The facial nerve is identified at its exit from the temporal bone. The main trunk is found at the perpendicular bisection of a line joining the cartilaginous pointer to the mastoid tip. The main trunk is traced in the parotid until the proximal parts of the temporal and zygomatic branches are identified.
4. The posterior belly of the digastric muscle and the sternocleidomastoid muscle are divided close to their origin. The internal jugular vein and the external and internal carotid arteries are identified in the neck. The vessels are marked with vessel loops.

5. The skin of the external auditory canal, the tympanic membrane, the malleus, and incus is removed.
6. A canal wall–down mastoidectomy is performed, with removal of the bone anterior and posterior to the sigmoid sinus. The facial nerve is skeletonized from the stylomastoid foramen to the geniculate ganglion. The last shell of bone is removed using a double-curved raspatory. The suprastructure of the stapes is preferably removed after cutting its crura with microscissors.
7. The inferior tympanic bone is widely removed, and the mastoid tip is amputated using a rongeur. A new bony canal is drilled in the root of the zygoma superior to the eustachian tube.
8. The facial nerve is freed at the level of the stylomastoid foramen using strong scissors. The soft tissues at this level are not separated from the nerve.
9. The mastoid segment is next elevated using a Beaver knife to cut the fibrous attachments between the nerve and the fallopian canal. The tympanic segment of the nerve is elevated carefully, using a curved raspatory, until the level of the

geniculate ganglion is reached. A nontoothed forceps is used to hold the soft tissue surrounding the nerve at the stylomastoid foramen, and anterior rerouting is carried out.

10. A tunnel is created in the parotid gland to lodge the transposed nerve. The tunnel is closed around the nerve using two sutures. The nerve is then fixed to the new bony canal, just superior to the eustachian tube, using fibrin glue.

11. Drilling of the infralabyrinthine cells is completed, and the vertical portion of the ICA is identified.

12. The mandibular condyle is separated from the anterior wall of the external auditory canal using a large septal raspatory. The Fisch infratemporal fossa retractor is applied, and the mandibular condyle is anteriorly displaced, with care being taken not to injure the facial nerve. The anterior wall of the external auditory canal is further drilled, thus completing the exposure of the vertical portion of the ICA. A small incision is made in the posterior fossa dura just behind the sigmoid sinus, through which an aneurysm needle is passed. Another incision is made just anterior to the sinus to allow for the exit of the needle.

13. The sinus is closed by double ligation with a Vicryl suture. Suture closure of the sinus, however, may lead to gaps in the dural incision, with a higher risk of cerebrospinal fluid (CSF) leakage postoperatively. Alternatively, the sigmoid sinus can be closed with extraluminal Surgicel packing.

14. The structures attached to the styloid process are severed. The styloid is fractured using a rongeur, and is then cut with strong scissors.

15. The remaining tough fibrous tissue surrounding the ICA at its ingress into the skull base is carefully removed using scissors.

16. The internal jugular vein in the neck is double ligated and cut or closed with vascular clips (the easier and faster method).

17. The vein is elevated superiorly, with care being taken not to injure the related lower cranial nerves. In cases in which the eleventh nerve passes laterally, the vein has to be pulled under the nerve carefully to prevent it from being damaged.

18. If necessary, the lateral wall of the sigmoid sinus can be removed. Removal continues down to the level of the jugular bulb.

19. The lateral wall of the jugular bulb is opened. Bleeding usually occurs from the apertures of the inferior petrosal sinus and the condylar emissary vein. This is controlled with Surgicel packing.

20. If there is limited intradural extension, the dura is opened without injury to the endolymphatic sac.

21. At the end of the procedure, the eustachian tube is closed with a piece of muscle. The dural opening is closed with a muscle plug or with only abdominal fat. We never use a rotated temporalis muscle flap (as suggested by Fisch), so as to avoid aesthetic problems, but the sternocleidomastoid muscle and the digastric muscle are sutured together and the temporalis muscle is left in its place.

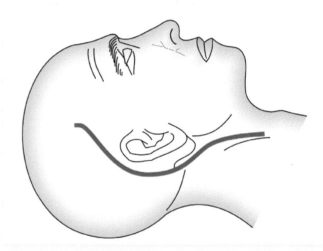

Fig. 10.8 Incision for infratemporal fossa approach type A.

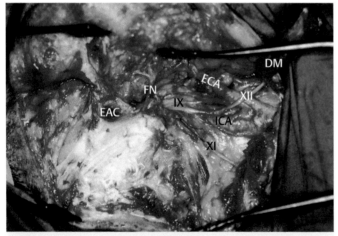

Fig. 10.9 The posterior belly of the digastric muscle and the sternocleidomastoid muscle are divided close to their origin. The internal jugular vein and the external and internal carotid arteries are identified in the neck. DM, digastric muscle; EAC, external auditory canal; ECA, external carotid artery; FN, facial nerve; ICA, internal carotid artery; IX, glossopharyngeal nerve; XI, spinal accessory nerve; XII, hypoglossal nerve.

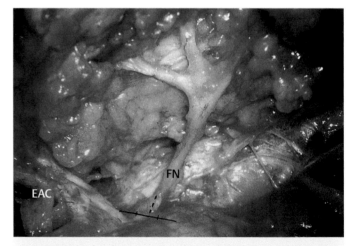

Fig. 10.10 The facial nerve is identified at its exit from the temporal bone. EAC, external auditory canal; FN, facial nerve.

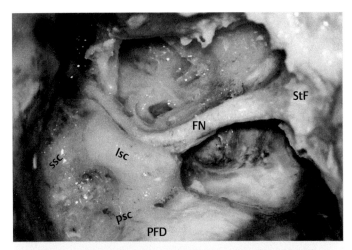

Fig. 10.11 A canal wall–down mastoidectomy is performed, with removal of the bone anterior and posterior to the sigmoid sinus. The facial nerve is decompressed from the stylomastoid foramen to the geniculate ganglion. FN, facial nerve; lsc, lateral semicircular canal; PFD, posterior fossa dura; psc, posterior semicircular canal; ssc, superior semicircular canal; StF, stylomastoid foramen.

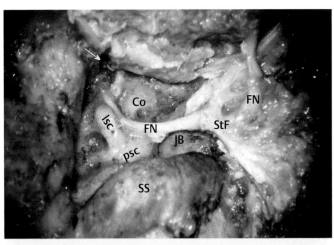

Fig. 10.12 The inferior tympanic bone is widely removed, and the mastoid tip is amputated using a rongeur. A new bony canal (*arrow*) is drilled in the root of the zygoma superior to the eustachian tube. Co, cochlea; FN, facial nerve; JB, jugular bulb; lsc, lateral semicircular canal; PFD, posterior fossa dura; psc, posterior semicircular canal; StF, stylomastoid foramen.

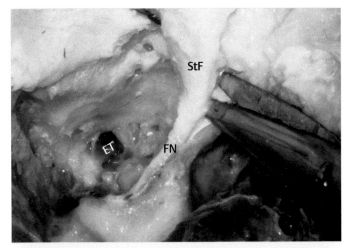

Fig. 10.13 The facial nerve is freed at the level of the stylomastoid foramen using strong scissors. The soft tissues at this level are not separated from the nerve. ET, eustachian tube; FN, facial nerve; StF, stylomastoid foramen.

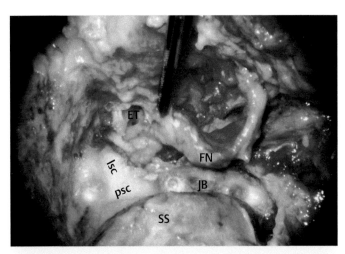

Fig. 10.14 The facial nerve is freed at the level of the stylomastoid foramen using strong scissors. The soft tissues at this level are not separated from the nerve. ET, eustachian tube; FN, facial nerve; StF, stylomastoid foramen.

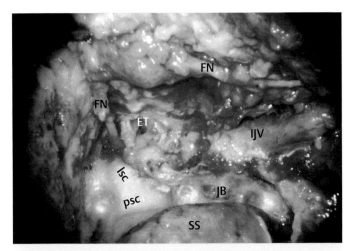

Fig. 10.15 A tunnel is created in the parotid gland to lodge the transposed nerve. ET, eustachian tube; FN, facial nerve; IJV, internal jugular vein; JB, jugular bulb; lsc, lateral semicircular canal; psc, posterior semicircular canal; SS, sigmoid sinus.

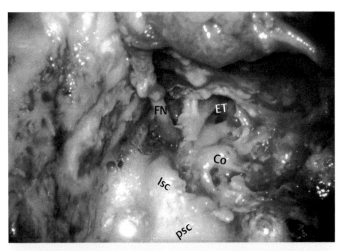

Fig. 10.16 The facial nerve is in its new bony canal, just superior to the eustachian tube. The nerve is fixed to the new bony canal using fibrin glue. Co, cochlea; ET, eustachian tube; FN, facial nerve; lsc, lateral semicircular canal; psc, posterior semicircular canal.

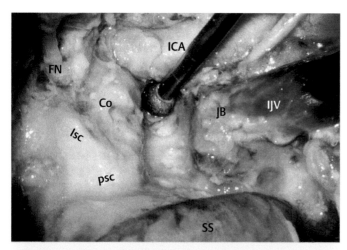

Fig. 10.17 Drilling of the infralabyrinthine cells is completed, and the vertical portion of the ICA is identified. Co, cochlea; FN, facial nerve; ICA, internal carotid artery; IJV, internal jugular vein; JB, jugular bulb; lsc, lateral semicircular canal; psc, posterior semicircular canal; SS, sigmoid sinus.

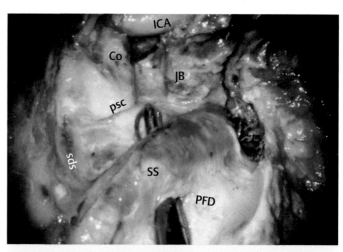

Fig. 10.18 Closure of the sigmoid sinus (SS) is starting. Up to now we prefer extraluminal packing of the SS with Surgicel instead of ligation to avoid CSF leakage from the posterior fossa dura. Co, cochlea; ICA, internal carotid artery; JB, jugular bulb; PFD, posterior fossa dura; psc, posterior semicircular canal; sps, superior petrosal sinus.

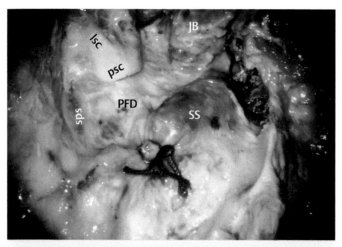

Fig. 10.19 The sigmoid sinus is closed by double ligation with a Vicryl suture. JB, jugular bulb; lsc, lateral semicircular canal; PFD, posterior fossa dura; psc, posterior semicircular canal; sps, superior petrosal sinus; SS, sigmoid sinus.

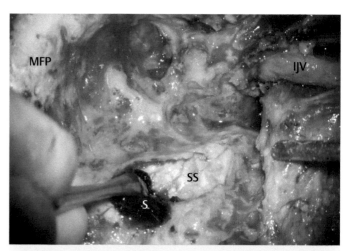

Fig. 10.20 Surgical view. This is the technique of extraluminal closure of the sigmoid sinus to avoid the risk of CSF leakage with suture of the sigmoid sinus. IJV, internal jugular vein; MFD, middle fossa plate; S, Surgicel; SS, sigmoid sinus.

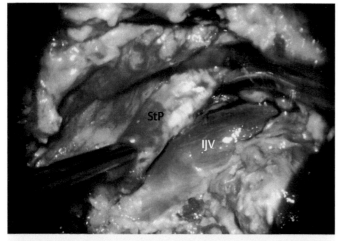

Fig. 10.21 The structures attached to the styloid process are severed. The styloid is fractured using a rongeur, and is then cut with strong scissors. IJV, internal jugular vein; StP, styloid process.

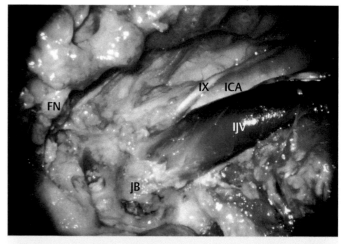

Fig. 10.22 After removal of the styloid process the internal carotid artery (ICA) could be controlled from the neck to its entrance at the base of the skull. FN, facial nerve; IJV, internal jugular vein; JB, jugular bulb; IX, glossopharyngeal nerve.

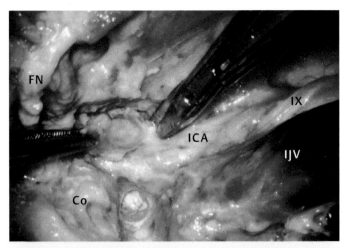

Fig. 10.23 The remaining tough fibrous tissue surrounding the ICA at its ingress into the skull base is carefully removed using scissors. Co, cochlea; FN, facial nerve; ICA, internal carotid artery; IJV, internal jugular vein; IX, glossopharyngeal nerve.

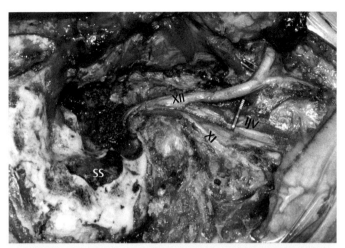

Fig. 10.24 Surgical view. The internal jugular vein in the neck is double ligated and cut or closed with vascular clips. IJV, internal jugular vein; SS, sigmoid sinus; XI, spinal accessory nerve; XII, hypoglossal nerve.

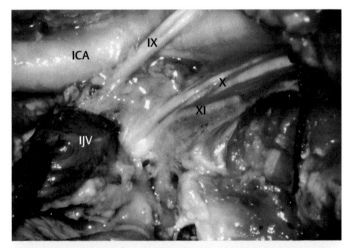

Fig. 10.25 The vein is elevated superiorly, with care being taken not to injure the related lower cranial nerves. ICA, internal carotid artery; IJV, internal jugular vein; IX, glossopharyngeal nerve; X, vagus nerve; XI, accessory nerve.

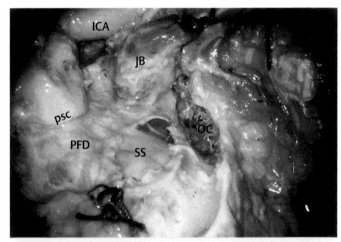

Fig. 10.26 If necessary, the lateral wall of the sigmoid sinus can be removed. Removal continues down to the level of the jugular bulb. ICA, internal carotid artery; JB, jugular bulb; OC, occipital condyle; PFD, posterior fossa dura; psc, posterior semicircular canal; SS, sigmoid sinus.

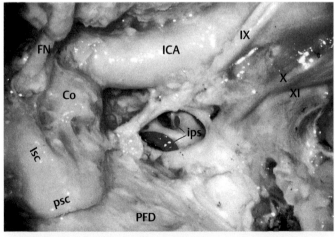

Fig. 10.27 The lateral wall of the jugular bulb is opened. Bleeding usually occurs from the apertures of the inferior petrosal sinus and the condylar emissary vein. This is controlled with Surgicel packing. Co, cochlea; FN, facial nerve; ICA, internal carotid artery; ips, inferior petrosal sinus; lsc, lateral semicircular canal; PFD, posterior fossa dura; psc, posterior semicircular canal; IX, glossopharyngeal nerve; X, vagus nerve; XI, accessory nerve.

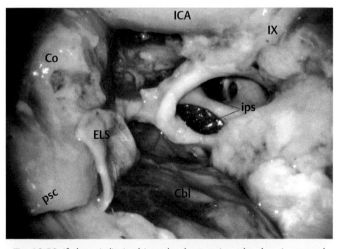

Fig. 10.28 If there is limited intradural extension, the dura is opened without injury to the endolymphatic sac. Cbl, cerebellum; Co, cochlea; ELS, endolymphatic sac; ICA, internal carotid artery; ips, inferior petrosal sinus; psc, posterior semicircular canal; IX, glossopharyngeal nerve.

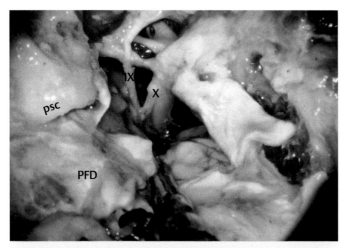

Fig. 10.29 View of the intradural space after opening of the posterior fossa dura. The glossopharyngeal and vagus nerves are well identified in the cerebellomedullary cistern before entering the jugular foramen. PFD, posterior fossa dura; psc, posterior semicircular canal; IX, glossopharyngeal nerve; X, vagus nerve.

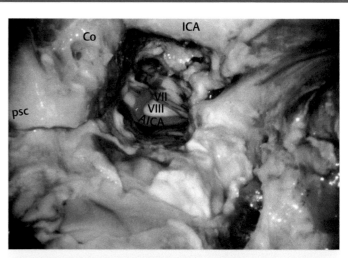

Fig. 10.30 The facial and vestibulocochlear nerves and the anterior inferior cerebellar artery are visible. AICA, anterior inferior cerebellar artery; Co, cochlea; ICA, internal carotid artery; psc, posterior semicircular canal; VII, facial nerve; VIII, vestibulocochlear nerve.

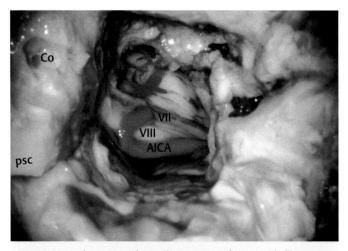

Fig. 10.31 A closer view shows the anterior inferior cerebellar artery passing between the seventh and eighth nerves. AICA, anterior inferior cerebellar artery; Co, cochlea; psc, posterior semicircular canal; VII, facial nerve; VIII, vestibulocochlear nerve.

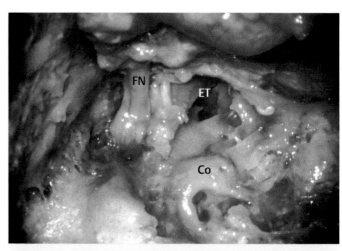

Fig. 10.32 The eustachian tube (ET) and the rerouted facial nerve (FN) are visible. Co, cochlea.

10.1.4 Transcondylar–Transtubercular Extension of the Infratemporal Fossa Type A Approach

The classic infratemporal fossa approach type A of Fisch permits only superior and anterior exposure of the jugular bulb and is indicated for TJPs class C1 and certain class C2. For larger tumor such as class C2, C3, and C4 tumors involving the lower cranial nerves, a transcondylar–transtubercular extension is required in addition to the classic ITFA. This extension facilitates inferomedial access to the jugular bulb above the lateral mass of the atlas and occipital condyle. This is shown in ▶ Fig. 10.33, ▶ Fig. 10.34, ▶ Fig. 10.35, ▶ Fig. 10.36, ▶ Fig. 10.37, ▶ Fig. 10.38, ▶ Fig. 10.39, ▶ Fig. 10.40, ▶ Fig. 10.41.

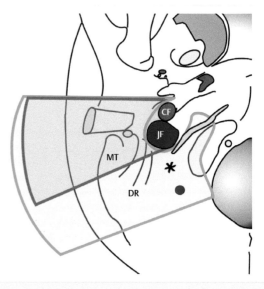

Fig. 10.33 Comparison of classic ITFA (zone delimited by the red line) and ITFA with transcondylar–transtubercular extension (zone delimited by the blue line). *, jugular process of the occipital condyle; CF, carotid foramen; DR, digastric ridge; JF, jugular foramen; MT, mastoid tip.

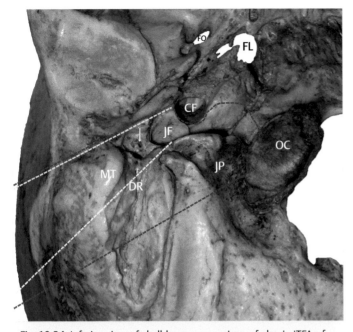

Fig. 10.34 Inferior view of skull base, comparison of classic ITFA of Fisch and modified ITFA with transcondylar–transtubercular extension. In addition to removal of bone in classic ITFA of Fisch, drilling of the jugular process of the occipital bone and even some of the occipital condyle facilitates control of the area of the jugular bulb. Arrow, stylomastoid foramen; blue dashed line, modified ITFA with transcondylar–transtubercular extension; CF, carotid foramen; DR, digastric ridge; FL, foramen lacerum; FO, foramen ovale; JF, jugular foramen; JP, jugular process of the occipital bone; MT, mastoid tip; OC, occipital condyle; Yellow dashed line, classic ITFA of Fisch.

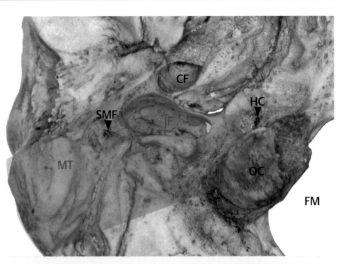

Fig. 10.35 At higher magnified view, note the amount of the bone removed in ITFA with transcondylar–transtubercular approach. CF, carotid foramen; FM, foramen magnum; HC, hypoglossal canal; JF, jugular foramen; MT, mastoid tip; OC, occipital condyle; SMF, stylomastoid foramen.

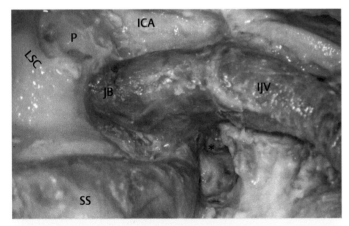

Fig. 10.36 The jugular process and the portion of the occipital condyle have been drilled out. The left occipital condyle is identified below the jugular bulb and posterior to the internal jugular vein. *, occipital condyle; ICA, internal carotid artery; IJV, internal jugular vein; JB, jugular bulb; LSC, lateral semicircular canal; P, promontory; SS, sigmoid sinus.

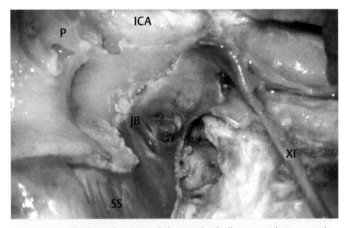

Fig. 10.37 The lateral aspect of the jugular bulb, sigmoid sinus, and internal jugular vein has been removed. On the medial wall of the jugular bulb the inferior petrosal sinus is identified. The opening of the posterior condylar vein is seen. *, occipital condyle; ICA, internal carotid artery; JB, jugular bulb; P, promontory; SS, sigmoid sinus.

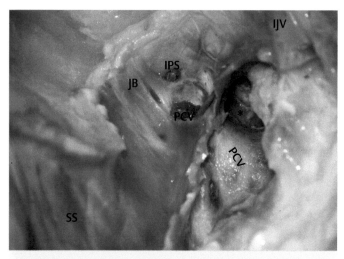

Fig. 10.38 Closer view. *, occipital condyle; IJV, internal jugular vein; IPS, inferior petrosal sinus; JB, jugular vein; PCV, posterior condylar vein; SS, sigmoid sinus.

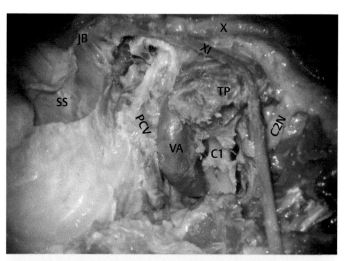

Fig. 10.39 Note the relationship among the sigmoid sinus, jugular bulb, posterior condylar vein, vertebral artery, and lower cranial nerves. C1, atlas; C2N, C2 nerve; JB, jugular bulb; PCV, posterior condylar vein; SS, sigmoid sinus; TP, transverse process of C1; VA, vertebral artery; X, vagus nerve; XI, spinal accessory nerve.

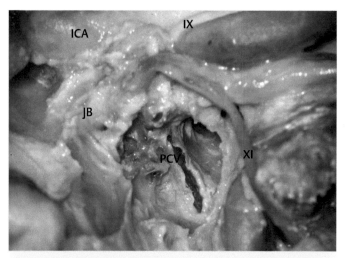

Fig. 10.40 The posterior condylar vein crossing the occipital condyle is noted. ICA, internal carotid artery; JB, jugular bulb; PCV, posterior condylar vein; IX, glossopharyngeal nerve; XI, spinal accessory nerve.

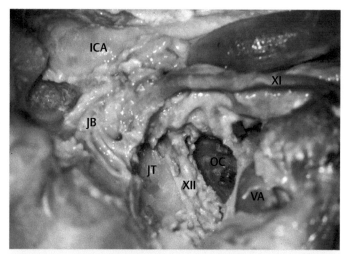

Fig. 10.41 After removal of the posterior condylar vein and further removal of the occipital condyle (OC), the hypoglossal nerve (XII) is noted. ICA, internal carotid artery; JB, jugular bulb; JT, jugular tubercle; VA, vertebral artery; XI, spinal accessory nerve; XII, hypoglossal nerve.

Left Ear

Refer to ▸ Fig. 10.42, ▸ Fig. 10.43, ▸ Fig. 10.44, ▸ Fig. 10.45, ▸ Fig. 10.46, ▸ Fig. 10.47, ▸ Fig. 10.48, ▸ Fig. 10.49, ▸ Fig. 10.50, ▸ Fig. 10.51, ▸ Fig. 10.52, ▸ Fig. 10.53, ▸ Fig. 10.54, ▸ Fig. 10.55, ▸ Fig. 10.56, ▸ Fig. 10.57, ▸ Fig. 10.58, ▸ Fig. 10.59, ▸ Fig. 10.60, ▸ Fig. 10.61, ▸ Fig. 10.62, ▸ Fig. 10.63, ▸ Fig. 10.64, ▸ Fig. 10.65, ▸ Fig. 10.66, ▸ Fig. 10.67, ▸ Fig. 10.68, ▸ Fig. 10.69, ▸ Fig. 10.70, ▸ Fig. 10.71, ▸ Fig. 10.72, ▸ Fig. 10.73, ▸ Fig. 10.74, ▸ Fig. 10.75, ▸ Fig. 10.76, ▸ Fig. 10.77, ▸ Fig. 10.78.

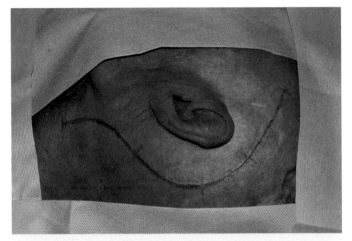

Fig. 10.42 Craniotemporal–cervical incision is made.

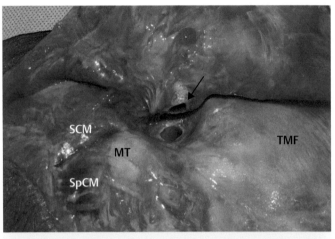

Fig. 10.43 The external auditory canal (*arrow*) is transected for further blind-sac closure. MT, mastoid tip; TMF, temporalis muscle fascia; SCM, sternocleidomastoid muscle; SpCM, splenius capitis muscle.

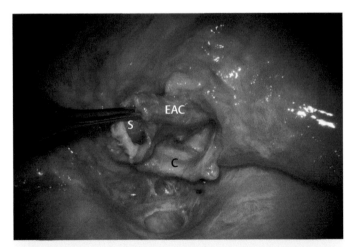

Fig. 10.44 Microscopic view. The skin (S) and soft tissues of the external auditory canal (EAC) are dissected from the underlying cartilage (C).

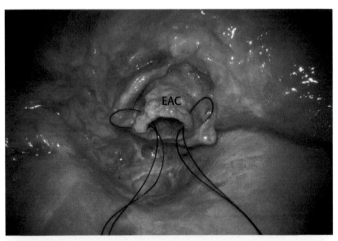

Fig. 10.45 The external auditory canal has been dissected form the cartilage. Two silk sutures are placed on the corners of the EAC to allow complete eversion of the skin.

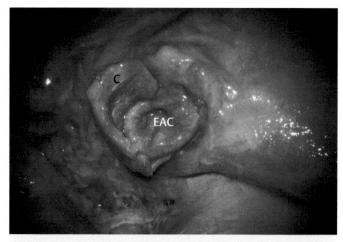

Fig. 10.46 The external auditory canal (EAC) has been completely everted and no skin can be seen on its medial surface. C, cartilage.

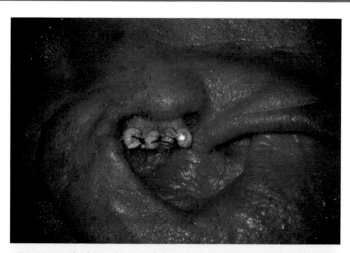

Fig. 10.47 Blind-sac closure of the external auditory canal starts with the skin layer.

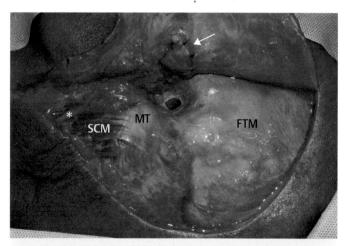

Fig. 10.48 Blind-sac closure of the external auditory canal ends with the suture of the cartilage layer (*arrow*). This is very important is case of cerebrospinal fluid leakage. *, greater auricular nerve; FTM, fascia of the temporalis muscle; MT, mastoid tip; SCM, sternocleidomastoid muscle.

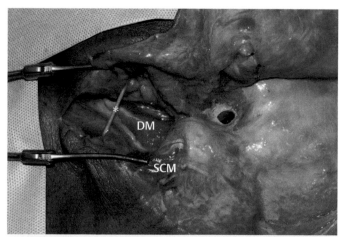

Fig. 10.49 The sternocleidomastoid muscle (SCM) is retracted posteriorly to show the posterior belly of the digastric muscle (DM). *, greater auricular nerve.

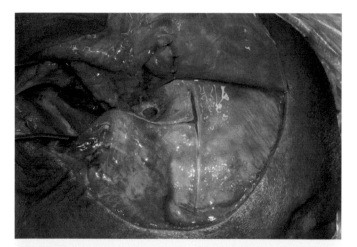

Fig. 10.50 A T-shape musculoperiosteal flap is performed.

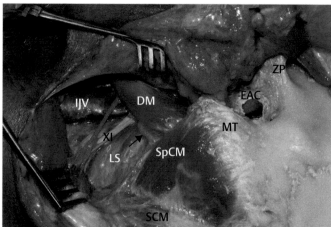

Fig. 10.51 Closer view. Arrow, occipital artey; DM, posterior belly of the digastric muscle; EAC, external auditory canal; IJV, internal jugular vein; LS, levator scapulae muscle; MT, mastoid tip; SCM, sternocleidomastoid muscle (cut and posteriorly retracted); SpCM, splenius capitis muscle; XI, spinal accessory nerve; ZP, zygomatic process.

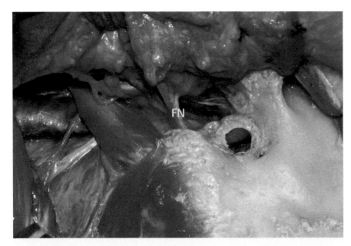

Fig. 10.52 The main trunk of the extratemporal facial nerve (FN) is identified at its exit from the temporal bone.

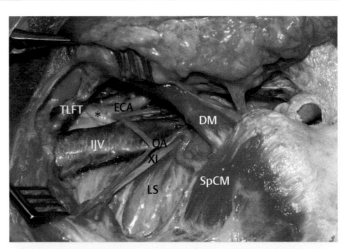

Fig. 10.53 The posterior belly of the digastric muscle is further retracted anteriorly. The internal jugular vein (IJV), external carotid artery (ECA), hypoglossal nerve (*), occipital artery (OA), and spinal accessory nerve (XI) can be seen. LS, levator scapulae muscle; SpCM, splenius capitis muscle TLFT, thyrolinguofacial venous trunk.

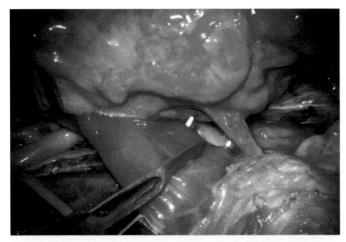

Fig. 10.54 The posterior belly of the digastric muscle (DM) is cut.

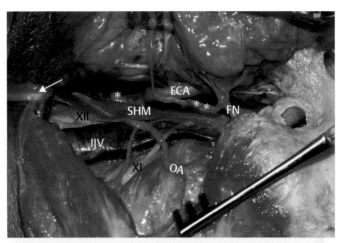

Fig. 10.55 The posterior belly of the digastric muscle has been cut and retracted inferiorly (arrow). * facial artery; **, stylomastoid artery; ECA, external carotid artery; FN, facial nerve (main trunk); IJV, internal jugular vein; OA, occipital artery; SHM, stylohyoid muscle; XI, spinal accessory nerve; XII, hypoglossal nerve.

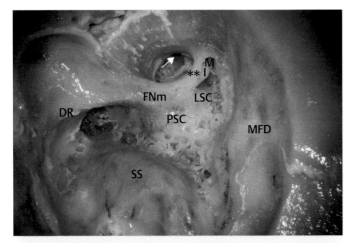

Fig. 10.56 Mastoidectomy has been performed. All the skin of the external auditory canal, tympanic membrane, and ossicles should be removed. **, posterior canal wall (facial bridge); arrow, eustachian tube; DR, digastric ridge; FN(m), mastoid portion of the facial nerve; I, incus; LSC, lateral semicircular canal; M, malleus; MFD, middle fossa dura; PSC, posterior semicircular canal; SS, sigmoid sinus.

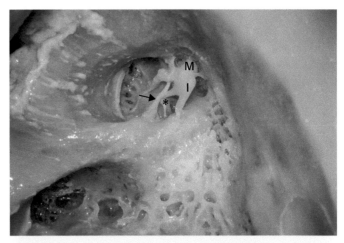

Fig. 10.57 Closer view. The posterior canal wall has been removed, exposing the ossicles. *, stapes; arrow, chorda tympani; I, incus; M, malleus.

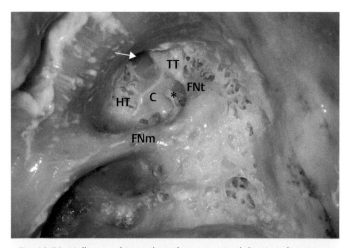

Fig. 10.58 Malleus and incus have been removed, leaving the stapes. The facial nerve is starting to be decompressed. Arrow, eustachian tube; C, cochlea (promontory); FN(m), mastoid portion of the facial nerve; FN(t), tympanic portion of the facial nerve; HT, hypotympanum; LSC, lateral semicircular canal; TT, tensor tympani muscle with cochleariform process.

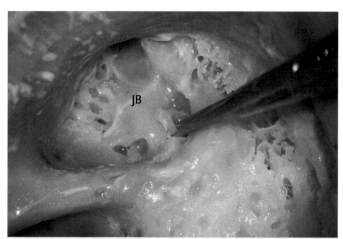

Fig. 10.59 The stapes superstructure is removed. JB, Jacobson's nerve.

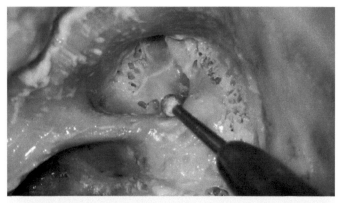

Fig. 10.60 The facial nerve is decompressed.

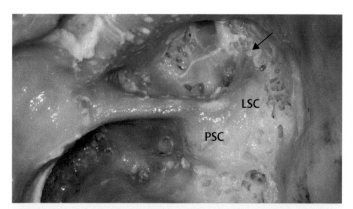

Fig. 10.61 Decompression of the mastoid and tympanic portions of the facial nerve has been performed. Further bone removal has to be performed in the area of the geniculate ganglion (arrow). LSC, lateral semicircular canal; PSC, posterior semicircular canal.

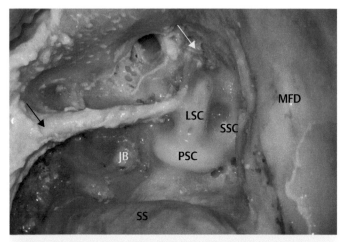

Fig. 10.62 Decompression of the facial nerve has been performed from the area of the stylomastoid foramen (black arrow) to the area of the geniculate ganglion (yellow arrow). All the semicircular canals have been skeletonized, as well as the jugular bulb (JB). LSC, lateral semicircular canal; MFD, middle fossa dura; PSC, posterior semicircular canal; SSC, superior semicircular canal; SS, sigmoid sinus.

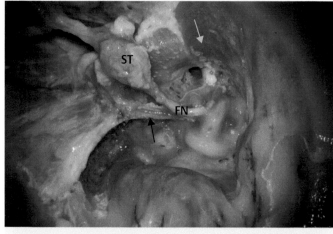

Fig. 10.63 Anterior rerouting of the facial nerve (FN) is starting. A new bony canal (green arrow) is drilled in the root of the zygoma superior to the eustachian tube. The soft tissues (ST) at the level of the stylomastoid foramen are not separated from the nerve. Note that the bone of the fallopian canal under the facial nerve has not been drilled yet (black arrow).

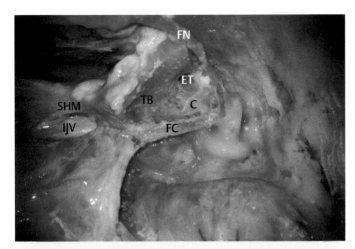

Fig. 10.64 Anterior rerouting of the facial nerve (FN) has been completed. The facial nerve is in its new bony canal, just superior to the eustachian tube (ET). In live surgery, the nerve is fixed to the new bony canal using fibrin glue. C, cochlea (promontory); FC, fallopian canal; IJV, internal jugular vein; SHM, stylohyoid muscle; TB, tympanic bone.

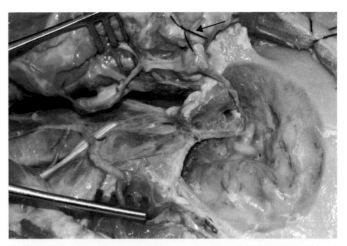

Fig. 10.65 A tunnel is also created in the parotid gland to lodge the transposed nerve, which is fixed with a suture (*arrow*).

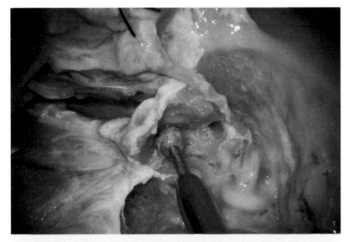

Fig. 10.66 Drilling of the anterior and inferior tympanic bone continues. This is a very important step to get complete control of the jugular foramen area and the vertical portion of the petrous internal carotid artery.

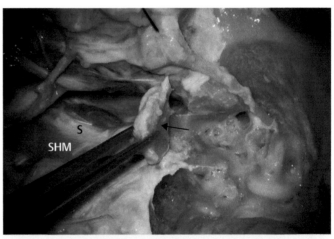

Fig. 10.67 The inferior tympanic bone and mastoid tip are removed (*arrow*). The structures attached to the styloid process are severed. The styloid is fractured using a rongeur, and is then cut with strong scissors. S, styloid; SHM, stylohyoid muscle.

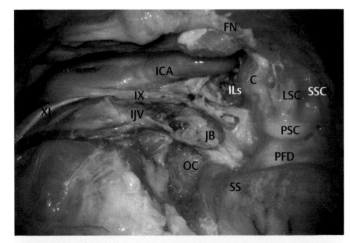

Fig. 10.68 After removal of the tympanic bone and styloid, all the vertical portion of the petrous internal carotid artery (ICA) can be appreciated. C, cochlea; FN, rerouted facial nerve; ILs, infralabyrinthine cells; IJV, internal jugular vein; IX, glossopharyngeal nerve; JB, jugular bulb; LSC, lateral semicircular canal; OC, occipital condyle; PFD, posterior fossa dura; PSC, posterior semicircular canal; SS, sigmoid sinus; SSC, superior semicircular canal; XI, accessory nerve.

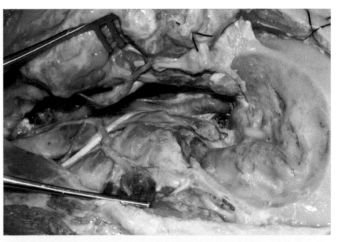

Fig. 10.69 Note the extent of the approach at smaller magnification.

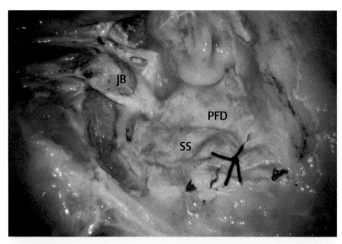

Fig. 10.70 The sigmoid sinus (SS) is closed by ligation. Alternatively, it can be closed extraluminally with Surgicel, to avoid the risk of CSF leakage. JB, jugular bulb; PFD, posterior fossa dura.

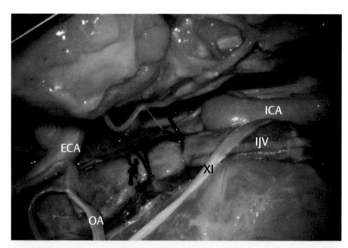

Fig. 10.71 The internal jugular vein (IJV) in the neck is double ligated and cut. ECA, external carotid artery; ICA, internal carotid artery; OA, occipital artery; XI, accessory nerve.

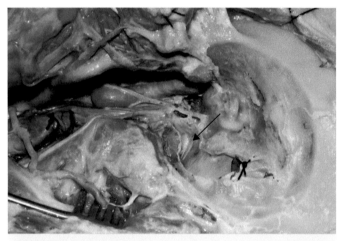

Fig. 10.72 The internal jugular vein and the lateral wall of the jugular bulb and sigmoid sinus have been removed, leaving the medial wall (*arrow*) in place.

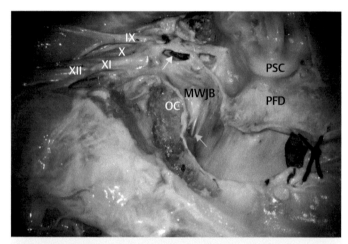

Fig. 10.73 Closer view. After opening the lateral wall of the jugular bulb, the openings of the inferior petrosal sinus (*yellow arrow*) and condylar emissary vein (*green arrow*) can be appreciated.
IX, glossopharyngeal nerve; MWJB, medial wall of the jugular bulb; OC, occipital condyle; PFD, posterior fossa dura; PSC, posterior semicircular canal; X, vagus nerve; XI, accessory nerve; XII, hypoglossal nerve.

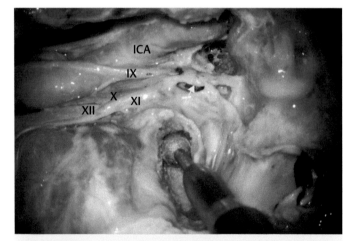

Fig. 10.74 The occipital condyle is starting to be drilled for the transcondylar–transtubercular extension of the approach. Note the close relationship between the inferior petrosal sinus (*arrow*) and the lower cranial nerves. This is very important during surgery, because extensive packing of the sinus with Surgicel could lead to paralysis of the aforementioned nerves. ICA, internal carotid artery; IX, glossopharyngeal nerve; X, vagus nerve; XI, accessory nerve; XII, hypoglossal nerve.

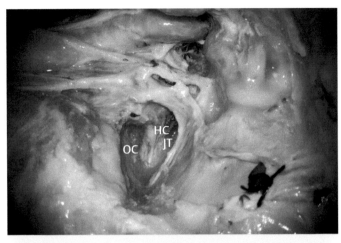

Fig. 10.75 The jugular tubercle (JT) has been partially drilled and the hypoglossal canal (HC) could be appreciated. OC, occipital condyle.

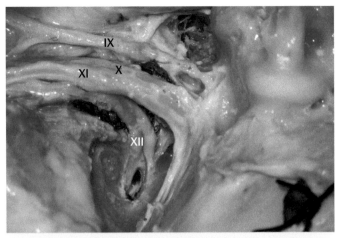

Fig. 10.76 The occipital condyle and jugular tubercle are further drilled and the hypoglossal canal is opened, so the hypoglossal nerve (XII) can be seen. IX, glossopharyngeal nerve; X, vagus nerve; XI, accessory nerve.

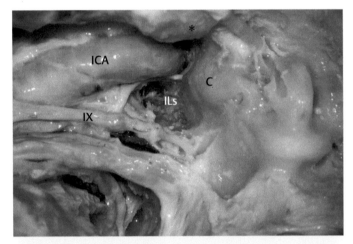

Fig. 10.77 The infralabyrinthine cells (ILs) and the anterior tympanic bone (*) are starting to be removed. C, cochlea; ICA, internal carotid artery; IX, glossopharyngeal nerve.

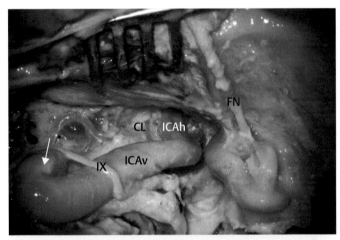

Fig. 10.78 Drilling of the infralabyrinthine cells, anterior tympanic bone, and clivus (CL) exposes the horizontal portion of the petrous internal carotid artery (ICA[h]). arrow, kinking of the internal carotid artery; FN, facial nerve (rerouted); ICA(v), vertical portion of the petrous internal carotid artery; IX, glossopharyngeal nerve.

Right Ear

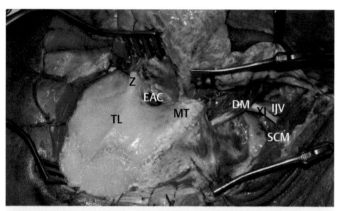

Fig. 10.79 Right ear. Infratemporal fossa approach type A. Skin incision, musculoperiosteal flap and blind-sac closure of the external auditory canal have been previously performed. The sternocleidomastoid muscle has been cut and posteriorly retracted (see ▶ Fig. 10.80 for illustration). DM, posterior belly of the digastric muscle; EAC, external auditory canal; IJV, internal jugular vein; MT, mastoid tip; TL, temporalis line; XI, accessory nerve; Z, zygoma.

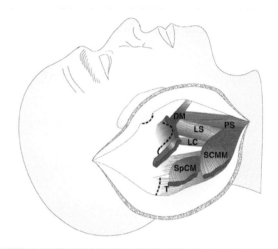

Fig. 10.80 Posterior neck muscles. The muscles in this region can be grouped into three levels. The sternocleidomastoid is the most superficial. More medially, and perpendicular to the sternocleidomastoid, lies the splenius capitis and attached to its medial surface lies the slender longissimus capitis. DM, posterior belly of the digastric muscle; LC, longissimus capitis muscle; LS, levator scapulae muscle; PS, posterior scalene muscle; SCMM, sternocleidomastoid muscle; SpCM, splenius capitis muscle; T, trapezius muscle.

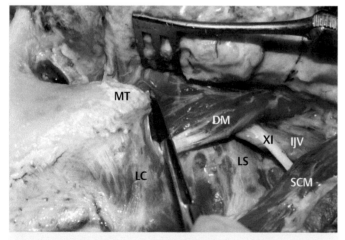

Fig. 10.81 The posterior belly of the digastric muscle (DM) is cut. The splenius capitis muscle has been previously cut. IJV, internal jugular vein; LC, longissimus capitis muscle; LS, levator scapulae muscle; MT, mastoid tip; SCM, sternocleidomastoid muscle; XI, accessory nerve.

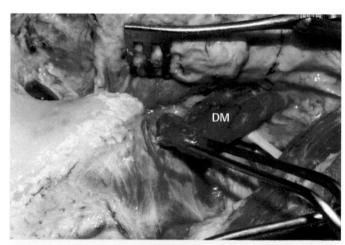

Fig. 10.82 The posterior belly of the digastric muscle (DM) is displaced.

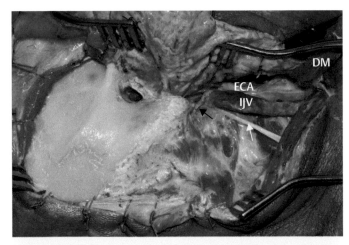

Fig. 10.83 Inferior transposition of the posterior belly of the digastric muscle (DM) allows exposure of the external carotid artery (ECA). black arrow, occipital artery; yellow arrow, accessory nerve.

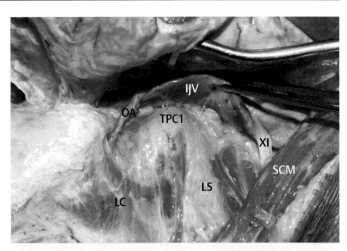

Fig. 10.84 Note that the internal jugular vein (IJV) lies just anterior to the transverse process of the atlas (TPC1). LC, longissimus capitis muscle; LS, levator scapulae muscle; OA, occipital artery; SCM, sternocleidomastoid muscle; XI, accessory nerve.

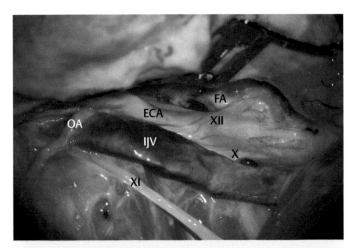

Fig. 10.85 Microscopic view. ECA, external carotid artery; FA, facial artery; IJV, internal jugular vein; OA, occipital artery; X, vagus nerve; XI, accessory nerve; XII, hypoglossal nerve.

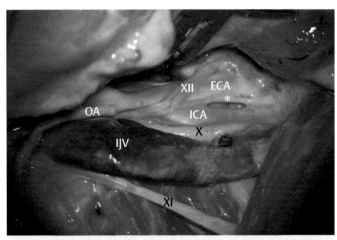

Fig. 10.86 Further dissection with exposure of the internal carotid artery (ICA). *, descending branch of the hypoglossal nerve; ECA, external carotid artery; IJV, internal jugular vein; OA, occipital artery; X, vagus nerve; XI, accessory nerve; XII, hypoglossal nerve.

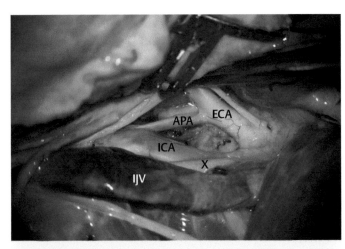

Fig. 10.87 Anterior displacement of the external carotid artery (ECA) with exposure of the ascending pharyngeal artery (APA). ICA, internal carotid artery; IJV, internal jugular vein; X, vagus nerve.

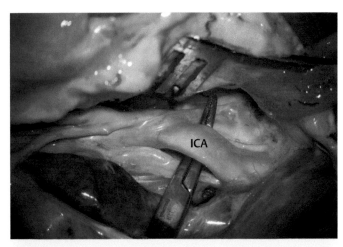

Fig. 10.88 The internal carotid artery (ICA) is isolated and marked with umbilical tape.

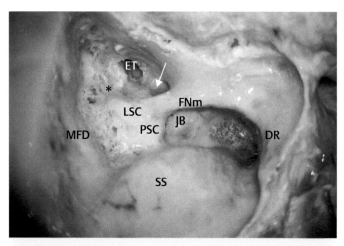

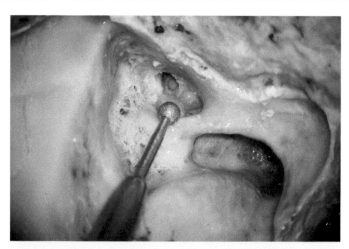

Fig. 10.89 Canal wall–down mastoidectomy has been completed. All the skin of the external auditory canal, tympanic membrane, malleus, and incus have been removed. *, tympanic portion of the facial nerve; arrow, internal carotid artery; C, cochlea (promontory); DR, digastric ridge; ET, eustachian tube; FN(m), mastoid portion of the facial nerve; JB, jugular bulb; LSC, lateral semicircular canal; MFD, middle fossa dura; SS, sigmoid sinus.

Fig. 10.90 Decompression of the facial nerve is started.

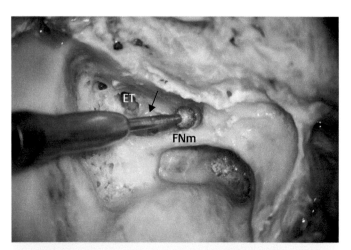

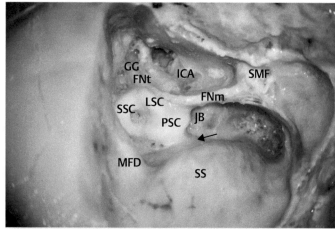

Fig. 10.91 The tympanic bone between the internal carotid artery (*arrow*) and the mastoid portion of the facial nerve (FN[m]) is drilled. ET, eustachian tube.

Fig. 10.92 The facial nerve has been decompressed from the stylomastoid foramen (SMF) to the geniculate ganglion (GG). arrow, endolymphatic duct and sac; FN(m), mastoid portion of the facial nerve; FN(t), tympanic portion of the facial nerve; ICA, internal carotid artery; JB, jugular bulb; LSC, lateral semicircular canal; MFD, middle fossa dura; PSC, posterior semicircular canal; SS, sigmoid sinus; SSC, superior semicircular canal.

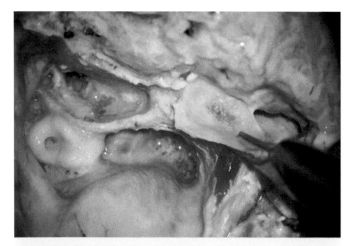

Fig. 10.93 The mastoid tip is removed.

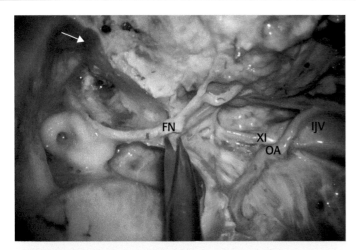

Fig. 10.94 The facial nerve (FN) is freed at the level of the stylomastoid foramen using strong scissors. A new bony canal (*arrow*) has been previously created superior to the eustachian tube for the rerouted facial nerve. IJV, internal jugular vein; OA, occipital artery; XI, accessory nerve.

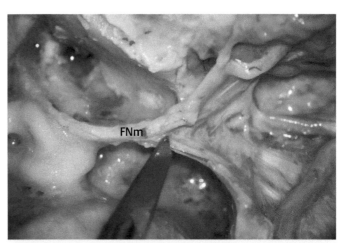

Fig. 10.95 The mastoid segment of the facial nerve (FN[m]) is elevated using a Beaver knife to cut the fibrous attachments between the nerve and the fallopian canal. The tympanic segment of the nerve is elevated carefully, using a curved raspatory, until the level of the geniculate ganglion is reached.

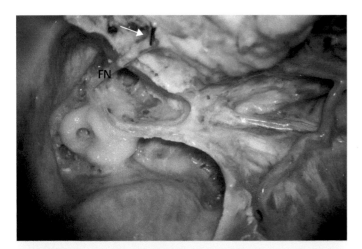

Fig. 10.96 The facial nerve (FN) has been completely rerouted and sutured to the parotid gland (*arrow*).

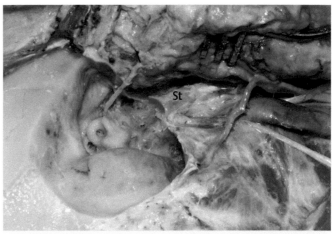

Fig. 10.97 Note the extent of the approach at smaller magnification. The remaining part of the inferior tympanic bone and the styloid (St) has to be removed to allow control of the internal carotid artery on its entrance in the skull base.

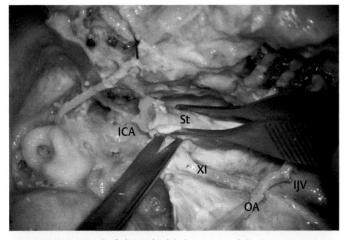

Fig. 10.98 Removal of the styloid (St) is accomplished. ICA, petrous portion of the internal carotid artery; IJV, internal jugular vein; OA, occipital artery; XI, accessory nerve.

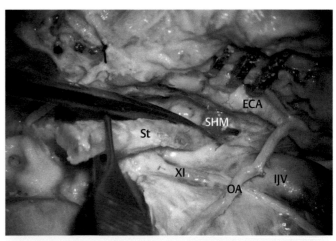

Fig. 10.99 The stylohyoid muscle (SHM) is cut to free the styloid (St). ECA, external carotid artery; IJV, internal jugular vein; OA, occipital artery; XI, accessory nerve.

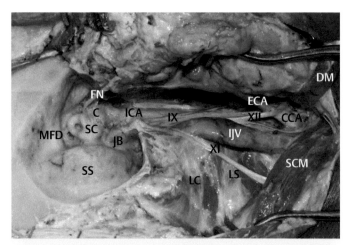

Fig. 10.100 After removal of the styloid, the internal carotid artery (ICA) can be controlled from the neck to the skull base. C, cochlea; CCA, common carotid artery; DM, posterior belly of the digastric muscle; ECA, external carotid artery; FN, facial nerve (rerouted); IJV, internal jugular vein; IX, glossopharyngeal nerve; JB, jugular bulb; LC, longissimus capitis muscle; LS, levator scapulae muscle; MFD, middle fossa dura; SC, semicircular canal; SCM, sternocleidomastoid muscle; SS, sigmoid sinus; XI, accessory nerve; XII, hypoglossal nerve.

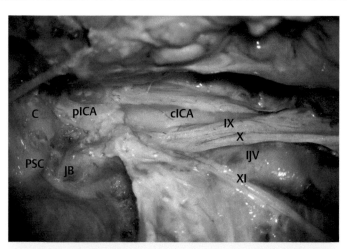

Fig. 10.101 Closer view. C, cochlea; cICA, cervical portion of the internal carotid artery; IJV, internal jugular vein; IX, glossopharyngeal nerve; JB, jugular bulb; pICA, petrous portion of the internal carotid artery; PSC, posterior semicircular canal; X, vagus nerve; XI, accessory nerve.

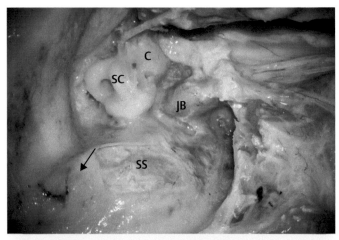

Fig. 10.102 The sigmoid sinus (SS) is partially decompressed. A shell of bone is left toward the transverse sinus (*arrow*) to allow extraluminal packing of the SS. C, cochlea; JB, jugular bulb; SC, semicircular canals.

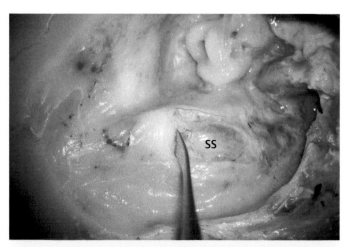

Fig. 10.103 The sigmoid sinus (SS) is packed extraluminally with Surgicel.

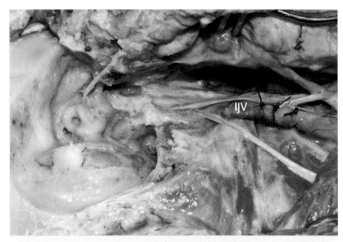

Fig. 10.104 The internal jugular vein (IJV) is ligated.

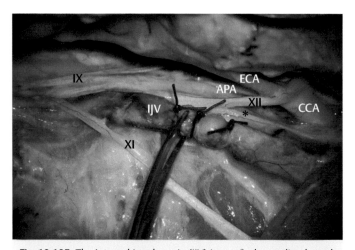

Fig. 10.105 The internal jugular vein (IJV) is cut. *, descending branch of the hypoglossal nerve; APA, ascending pharyngeal artery; CCA, common carotid artery; ECA, external carotid artery; IX, glossopharyngeal nerve; XI, accessory nerve; XII hypoglossal nerve.

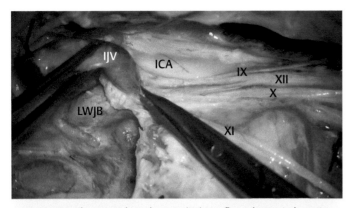

Fig. 10.106 The internal jugular vein (IJV) is reflected superiorly paying attention not to damage the accessory nerve (XI). Then, it is removed with the lateral wall of the jugular bulb (LWJB). ICA, internal carotid artery; IX, glossopharyngeal nerve; X, vagus nerve; XII, hypoglossal nerve.

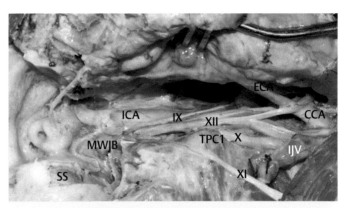

Fig. 10.107 The distal part of the internal jugular vein (IJV) and the medial wall of the jugular bulb (MWJB) can be appreciated. CCA, common carotid artery; ECA, external carotid artery; ICA, internal carotid artery; IX, glossopharyngeal nerve; SS, sigmoid sinus; TPC1, transverse process of the atlas; X, vagus nerve; XI, accessory nerve; XII, hypoglossal nerve.

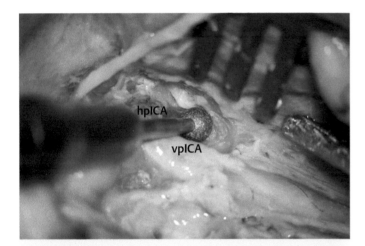

Fig. 10.108 The petrous bone in the area of the petrous apex is drilled to control the horizontal portion of the petrous internal carotid artery (hpICA). vpICA, vertical portion of the petrous internal carotid artery.

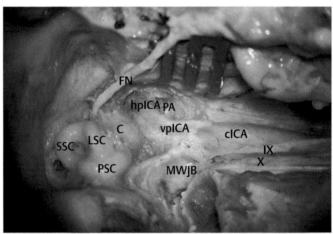

Fig. 10.109 The horizontal portion of the petrous internal carotid artery (hpICA) is under control. C, cochlea; cICA, cervical internal carotid artery; FN, facial nerve (rerouted); IX, glossopharyngeal nerve; LSC, lateral semicircular canal; MWJB, medial wall of the jugular bulb; PA, petrous apex; PSC, posterior semicircular canal; SSC, superior semicircular canal; vpICA, vertical portion of the internal carotid artery; X, vagus nerve.

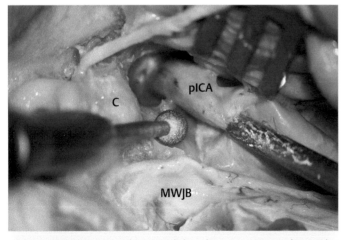

Fig. 10.110 The petrous bone medial to the petrous internal carotid artery (pICA) is drilled to reach the clivus. C, cochlea; MWJB, medial wall of the jugular bulb.

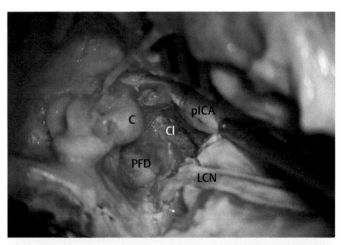

Fig. 10.111 The clivus (Cl) is under view. C, cochlea; LCN, lower cranial nerve; PFD, posterior fossa dura; pICA, petrous internal carotid artery.

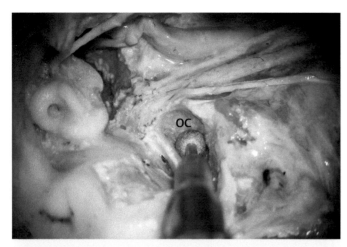

Fig. 10.112 Drilling of the occipital condyle (OC) is starting.

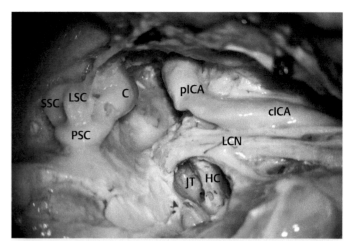

Fig. 10.113 Drilling of the occipital condyle exposes the hypoglossal canal (HC). C, cochlea; cICA, cervical internal carotid artery; JT, jugular tubercle; LCN, lower cranial nerve; LSC, lateral semicircular canal; pICA, petrous internal carotid artery; PSC, posterior semicircular canal; SSC, superior semicircular canal.

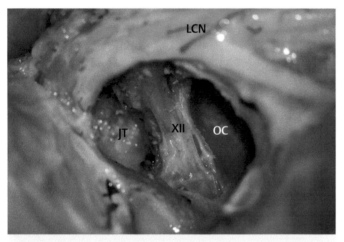

Fig. 10.114 The hypoglossal nerve (XII) is under view. JT, jugular tubercle; LCN, lower cranial nerve; OC, occipital condyle.

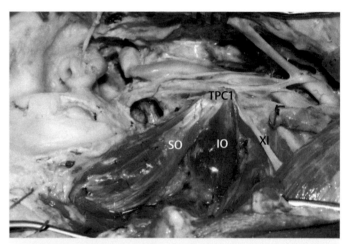

Fig. 10.115 The longissimus capitis and levator scapulae muscles have been removed. IO inferior oblique muscle; SO, superior oblique muscle; TPC1, transverse process of the atlas; XI, accessory nerve.

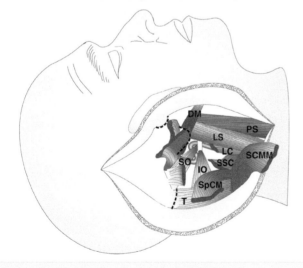

Fig. 10.116 Illustration of deeper posterior neck muscles. DM, posterior belly of the digastric muscle; IO, inferior oblique muscle; LC, longissimus capitis muscle; LS, levator scapulae muscle; PS, posterior scalene muscle; SCMM, sternocleidomastoid muscle; SO, superior oblique muscle; SpCM, splenius capitis muscle; SSC, semispinalis capitis muscle; T, trapezius muscle.

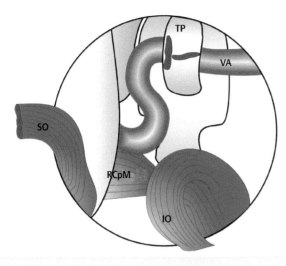

Fig. 10.117 Magnified view during an extreme lateral extension of the approach. The transverse process of the atlas (TP) is an important landmark. It provides attachment to the levator scapulae as well as the superior (SO) and inferior oblique (IO) muscles. The vertebral artery (VA) bends sideway after leaving the transverse process of the axis, ascends to enter the transverse foramen of the atlas, and then curves backward and medially to cross over the posterior arch of atlas. RCpM, rectus capitis muscle.

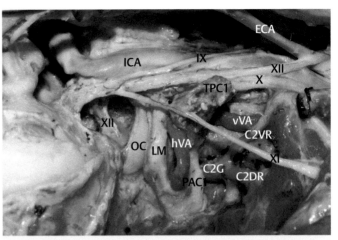

Fig. 10.118 View after removal of the posterior neck muscles attached to the transverse process of the atlas (TPC1). The vertebral artery (VA) can be visible. The C2 nerve root crosses the VA between C1 and C2. The VA passes anteriorly and medially to pierce the dura posteromedial to the occipital condyle. C1, atlas; C2DR, C2 dorsal ramus; C2G, C2 ganglion; C2VR, C2 ventral ramus; ECA, external carotid artery; hVA, horizontal vertebral artery; ICA, internal carotid artery; IX, glossopharyngeal nerve; LM, lateral mass; OC, occipital condyle; PAC1, posterior arch of the atlas; vVA, vertical vertebral artery; X, vagus nerve; XI, accessory nerve; XII, hypoglossal nerve.

10.2 Infratemporal Fossa Approach Type B

This approach is mainly designed for extradural petrous apex and midclival tumors, with preservation of the inner ear function.

10.2.1 Indications

- Petrous apex lesions, such as petrous bone cholesteatoma of the apical and infralabyrinthine types and cholesterol granuloma.
- Clival lesions, such as chordoma, chondrosarcoma, and extensive glomus tumors invading the clivus.
- Other rare lesions involving the infratemporal fossa, such as choristomas of the eustachian tube and giant cell tumors of the petrous bone.

10.2.2 Surgical Steps

1. After the skin flap has been created and cul de sac closure of the external auditory canal skin has been carried out, the extratemporal facial nerve is exposed in the parotid, and the frontal branch of the nerve is followed until it crosses the zygomatic arch.
2. The temporalis muscle is detached from its bed and reflected anteriorly. The zygomatic arch is exposed, with care being taken not to injure the frontal branch of the facial nerve. The periosteum of the zygomatic arch is incised.
3. The arch is transected after two burr holes have been created for further refixation at the end of the procedure in live surgery.
4. The skin of the external auditory canal, the tympanic membrane, the malleus, and the incus is removed after disarticulation of the incudostapedial joint.

5. A subtotal petrosectomy is performed. The facial nerve is skeletonized and the inner ear is preserved.
6. The anterior wall of the external auditory canal is drilled. The vertical segment of the internal carotid artery is identified and skeletonized. The capsule of the temporomandibular joint is detached and cut using strong scissors. The articular disk is removed, exposing the mandibular condyle.
7. A small minicraniotomy is created, and a retractor is applied to displace the head of the mandible inferiorly.
8. The glenoid fossa is drilled. The sphenoid spine serves as a landmark for the middle meningeal artery. The artery is completely exposed, bipolarly coagulated, and cut.
9. With further drilling, the mandibular nerve is identified and cut after bipolar coagulation in live surgery.
10. The bony eustachian tube is drilled, and the horizontal carotid artery is further identified. Tumor removal follows next.
11. At the end of the procedure in live surgery, the eustachian tube is sutured, the zygomatic process is refixed into place, the temporalis muscle is used to obliterate the cavity, and the wound is closed in layers. A drain is inserted.

The surgical steps have been shown in subsequent figures of this chapter (▶ Fig. 10.119, ▶ Fig. 10.120, ▶ Fig. 10.121, ▶ Fig. 10.122, ▶ Fig. 10.123, ▶ Fig. 10.124, ▶ Fig. 10.125, ▶ Fig. 10.126, ▶ Fig. 10.127, ▶ Fig. 10.128, ▶ Fig. 10.129, ▶ Fig. 10.130, ▶ Fig. 10.131, ▶ Fig. 10.132, ▶ Fig. 10.133, ▶ Fig. 10.134, ▶ Fig. 10.135, ▶ Fig. 10.136, ▶ Fig. 10.137, ▶ Fig. 10.138, ▶ Fig. 10.139, ▶ Fig. 10.140, ▶ Fig. 10.141, ▶ Fig. 10.142, ▶ Fig. 10.143, ▶ Fig. 10.144, ▶ Fig. 10.145, ▶ Fig. 10.146, ▶ Fig. 10.147, ▶ Fig. 10.148, ▶ Fig. 10.149, ▶ Fig. 10.150, ▶ Fig. 10.151, ▶ Fig. 10.152, ▶ Fig. 10.153, ▶ Fig. 10.154, ▶ Fig. 10.155, ▶ Fig. 10.156, ▶ Fig. 10.157).

10.2.3 Hints and Pitfalls

- Exposure of the extratemporal portion of the facial nerve is useful in preventing overstretching of the nerve during the application of the infratemporal fossa retractor.
- The sphenoid spine serves as a landmark for the middle meningeal artery, which lies immediately anterior to it.
- Before the mandibular nerve is transacted in live surgery, bipolar coagulation helps reduce bleeding from the venus plexus surrounding the nerve.
- Drilling should always be parallel to the course of the internal carotid artery in order to reduce the risk of tearing the artery wall.
- Bleeding from the veins within the carotid sheath may easily be controlled by Surgicel packing.
- Bleeding from the inferior petrosal sinus can be controlled by intraluminal packing.

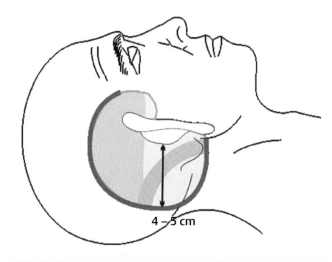

Fig. 10.120 Skin incision for the Infratemporal fossa, type B approach.

Left Ear

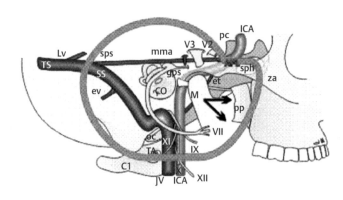

Fig. 10.119 The structures controlled by the type B infratemporal fossa approach. VII, facial nerve; IX, glossopharyngeal nerve; X, vagus nerve; XI, accessory nerve; XII, hypoglossal nerve; AFL, anterior foramen lacerum; C1, atlas; CO, cochlea; et, eustachian tube; ev, emissary vein; gps, greater superficial petrosal nerve; ICA, internal carotid artery; JV, jugular vein; Lv, Labbé's vein; M, mandible; mma, middle meningeal artery; oc, occipital condyle; pp, pterygoid process; sph, sphenoid sinus; sps, superior petrosal sinus; SS, sigmoid sinus; TA, lateral process of the atlas; TS, transverse sinus; V2, second division of the trigeminal nerve; V3, third division of the trigeminal nerve; za, zygomatic arch.

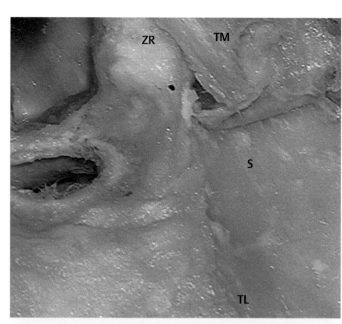

Fig. 10.121 The temporalis muscle (TM) of a left temporal bone has been reflected anteriorly after it has been dissected from the squamous bone (S). TL, temporalis line; ZR, root of the zygomatic process.

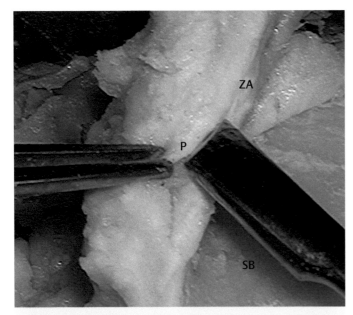

Fig. 10.122 The periosteum (P) overlying the zygomatic arch (ZA) is being dissected away. This step helps avoid the laterally lying frontal branch of the facial nerve. SB, squamous bone.

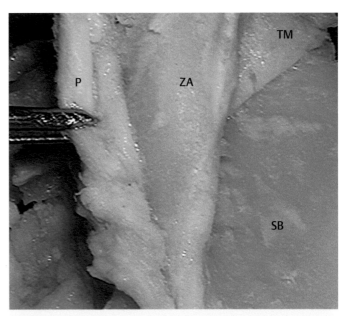

Fig. 10.123 The view after dissection of the periosteum (P) from the zygomatic arch (ZA). SB, squamous bone; TM, temporalis muscle.

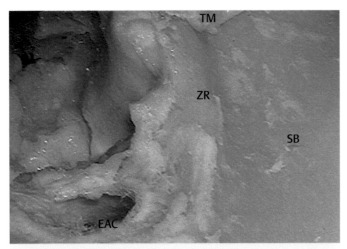

Fig. 10.124 The zygomatic arch has been transected. EAC, external auditory canal; SB, squamous bone; TM, temporalis muscle; ZR, zygomatic root.

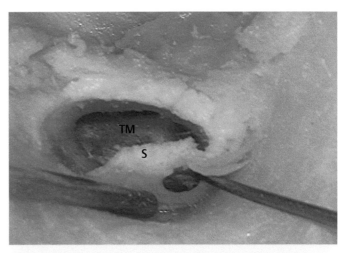

Fig. 10.125 The skin of the external auditory canal (S) is being dissected away under the microscope. TM, tympanic membrane.

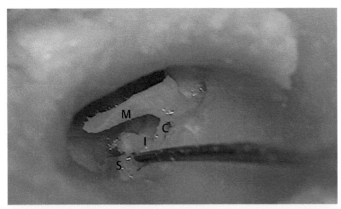

Fig. 10.126 After complete removal of the external auditory canal skin and tympanic membrane, the incudostapedial joint is disarticulated in order to remove the ossicular chain. C, chorda tympani; I, Incus; M, malleus; S, stapes.

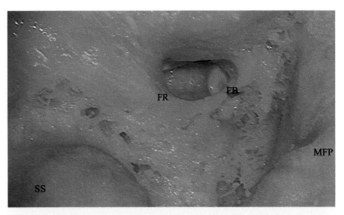

Fig. 10.127 The mastoid cavity and the posterior and superior walls of the external auditory canal have been partially drilled. FB, facial bridge; FR, facial ridge; MFP, middle fossa plate; SS, sigmoid sinus.

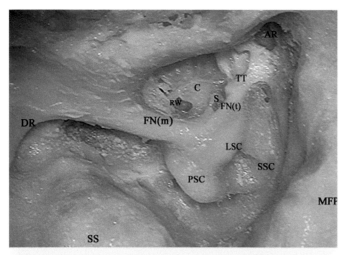

Fig. 10.128 A radical mastoidectomy has been carried out, and the facial nerve has been skeletonized. AR, anterior attic recess; C, basal turn of the cochlea (promontory); DR, digastric ridge; FN(m), mastoid segment of the facial nerve; FN(t), tympanic segment of the facial nerve; LSC, lateral semicircular canal; MFP, middle fossa plate; PSC, posterior semicircular canal; RW, round window; S, stapes; SS, sigmoid sinus; SSC, superior semicircular canal; TT, tensor tympani.

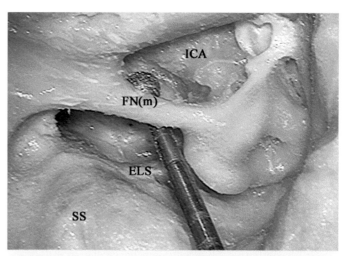

Fig. 10.129 The retrofacial and infralabyrinthine air cells are being drilled using an appropriately sized diamond drill. Attention must be paid during this step to avoid injuring the laterally lying facial nerve with the burr or the shaft. ELS, endolymphatic sac; FN(m), mastoid segment of the facial nerve; ICA, internal carotid artery; SS, sigmoid sinus.

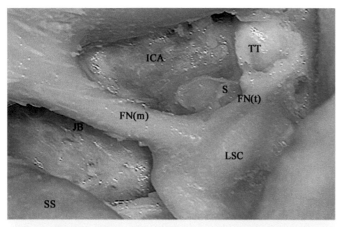

Fig. 10.130 The anterior wall of the external auditory canal has been partially drilled, and the vertical segment of the internal carotid artery (ICA) has been identified. FN(m), mastoid segment of the facial nerve; FN(t), tympanic segment of the facial nerve; JB, jugular bulb; LSC, lateral semicircular canal; S, stapes; SS, sigmoid sinus; TT, tensor tympani.

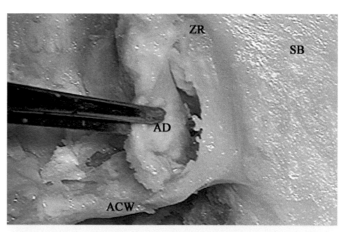

Fig. 10.131 Dissecting the articular disk (AD) of the temporomandibular joint. ACW, anterior canal wall; SB, squamous bone; ZR, zygomatic root.

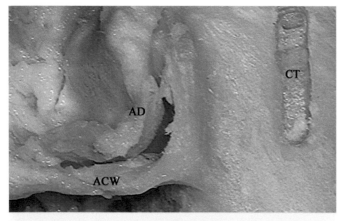

Fig. 10.132 A small craniotomy (CT) has been created in the squamous bone. ACW, anterior canal wall; AD, articular disk.

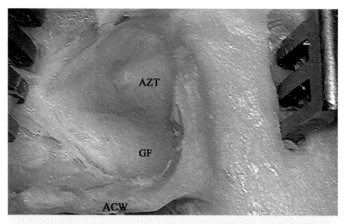

Fig. 10.133 A self-retaining retractor is used to keep the mandible retracted inferiorly. ACW, anterior canal wall; AZT, anterior zygomatic tubercle; GF, glenoid fossa.

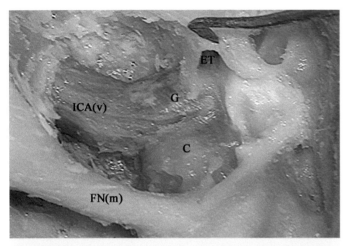

Fig. 10.134 The rest of the anterior canal wall has been drilled away, and the internal carotid artery is better skeletonized. C, basal turn of the cochlea (promontory); ET, eustachian tube; FN(m), mastoid segment of the facial nerve; G, genu of the internal carotid artery; ICA(v), vertical segment of the internal carotid artery.

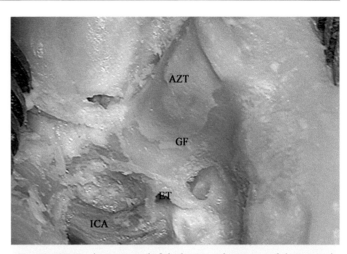

Fig. 10.135 To obtain control of the horizontal segment of the internal carotid artery, the eustachian tube (ET), glenoid fossa bone (GF), and the anterior zygomatic tubercle (AZT) have to be carefully drilled away. ICA, vertical segment of the internal carotid artery.

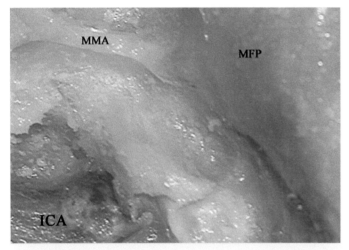

Fig. 10.136 In live surgery, the middle meningeal artery (MMA) should be coagulated to prevent bleeding. ICA, internal carotid artery; MFP, middle fossa plate.

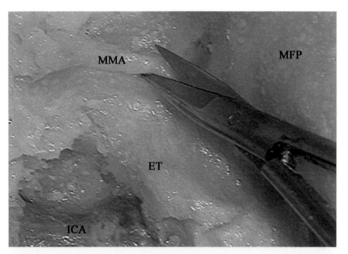

Fig. 10.137 The middle meningeal artery (MMA) is being sharply cut. ET, eustachian tube; ICA, internal carotid artery; MFP, middle fossa plate.

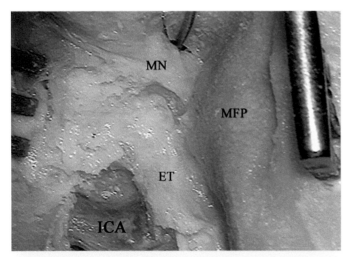

Fig. 10.138 Further anterior drilling uncovers the mandibular nerve (MN). This nerve also has to be coagulated in live surgery before it is cut. ET, eustachian tube; ICA, internal carotid artery; MFP, middle fossa plate.

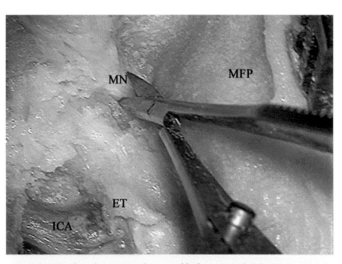

Fig. 10.139 Sharply cutting the mandibular nerve (MN). ET, eustachian tube; ICA, internal carotid artery; MFP, middle fossa plate.

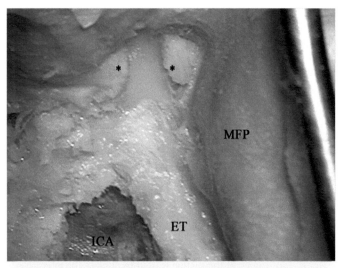

Fig. 10.140 The stumps of the mandibular nerve (*). ET, eustachian tube; ICA, internal carotid artery; MFP, middle fossa plate.

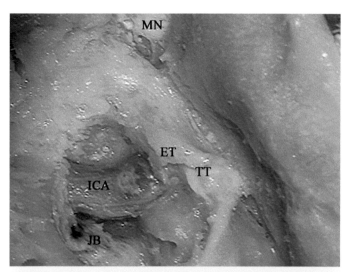

Fig. 10.141 The eustachian tube (ET) and tensor tympani muscles (TT) are the last structures lying lateral to the horizontal segment of the facial nerve and should be removed. ICA, internal carotid artery; JB, jugular bulb; MN, the cut end of the mandibular nerve.

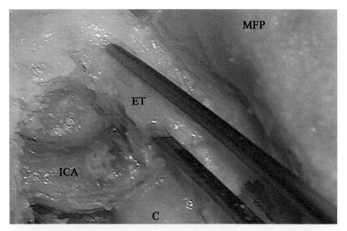

Fig. 10.142 The lateral, thin part of the eustachian tube (ET) that remains can be removed with forceps. C, basal turn of the cochlea (promontory); ICA, internal carotid artery; MFP, middle fossa plate.

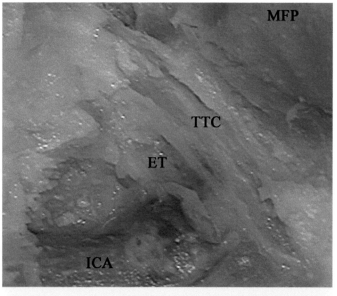

Fig. 10.143 The tensor tympani muscle has been dissected away from its canal (TTC). ET, medial wall of the eustachian tube; ICA, internal carotid artery; MFP, middle fossa plate.

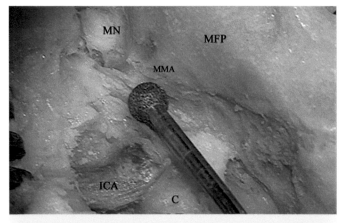

Fig. 10.144 A large diamond burr is used to remove the remaining bone overlying the horizontal segment of the internal carotid artery. C, basal turn of the cochlea (promontory); ICA, vertical segment of the internal carotid artery; MFP, middle fossa plate; MMA, stump of the middle meningeal artery; MN, stump of the mandibular nerve.

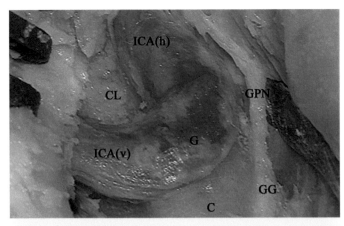

Fig. 10.145 The horizontal segment of the internal carotid artery (ICA [h]) has been skeletonized. Note that the greater petrosal nerve (GPN) is adherent to the dura, and that retracting the dura will lead to stress on the facial nerve at the geniculate ganglion (GG) level. Thus, if dural retraction is needed, cutting the petrosal nerve will prevent this injury. C, basal turn of the cochlea (promontory); CL, clivus bone; G, genu; ICA(v), vertical segment of the internal carotid artery.

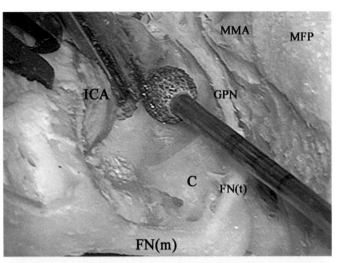

Fig. 10.146 The tip of the suction is used to displace the internal carotid artery (ICA) laterally while the medially lying bone is being drilled. C, basal turn of the cochlea (promontory); FN(m), mastoid segment of the facial nerve; FN(t), tympanic segment of the facial nerve; GPN, greater petrosal nerve; MFP, middle fossa plate; MMA, middle meningeal artery stump.

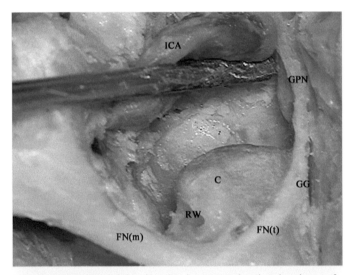

Fig. 10.147 Drilling of the clivus has been completed. C, basal turn of the cochlea (promontory); FN(m), mastoid segment of the facial nerve; FN(t), tympanic segment of the facial nerve; GG, geniculate ganglion; GPN, greater petrosal nerve; ICA, internal carotid artery; RW, round window.

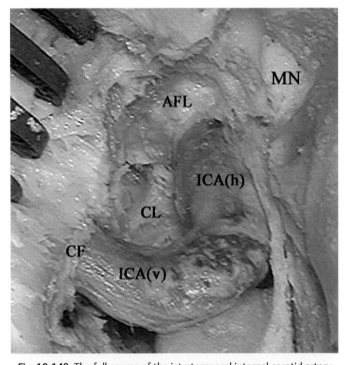

Fig. 10.148 The full course of the intratemporal internal carotid artery has been freed. AFL, anterior foramen lacerum; CF, carotid foramen; CL, dura overlying the clivus area; ICA(h), horizontal segment of the internal carotid artery; ICA(v), vertical segment of the internal carotid artery; MN, stump of the mandibular nerve.

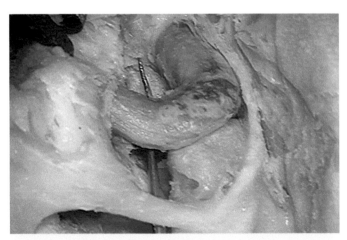

Fig. 10.149 The view after completion of the approach.

Right Ear

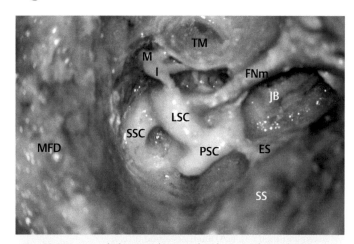

Fig. 10.150 Extended mastoidectomy has been performed. The middle fossa dura (MFD), the sigmoid sinus (SS), mastoid portion of the facial nerve (FN[m]), jugular bulb (JB), and labyrinth are under view. The tympanic membrane (TM) and ossicles have been left in place to understand the relationship with the petrous internal carotid artery. ES, endolymphatic duct and sac; I, incus; LSC, lateral semicircular canal; M, malleus; PSC, posterior semicircular canal; SSC, superior semicircular canal.

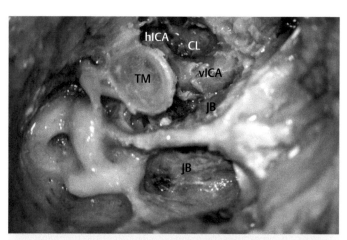

Fig. 10.151 The vertical (vICA) and horizontal (hICA) portions of the petrous internal carotid artery have been skeletonized. All the retrofacial air cells have been removed and the jugular bulb (JB) anterior and posterior to the facial nerve is visible. All the tympanic bone has been drilled and the temporomandibular joint displaced anteroinferiorly. Note the relationship between the ICA, the tympanic membrane (TM), and the JB. CL, clivus.

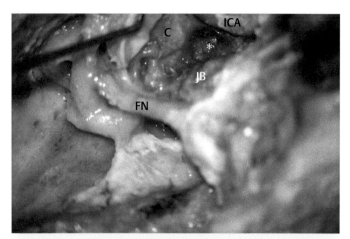

Fig. 10.152 Infracochlear cells (*) are between the internal carotid artery (ICA), the jugular bulb (JB) anterior to the facial nerve (FN), and the cochlea (C). Drilling of these cells can lead to the petrous apex.

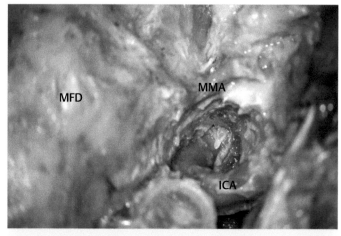

Fig. 10.153 The middle meningeal artery (MMA) has been identified. ICA, internal carotid artery; MFD, middle fossa dura.

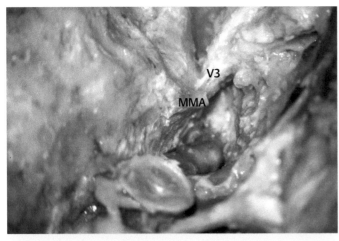

Fig. 10.154 The middle meningeal artery (MMA) has been cut. Further anterior drilling exposes the mandibular branch of the trigeminal nerve (V3).

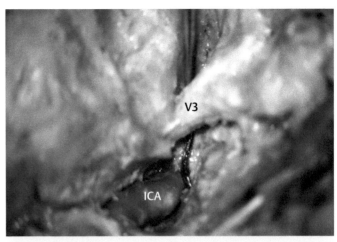

Fig. 10.155 The mandibular branch of the trigeminal nerve (V3) is isolated and then cut. ICA, internal carotid artery.

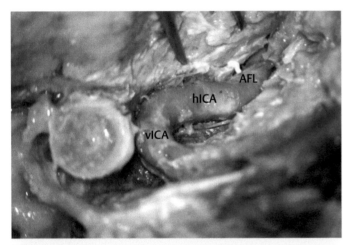

Fig. 10.156 Further anterior drilling exposes the petrous internal carotid artery (ICA[h]—horizontal, ICA[v]—vertical) at the level of the anterior foramen lacerum (AFL).

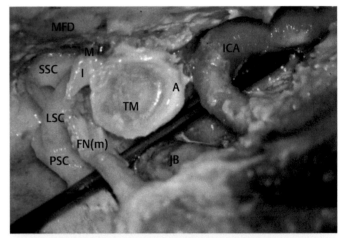

Fig. 10.157 Note the relationship of the internal carotid artery (ICA) to the tympanic membrane (TM) and middle ear. A, annulus; FN(m), mastoid segment of the facial nerve; I, incus; JB, jugular bulb; LSC, lateral semicircular canal; M, malleus; MFD, middle fossa dura; PSC, posterior semicircular canal; SSC, superior semicircular canal.

Bibliography

[1] Ahmad RA, Sivalingam S, Topsakal V, Russo A, Taibah A, Sanna M. Rate of recurrent vestibular schwannoma after total removal via different surgical approaches. Ann Otol Rhinol Laryngol. 2012; 121(3):156–161

[2] Al-Mefty O, Fox JL, Smith RR. Petrosal approach for petroclival meningiomas. Neurosurgery. 1988; 22(3):510–517

[3] Angeli RD, Ben Ammar M, Sanna M. Perioperative complications after translabyrinthine removal of large or giant vestibular schwannoma: outcomes for 123 patients. Acta Otolaryngol. 2011; 131(11):1237–1238

[4] Angeli RD, Piccirillo E, Di Trapani G, Sequino G, Taibah A, Sanna M. Enlarged translabyrinthine approach with transapical extension in the management of giant vestibular schwannomas: personal experience and review of literature. Otol Neurotol. 2011; 32(1):125–131

[5] Arìstegui M, Cokkeser Y, Saleh E, et al. Surgical anatomy of the extended middle cranial fossa approach. Skull Base Surg. 1994; 4(4):181–188

[6] Arriaga MA, Brackmann DE, Hitselberger WE. Extended middle fossa resection of petroclival and cavernous sinus neoplasms. Laryngoscope. 1993; 103 (6):693–698

[7] Aslan A, Balyan FR, Taibah A, Sanna M. Anatomic relationships between surgical landmarks in type b and type c infratemporal fossa approaches. Eur Arch Otorhinolaryngol. 1998; 255(5):259–264

[8] Aslan A, Falcioni M, Balyan FR, et al. The cochlear aqueduct: an important landmark in lateral skull base surgery. Otolaryngol Head Neck Surg. 1998; 118(4):532–536

[9] Aslan A, Falcioni M, Russo A, et al. Anatomical considerations of high jugular bulb in lateral skull base surgery. J Laryngol Otol. 1997; 111(4):333–336

[10] Bacciu A, Ait Mimoune H, D'Orazio F, Vitullo F, Russo A, Sanna M. Management of facial nerve in surgical treatment of previously untreated Fisch class C tympanojugular paragangliomas: long-term results. J Neurol Surg B Skull Base. 2014; 75(1):1–7

[11] Bacciu A, Clemente IA, Piccirillo E, Ferrari S, Sanna M. Guidelines for treating temporal bone carcinoma based on long-term outcomes. Otol Neurotol. 2013; 34(5):898–907

[12] Bacciu A, Di Lella F, Ventura E, Pasanisi E, Russo A, Sanna M. Lipomas of the internal auditory canal and cerebellopontine angle. Ann Otol Rhinol Laryngol. 2014; 123(1):58–64

[13] Bacciu A, Medina M, Ait Mimoune H, et al. Lower cranial nerves function after surgical treatment of Fisch Class C and D tympanojugular paragangliomas. Eur Arch Otorhinolaryngol. 2015; 272(2):311–319

[14] Bacciu A, Medina M, Ben Ammar M, et al. Intraoperatively diagnosed cerebellopontine angle facial nerve schwannoma: how to deal with it. Ann Otol Rhinol Laryngol. 2014; 123(9):647–653

[15] Bacciu A, Nusier A, Lauda L, Falcioni M, Russo A, Sanna M. Are the current treatment strategies for facial nerve schwannoma appropriate also for complex cases? Audiol Neurootol. 2013; 18(3):184–191

[16] Balyan FR, Celikkanat S, Aslan A, Taibah A, Russo A, Sanna M. Mastoidectomy in noncholesteatomatous chronic suppurative otitis media: is it necessary? Otolaryngol Head Neck Surg. 1997; 117(6):592–595

[17] Ben Ammar M, Piccirillo E, Topsakal V, Taibah A, Sanna M. Surgical results and technical refinements in translabyrinthine excision of vestibular schwannomas: the Gruppo Otologico experience. Neurosurgery. 2012; 70 (6):1481–1491, discussion 1491

[18] Bhatia S, Karmarkar S, De Donato G, et al. Canal wall down mastoidectomy: causes of failure, pitfalls and their management. J Laryngol Otol. 1995; 109 (7):583–589

[19] Cama A, Verginelli F, Lotti LV, et al. Integrative genetic, epigenetic and pathological analysis of paraganglioma reveals complex dysregulation of NOTCH signaling. Acta Neuropathol. 2013; 126(4):575–594

[20] Canalis RF, Black K, Martin N, Becker D. Extended retrolabyrinthine transtentorial approach to petroclival lesions. Laryngoscope. 1991; 101(1, Pt 1):6–13

[21] Cass SP, Sekhar LN, Pomeranz S, Hirsch BE, Snyderman CH. Excision of petroclival tumors by a total petrosectomy approach. Am J Otol. 1994; 15(4):474–484

[22] Caylan R, Falcioni M, De Donato G, et al. Intracanalicular meningiomas. Otolaryngol Head Neck Surg. 2000; 122(1):147–150

[23] Cokkeser Y, Aristegui M, Naguib MB, Saleh E, Taibah AK, Sanna M. Identification of internal acoustic canal in the middle cranial fossa approach: a safe technique. Otolaryngol Head Neck Surg. 2001; 124(1):94–98

[24] Daspit CP, Spetzler RF, Pappas CT. Combined approach for lesions involving the cerebellopontine angle and skull base: experience with 20 cases–preliminary report. Otolaryngol Head Neck Surg. 1991; 105(6):788–796

[25] Di Lella F, Merkus P, Di Trapani G, Taibah A, Guida M, Sanna M. Vestibular schwannoma in the only hearing ear: role of cochlear implants. Ann Otol Rhinol Laryngol. 2013; 122(2):91–99

[26] Falcioni M, De Donato G, Taibah A, Russo A, Sanna M. Modified body technique in the treatment of epithympanic cholesteatoma. Otologic group, Piacenza. Acta Otorhinolaryngol Ital. 1997; 17(5):325–328

[27] Falcioni M, Fois P, Taibah A, Sanna M. Facial nerve function after vestibular schwannoma surgery. J Neurosurg. 2011; 115(4):820–826

[28] Falcioni M, Mulder JJ, Taibah A, De Donato G, Sanna M. No cerebrospinal fluid leaks in translabyrinthine vestibular schwannoma removal: reappraisal of 200 consecutive patients. Am J Otol. 1999; 20(5):660–666

[29] Falcioni M, Piccioni LO, Taibah A, et al. Treatment of residual acoustic neurinomas. Acta Otorhinolaryngol Ital. 2000; 20(3):151–158

[30] Falcioni M, Russo A, Mancini F, et al. Enlarged translabyrinthine approach in large acoustic neurinomas. Acta Otorhinolaryngol Ital. 2001; 21(4):226–236

[31] Falcioni M, Russo A, Taibah A, Sanna M. Facial nerve tumors. Otol Neurotol. 2003; 24(6):942–947

[32] Falcioni M, Sanna M. Cerebrospinal fluid leak after acoustic surgery. J Neurosurg. 2001; 95(2):373–374

[33] Falcioni M, Taibah A, De Donato G, Russo A, Sanna M. Lateral approaches to the clivus . Acta Otorhinolaryngol Ital. 1997; 17(6) Suppl 57:3–16

[34] Falcioni M, Taibah A, Di Trapani G, Khrais T, Sanna M. Inner ear extension of vestibular schwannomas. Laryngoscope. 2003; 113(9):1605–1608

[35] Fisch U, Esslen E. Total intratemporal exposure of the facial nerve. Pathologic findings in Bell's palsy. Arch Otolaryngol. 1972; 95(4):335–341

[36] Fisch U, Mattox D. Microsurgery of the Skull Base. New York, NY: Thieme; 1988

[37] Fisch U. Infratemporal fossa approach for glomus tumors of the temporal bone. Ann Otol Rhinol Laryngol. 1982; 91(5, Pt 1):474–479

[38] Fisch U. Infratemporal fossa approach to tumours of the temporal bone and base of the skull. J Laryngol Otol. 1978; 92(11):949–967

[39] Fisch U. The infratemporal fossa approach for nasopharyngeal tumors. Laryngoscope. 1983; 93(1):36–44

[40] Gantz BJ, Fisch U. Modified transotic approach to the cerebellopontile angle. Arch Otolaryngol. 1983; 109(4):252–256

[41] Glasscock ME, III, Hays JW. The translabyrinthine removal of acoustic and other cerebellopontine angle tumors. Ann Otol Rhinol Laryngol. 1973; 82 (4):415–427

[42] Grinblat G, Prasad SC, Piras G, et al. Outcomes of drill canalplasty in exostoses and osteoma: analysis of 256 cases and literature review. Otol Neurotol. 2016; 37(10):1565–1572

[43] Hakuba A, Nishimura S, Jang BJ. A combined retroauricular and preauricular transpetrosal-transtentorial approach to clivus meningiomas. Surg Neurol. 1988; 30(2):108–116

[44] Hitselberger WE, Horn KL, Hankinson H, Brackmann DE, House WF. The middle fossa transpetrous approach for petroclival meningiomas. Skull Base Surg. 1993; 3(3):130–135

[45] House WF, Hitselberger WE. The transcochlear approach to the skull base. Arch Otolaryngol. 1976; 102(6):334–342

[46] House WF, Luetje CM, eds. Acoustic Tumors. Baltimore, MD: University Park Press; 1979

[47] House WF. Middle cranial fossa approach to the petrous pyramid: report of 50 cases. Arch Otolaryngol. 1963; 78:460–469

[48] House WF. Surgical exposure of the internal auditory canal and its contents through the middle, cranial fossa. Laryngoscope. 1961; 71:1363–1385

[49] House WF. Transtemporal bone microsurgical removal of acoustic neuromas. Arch Otolaryngol. 1964; 80:599–756

[50] Husseini ST, Piccirillo E, Taibah A, Paties CT, Almutair T, Sanna M. The Gruppo Otologico experience of endolymphatic sac tumor. Auris Nasus Larynx. 2013; 40(1):25–31

[51] Karmarkar S, Bhatia S, Saleh E, et al. Cholesteatoma surgery: the individualized technique. Ann Otol Rhinol Laryngol. 1995; 104(8):591–595

[52] Khrais T, Sanna M. Hearing preservation surgery in vestibular schwannoma. J Laryngol Otol. 2006; 120(5):366–370

[53] Khrais TH, Falcioni M, Taibah A, Agarwal M, Sanna M. Cerebrospinal fluid leak prevention after translabyrinthine removal of vestibular schwannoma. Laryngoscope. 2004; 114(6):1015–1020

[54] Kunimoto Y, Lauda L, Falcioni M, Taibah A, Hasegawa K, Sanna M. Staged resection for vestibular schwannoma. Acta Otolaryngol. 2015; 135(9):895–900

[55] Lope Ahmad RA, Sivalingam S, Konishi M, De Donato G, Sanna M. Oncologic outcome in surgical management of jugular paraganglioma and factors influencing outcomes. Head Neck. 2013; 35(4):527–534

[56] Mazzoni A, Sanna M. A posterolateral approach to the skull base: the petro-occipital transsigmoid approach. Skull Base Surg. 1995;5(3):157–167

[57] Mazzoni A. Internal auditory artery supply to the petrous bone. Ann Otol Rhinol Laryngol. 1972; 81(1):13–21

[58] Mazzoni A. Internal auditory canal arterial relations at the porus acusticus. Ann Otol Rhinol Laryngol. 1969; 78(4):797–814

[59] Mazzoni A. Jugulo-petrosectomy. Arch Ital Otol Rinol Laringol. 1974; 2:20–35

[60] Medina M, Di Lella F, Di Trapani G, et al. Cochlear implantation versus auditory brainstem implantation in bilateral total deafness after head trauma: personal experience and review of the literature. Otol Neurotol. 2014; 35(2):260–270

[61] Medina M, Prasad SC, Patnaik U, et al. The effects of tympanomastoid paragangliomas on hearing and the audiological outcomes after surgery over a long-term follow-up. Audiol Neurootol. 2014; 19(5):342–350

[62] Mutlu C, Khashaba A, Saleh E, et al. Surgical treatment of cholesteatoma in children. Otolaryngol Head Neck Surg. 1995; 113(1):56–60

[63] Naguib MB, Aristegui M, Saleh E, et al. Surgical anatomy of the petrous apex as it relates to the enlarged middle cranial fossa approaches. Otolaryngol Head Neck Surg. 1994; 111(4):488–493

[64] Naguib MB, Saleh E, Cokkeser Y, et al. The enlarged translabyrinthine approach for removal of large vestibular schwannomas. J Laryngol Otol. 1994; 108(7):545–550

[65] Naguib MB, Sanna M. Subtemporal exposure of the intrapetrous internal carotid artery. An anatomical study with surgical application. J Laryngol Otol. 1999; 113(8):717–720

[66] Nuseir A, Sequino G, De Donato G, Taibah A, Sanna M. Surgical management of vestibular schwannoma in elderly patients. Eur Arch Otorhinolaryngol. 2012; 269(1):17–23

[67] Odat HA, Piccirillo E, Sequino G, Taibah A, Sanna M. Management strategy of vestibular schwannoma in neurofibromatosis type 2. Otol Neurotol. 2011; 32(7):1163–1170

[68] Omran A, De Denato G, Piccirillo E, Leone O, Sanna M. Petrous bone cholesteatoma: management and outcomes. Laryngoscope. 2006; 116(4):619–626

[69] Pandya Y, Piccirillo E, Mancini F, Sanna M. Management of complex cases of petrous bone cholesteatoma. Ann Otol Rhinol Laryngol. 2010; 119(8):514–525

[70] Piazza P, Di Lella F, Bacciu A, Di Trapani G, Ait Mimoune H, Sanna M. Preoperative protective stenting of the internal carotid artery in the management of complex head and neck paragangliomas: long-term results. Audiol Neurootol. 2013; 18(6):345–352

[71] Piccirillo E, Agarwal M, Rohit, Khrais T, Sanna M. Management of temporal bone hemangiomas. Ann Otol Rhinol Laryngol. 2004; 113(6):431–437

[72] Piccirillo E, Wiet MR, Flanagan S, et al. Cystic vestibular schwannoma: classification, management, and facial nerve outcomes. Otol Neurotol. 2009; 30(6):826–834

[73] Polo R, Del Mar Medina M, Arístegui M, et al. Subtotal petrosectomy for cochlear implantation: lessons learned after 110 cases. Ann Otol Rhinol Laryngol. 2016; 125(6):485–494

[74] Prasad SC, Balasubramanian K, Piccirillo E, et al. Surgical technique and results of cable graft interpositioning of the facial nerve in lateral skull base surgeries: experience with 213 consecutive cases. J Neurosurg. 2017 Apr 7:1-8. epub ahead of print

[75] Prasad SC, D'Orazio F, Medina M, Bacciu A, Sanna M. State of the art in temporal bone malignancies. Curr Opin Otolaryngol Head Neck Surg. 2014; 22(2):154–165

[76] Prasad SC, Giannuzzi A, Nahleh EA, Donato GD, Russo A, Sanna M. Is endoscopic ear surgery an alternative to the modified Bondy technique for limited epitympanic cholesteatoma? Eur Arch Otorhinolaryngol. 2016; 273(9):2533–2540

[77] Prasad SC, Mimoune HA, D'Orazio F, et al. The role of wait-and-scan and the efficacy of radiotherapy in the treatment of temporal bone paragangliomas. Otol Neurotol. 2014; 35(5):922–931

[78] Prasad SC, Mimoune HA, Khardaly M, Piazza P, Russo A, Sanna M. Strategies and long-term outcomes in the surgical management of tympanojugular paragangliomas. Head Neck. 2016; 38(6):871–885

[79] Prasad SC, Piccirillo E, Chovanec M, La Melia C, De Donato G, Sanna M. Lateral skull base approaches in the management of benign parapharyngeal space tumors. Auris Nasus Larynx. 2015; 42(3):189–198

[80] Prasad SC, Piccirillo E, Nuseir A, et al. Giant cell tumors of the skull base: case series and current concepts. Audiol Neurootol. 2014; 19(1):12–21

[81] Prasad SC, Piras G, Piccirillo E, et al. Surgical strategy and facial nerve outcomes in petrous bone cholesteatoma. Audiol Neurootol. 2016; 21(5):275–285

[82] Prasad SC, Roustan V, Piras G, Caruso A, Lauda L, Sanna M. Subtotal petrosectomy: Surgical technique, indications, outcomes, and comprehensive review of literature. Laryngoscope. 2017 Mar 27; epub ahead of print

[83] Prasad SC, Shin SH, Russo A, Di Trapani G, Sanna M. Current trends in the management of the complications of chronic otitis media with cholesteatoma. Curr Opin Otolaryngol Head Neck Surg. 2013; 21(5):446–454

[84] Rabelo de Freitas M, Russo A, Sequino G, Piccirillo E, Sanna M. Analysis of hearing preservation and facial nerve function for patients undergoing vestibular schwannoma surgery: the middle cranial fossa approach versus the retrosigmoid approach–personal experience and literature review. Audiol Neurootol. 2012; 17(2):71–81

[85] Rohit, Jain Y, Caruso A, Russo A, Sanna M. Glomus tympanicum tumour: an alternative surgical technique. J Laryngol Otol. 2003; 117(6):462–466

[86] Russo A, Piccirillo E, De Donato G, Agarwal M, Sanna M. Anterior and posterior facial nerve rerouting: a comparative study. Skull Base. 2003; 13(3):123–130

[87] Saleh E, Achilli V, Naguib M, et al. Facial nerve neuromas: diagnosis and management. Am J Otol. 1995; 16(4):521–526

[88] Saleh E, Naguib M, Aristegui M, Cokkeser Y, Russo A, Sanna M. Surgical anatomy of the jugular foramen area. In: Mazzoni A, Sanna M, ed. Skull Base Surgery Update. Vol 1. Amsterdam: Kugler; 1995:3–8

[89] Samii M, Ammirati M. The combined supra-infratentorial pre-sigmoid sinus avenue to the petro-clival region. Surgical technique and clinical applications. Acta Neurochir (Wien). 1988; 95(1–2):6–12

[90] Sanna M, Saleh E, Khrais T, et al. Atlas of Microsurgery of the Lateral Skull Base. 2nd ed. Stuttgart: Thieme; 2008

[91] Sanna M, Piazza P, Shi SH, et al. Microsurgery of Skull Base Paragangliomas. Stuttgart: Thieme; 2013

[92] Sanna M, Sunose H, Mancini F, et al. Middle Ear and Mastoid Microsurgery. 2nd ed. Stuttgart: Thieme; 2012

[93] Sanna M, Merkus P, Free RH, Falcioni. Surgery for Cochlear Implant and Other auditory Implants. 1st ed. Stuttgart: Thieme; 2015

[94] Sanna M, Khrais T, Mancini F, Russo A, Taiba A The Facial Nerve in Temporal Bone and Lateral Skull Base Surgery. Stuttgart: Thieme; 2006

[95] Sanna M, Agarwal M, Jain Y, Russo A, Taibah AK. Transapical extension in difficult cerebellopontine angle tumours: preliminary report. J Laryngol Otol. 2003; 117(10):788–792

[96] Sanna M, Agarwal M, Khrais T, Di Trapani G. Modified Bondy's technique for epitympanic cholesteatoma. Laryngoscope. 2003; 113(12):2218–2221

[97] Sanna M, Agarwal M, Mancini F, Taibah A. Transapical extension in difficult cerebellopontine angle tumors. Ann Otol Rhinol Laryngol. 2004; 113(8):676–682

[98] Sanna M, Bacciu A, Falcioni M, Taibah A, Piazza P. Surgical management of jugular foramen meningiomas: a series of 13 cases and review of the literature. Laryngoscope. 2007; 117(10):1710–1719

[99] Sanna M, Bacciu A, Falcioni M, Taibah A. Surgical management of jugular foramen schwannomas with hearing and facial nerve function preservation: a series of 23 cases and review of the literature. Laryngoscope. 2006; 116(12):2191–2204

[100] Sanna M, Bacciu A, Pasanisi E, Piazza P, Fois P, Falcioni M. Chondrosarcomas of the jugular foramen. Laryngoscope. 2008; 118(10):1719–1728

[101] Sanna M, Bacciu A, Pasanisi E, Taibah A, Piazza P. Posterior petrous face meningiomas: an algorithm for surgical management. Otol Neurotol. 2007; 28(7):942–950

[102] Sanna M, De Donato G, Di Lella F, Falcioni M, Aggrawal N, Romano G. Nonvascular lesions of the jugular foramen: the Gruppo Otologico experience. Skull Base. 2009; 19(1):57–74

[103] Sanna M, De Donato G, Piazza P, Falcioni M. Revision glomus tumor surgery. Otolaryngol Clin North Am. 2006; 39(4):763–782, vii

[104] Sanna M, De Donato G, Taibah A, Russo A, Falcioni M, Mancini F. Infratemporal fossa approaches to the lateral skull base. Keio J Med. 1999; 48(4):189–200

[105] Sanna M, Dispenza F, Flanagan S, De Stefano A, Falcioni M. Management of chronic otitis by middle ear obliteration with blind sac closure of the external auditory canal. Otol Neurotol. 2008; 29(1):19–22

[106] Sanna M, Dispenza F, Mathur N, De Stefano A, De Donato G. Otoneurological management of petrous apex cholesterol granuloma. Am J Otolaryngol. 2009; 30(6):407–414

[107] Sanna M, Facharzt AA, Russo A, Lauda L, Pasanisi E, Bacciu A. Modified Bondy's technique: refinements of the surgical technique and long-term results. Otol Neurotol. 2009; 30(1):64–69

[108] Sanna M, Falcioni M, De Donato G, et al. Facial nerve identification in the translabyrinthine approach: an alternative method. Acta Otorhinolaryngol Ital. 1999; 19(1):1–5

[109] Sanna M, Falcioni M, Rohit. Cerebro-spinal fluid leak after acoustic neuroma surgery. Otol Neurotol. 2003; 24(3):524

[110] Sanna M, Falcioni M, Taibah A, De Donato G, Russo A, Piccirillo E. Treatment of residual vestibular schwannoma. Otol Neurotol. 2002; 23(6):980–987

[111] Sanna M, Falcioni M. Conservative facial nerve management in jugular foramen schwannomas. Am J Otol. 2000; 21(6):892

[112] Sanna M, Flanagan S. Surgical management of lesions of the internal carotid artery using a modified Fisch Type A infratemporal approach. Otol Neurotol. 2007; 28(7):994

[113] Sanna M, Flanagan S. The combined transmastoid retro- and infralabyrinthine transjugular transcondylar transtubercular high cervical approach for resection of glomus jugulare tumors. Neurosurgery. 2007; 61(6):E1340–, author reply E1340

[114] Sanna M, Fois P, Pasanisi E, Russo A, Bacciu A. Middle ear and mastoid glomus tumors (glomus tympanicum): an algorithm for the surgical management. Auris Nasus Larynx. 2010; 37(6):661–668

[115] Sanna M, Fois P, Russo A, Falcioni M. Management of meningoencephalic herniation of the temporal bone: personal experience and literature review. Laryngoscope. 2009; 119(8):1579–1585

[116] Sanna M, Gamoletti R, Bortesi G, Jemmi G, Zini C. Posterior canal wall atrophy after intact canal wall tympanoplasty. Am J Otol. 1986; 7(1):74–75

[117] Sanna M, Jain Y, De Donato G, Rohit, Lauda L, Taibah A. Management of jugular paragangliomas: the Gruppo Otologico experience. Otol Neurotol. 2004; 25(5):797–804

[118] Sanna M, Khrais T, Russo A, Piccirillo E, Augurio A. Hearing preservation surgery in vestibular schwannoma: the hidden truth. Ann Otol Rhinol Laryngol. 2004; 113(2):156–163

[119] Sanna M, Mazzoni A, Saleh E, Taibah A, Mancini F. The system of the modified transcochlear approach: a lateral avenue to the central skull base. Am J Otol. 1998; 19(1):88–97, discussion 97–98

[120] Sanna M, Mazzoni A, Saleh EA, Taibah AK, Russo A. Lateral approaches to the median skull base through the petrous bone: the system of the modified transcochlear approach. J Laryngol Otol. 1994; 108(12):1036–1044

[121] Sanna M, Mazzoni A, Taibah A, Russo A, Arístegui M. The modified transcochlear approach to the petroclival area and the prepontine cistern: indications, techniques and results. Acta Otorrinolaringol Esp. 1995; 46(4):259–267

[122] Sanna M, Mazzoni A, Taibah A, Saleh E, Russo A, Khashaba A. The modified transcochlear approaches to the skull base: results and indications. In: Mazzoni A, Sanna M, eds. Skull Base Surgery Update. Vol 1. Amsterdam: Kugler; 1995:315–323

[123] Sanna M, Mazzoni A. The modified transcochlear approach to the tumors of the petroclival area and prepontine cistern. Skull Base Surg. 1996;6(4):237-248

[124] Sanna M, Medina MD, Macak A, Rossi G, Sozzi V, Prasad SC. Vestibular schwannoma resection with ipsilateral simultaneous cochlear implantation in patients with normal contralateral hearing. Audiol Neurootol. 2016; 21(5):286–295

[125] Sanna M, Pandya Y, Mancini F, Sequino G, Piccirillo E. Petrous bone cholesteatoma: classification, management and review of the literature. Audiol Neurootol. 2011; 16(2):124–136

[126] Sanna M, Piazza P, De Donato G, Menozzi R, Falcioni M. Combined endovascular-surgical management of the internal carotid artery in complex tympanojugular paragangliomas. Skull Base. 2009; 19(1):26–42

[127] Sanna M, Piazza P, Ditrapani G, Agarwal M. Management of the internal carotid artery in tumors of the lateral skull base: preoperative permanent balloon occlusion without reconstruction. Otol Neurotol. 2004; 25(6):998–1005

[128] Sanna M, Rohit, Skinner LJ, Jain Y. Technique to prevent post-operative CSF leak in the translabyrinthine excision of vestibular schwannoma. J Laryngol Otol. 2003; 117(12):965–968

[129] Sanna M, Russo A, Khrais T, Jain Y, Augurio AM. Canalplasty for severe external auditory meatus exostoses. J Laryngol Otol. 2004; 118(8):607–611

[130] Sanna M, Russo A, Taibah A, Falcioni M, Agarwal M. Enlarged translabyrinthine approach for the management of large and giant acoustic neuromas: a report of 175 consecutive cases. Ann Otol Rhinol Laryngol. 2004; 113(4):319–328

[131] Sanna M, Saleh E, Russo A, Falcioni M. Identification of the facial nerve in the translabyrinthine approach: an alternative technique. Otolaryngol Head Neck Surg. 2001; 124(1):105–106

[132] Sanna M, Shin SH, De Donato G, et al. Management of complex tympanojugular paragangliomas including endovascular intervention. Laryngoscope. 2011; 121(7):1372–1382

[133] Sanna M, Shin SH, Piazza P, et al. Infratemporal fossa approach type a with transcondylar-transtubercular extension for Fisch type C2 to C4 tympanojugular paragangliomas. Head Neck. 2014; 36(11):1581–1588

[134] Sanna M, Zini C, Gamoletti R, et al. Surgical treatment of cholesteatoma in children. Adv Otorhinolaryngol. 1987; 37:110–116

[135] Sanna M, Zini C, Gamoletti R, et al. The surgical management of childhood cholesteatoma. J Laryngol Otol. 1987; 101(12):1221–1226

[136] Sanna M, Zini C, Gamoletti R, et al. Prevention of recurrent cholesteatoma in closed tympanoplasty. Ann Otol Rhinol Laryngol. 1987; 96(3, Pt 1):273–275

[137] Sanna M, Zini C, Gamoletti R, et al. Petrous bone cholesteatoma. Skull Base Surg. 1993; 3(4):201–213

[138] Sanna M, Zini C, Gamoletti R, Pasanisi E. Primary intratemporal tumours of the facial nerve: diagnosis and treatment. J Laryngol Otol. 1990; 104(10):765–771

[139] Sanna M, Zini C, Mazzoni A, et al. Hearing preservation in acoustic neuroma surgery. Middle fossa versus suboccipital approach. Am J Otol. 1987; 8(6):500–506

[140] Sanna M, Zini C, Scandellari R, Jemmi G. Residual and recurrent cholesteatoma in closed tympanoplasty. Am J Otol. 1984; 5(4):277–282

[141] Sanna M. Anatomy of the posterior mesotympanum. In: Zini C, Sheehy JL, Sanna M, eds. Microsurgery of Cholesteatoma of the Middle Ear. Milan: Ghedini; 1980:69–73

[142] Sanna M, Russo A, Caruso A Color Atlas of Endo-Otoscopy. 1st ed. Stuttgart: Thieme; 2017

[143] Sbaihat A, Bacciu A, Pasanisi E, Sanna M. Skull base chondrosarcomas: surgical treatment and results. Ann Otol Rhinol Laryngol. 2013; 122(12):763–770

[144] Shaan M, Landolfi M, Taibah A, Russo A, Szymanski M, Sanna M. Modified Bondy technique. Am J Otol. 1995; 16(5):695–697

[145] Shin SH, Piazza P, De Donato G, et al. Management of vagal paragangliomas including application of internal carotid artery stenting. Audiol Neurootol. 2012; 17(1):39–53

[146] Shin SH, Sivalingam S, De Donato G, Falcioni M, Piazza P, Sanna M. Vertebral artery involvement by tympanojugular paragangliomas: management and outcomes with a proposed addition to the Fisch classification. Audiol Neurootol. 2012; 17(2):92–104

[147] Sivalingam S, Konishi M, Shin SH, Lope Ahmed RA, Piazza P, Sanna M. Surgical management of tympanojugular paragangliomas with intradural extension, with a proposed revision of the Fisch classification. Audiol Neurootol. 2012; 17(4):243–255

[148] Tanbouzi Husseini S, Kumar DV, De Donato G, Almutair T, Sanna M. Facial reanimation after facial nerve injury using hypoglossal to facial nerve anastomosis: the Gruppo Otologico experience. Indian J Otolaryngol Head Neck Surg. 2013; 65(4):305–308

[149] Tos M, Thomsen J. Translabyrinthine Acoustic Neuroma Surgery: A Surgical Manual. Stuttgart: Thieme; 1991

[150] Zini C, Mazzoni A, Gandolfi A, Sanna M, Pasanisi E.. Retrolabyrinthine vs. middle fossa vestibular neurectomy. Am J Otol. 1984; 9:448–450

Index